Language Development from Theory to Practice

THIRD EDITION

Khara L. Pence Turnbull
Charlottesville, Virginia

Laura M. Justice
The Ohio State University

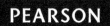
PEARSON

Boston   Columbus   Indianapolis   New York   San Francisco   Upper Saddle River
Amsterdam   Cape Town   Dubai   London   Madrid   Milan   Munich   Paris   Montréal   Toronto
Delhi   Mexico City   São Paulo   Sydney   Hong Kong   Seoul   Singapore   Taipei   Tokyo

Vice President and Editorial Director: Jeffery W. Johnston
Executive Editor: Ann Castel Davis
Editorial Assistant: Anne McAlpine
Executive Field Marketing Manager: Krista Clark
Senior Product Marketing Manager: Christopher Barry
Project Manager: Kerry Rubadue
Program Program Manager: Joe Sweeney
Operations Specialist: Carol Melville
Text Designer: Lumina

Cover Design Director: Diane Ernsberger
Cover Art: Getty Images
Media Producer: Autumn Benson
Full-Service Project Management: Lumina
Composition: Lumina
Printer/Binder: LSC Communications
Cover Printer: LSC Communications
Text Font: ITC Garamond Std

Library of Congress Cataloging-in-Publication Data

Names: Pence, Khara L. | Justice, Laura M., 1968-
Title: Language development from theory to practice / Khara L. Pence
  Turnbull, Charlottesville, Virginia ; Laura M. Justice, The Ohio State University.
Description: Third edition. | Upper Saddle River, New Jersey : Pearson
  Education, Inc., 2015. | Includes bibliographical references and index.
Identifiers: LCCN 2015028472| ISBN 9780134170428 (alk. paper) | ISBN
  0134170423 (alk. paper)
Subjects: LCSH: Language acquisition.
Classification: LCC P118 .P396 2015 | DDC 401/.93--dc23 LC record available at http://lccn.loc.gov/2015028472

Bound Book ISBN 10: 0-13-417042-3
ISBN 13: 978-0-13-417042-8
E-text Package ISBN 10: 0-13-441208-7
ISBN 13: 978-0-13-441208-5
Pearson E-text ISBN 10: 0-13-417067-9
ISBN 13: 978-0-13-417067-1

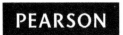

To the very special and sweet guys in my life,
Doug, Ian, and Murray
—K.P.T.

To Ian, Addie, and Griffin, for their unwavering
support, love, and thoughtfulness
—L.J.

Preface

The field of language development is an incredibly exciting area of study for college and university students in diverse disciplines, including allied health (e.g., speech–language pathology, audiology), liberal arts (e.g., linguistics, psychology), and education (e.g., elementary education, special education). For students in many preprofessional training programs, a basic course in language development is required at the undergraduate or graduate level. Yet, instructors teaching courses in language development commonly say that the language-development textbooks currently available do not address several important criteria:

- Integration of theory and practice, including discussion of how theories of language development influence state-of-the-art educational and clinical practices with children

- Discussion of individual differences in language development, including those of children who are developing language in diverse cultures or developing language atypically (e.g., children with disabilities)

- Descriptions of techniques that educators, clinicians, and researchers use to measure children's language achievements, including computer software

- Examination of language development from a multidisciplinary perspective, including its relevance to theory and practice in different disciplines

Language Development from Theory to Practice was designed to meet and exceed these criteria. This text provides a survey of key topics in language development, including research methods, theoretical perspectives, major language milestones from birth to adolescence and beyond, and language diversity and language disorders. The research base and the theoretical foundation this text provides are designed to prepare students for advanced study in subjects associated with language development, such as language disorders, psycholinguistics, instruction of English as a second or foreign language, and developmental psychology, among others. Although we do not adopt a single theoretical framework for how language phenomena are interpreted in the text, we attempt to summarize the various theoretical orientations that have guided research and practice in the relevant fields mentioned earlier.

NEW TO THIS EDITION

The purpose of this third edition is to build on the strengths of the first and second editions by making a number of enhancements in response to suggestions from the field. We have retained a number of features from the second edition that were well received. One such feature, *Beyond the Book*, presents opportunities to connect the text to students' own future experiences with language. Another such feature, *Apply Your Knowledge*, presents problems that allow students to apply their knowledge in a similar way as on exams such as the Praxis. We have also made it a priority to improve students' learning opportunities in each chapter through the use of advance organizers, self-check quizzes, and video clips relevant to chapter content. We learned that students and educators would like to see more detailed coverage of topics (e.g., theory of mind, bilingualism) that students should find particularly interesting. We have thus responded by expanding some topics and shortening others. We have also continued to strive to present material in an enjoyable and reader-friendly way. Finally, we received feedback that it would be helpful for students to have a general understanding of language development and language building blocks as well as language neuroanatomy and neurophysiology prior to introducing language-development theories, as language acquisition theories have risen from our understanding of language development and language neurology. We have responded by reorganizing the chapters to begin with an introduction to language development (Chapter 1), followed by language building blocks (Chapter 2), language neuroanatomy and neurophysiology (Chapter 3), and language-development science and theories (Chapter 4).

More specifically, the third edition of *Language Development from Theory to Practice* features the following changes to ensure that the material is current and comprehensive, while meeting the needs of students and educators:

- We have created *Learning Outcomes* for each chapter and linked each learning outcome to one main section within each chapter.

- We have also created a brief multiple-choice item within each chapter section called *Check Your Understanding*; this feature allows students to check their own responses and to receive immediate feedback before proceeding to the next section.

- We have also included a comprehensive *End of Chapter Quiz* with multiple-choice items assessing the chapter's learning outcomes. The *End of Chapter Quiz* allows students to check their own responses and receive immediate, detailed feedback.

- We have added a feature to each chapter called *Learn More About*. Each *Learn More About* margin note links to a video clip illustrating chapter content and provides a detailed description of the video. For example, videos of child language samples include a description of specific instances of language form, content, and use. As another example, videos of research paradigms include a description of the research stimuli and procedure.

- We have also provided more detailed coverage of topics that should be of interest to students. For example, we have expanded our discussion of areas such as language pragmatics, theory of mind, Spanish dialects used in the United States, and language disorders in children who are bilingual. With regard to language-development theories, we have expanded the categorization scheme (previously nurture-inspired theories and nature-inspired theories) to include a third category—interactionist theories, based on common categorization schemes in the language-development literature. We have also provided greater emphasis on the distinctions between the three categories of theories rather than the distinctions between the individual theories, and we have reduced the number of individual theories we discuss.

- Finally, in response to feedback, we have separated our discussion of *Language Diversity* and *Language Disorders in Children* into two separate chapters to allow a more thorough treatment of each of these topics.

ORGANIZATION OF THE TEXT

Language Development from Theory to Practice includes ten chapters. Chapters 1 through 4 provide a basis for understanding language development. Specifically, in Chapter 1, we define language and explain how it relates to the areas of speech, hearing, and communication. We also introduce the three domains of language—form, content, and use—and describe the features of language that make it so remarkable. Chapter 1 concludes with an introduction to language differences and language disorders. In Chapter 2, we introduce the building blocks of language: phonological, morphological, syntactic, semantic, and pragmatic development. Chapter 3 addresses the neuroanatomy and neurophysiology of language. We describe the major structures of the brain, explain how the brain processes and produces language, and discuss sensitive periods in neuroanatomical and neurophysiological development. In Chapter 4, we describe the many reasons different people study language development. We introduce some major approaches to studying language development as well as some major language-development theories; we reference these approaches and theories subsequently in several places in the text. We conclude Chapter 4 by describing how theories of language development contribute to practice in several areas.

Chapters 5 through 8 provide a developmental account of language acquisition for four age groups (infancy—Chapter 5; toddlerhood—Chapter 6; preschool age—Chapter 7; and school age and beyond—Chapter 8). More specifically, in each of these four chapters, we describe the major language-development milestones children achieve during the period in question; examine achievements in language form, content, and use; explain some of the intra- and inter-individual differences in language development; and discuss methods researchers and clinicians use to measure language development.

In Chapter 9 we explore language differences. We detail the connection between language and culture, explain how languages evolve and change, describe bilingualism and second language acquisition, and explain some theories of second language acquisition and their implications for practice.

Finally, in Chapter 10, we examine language disorders in childhood. We define the term *language disorder*, explain who identifies and treats children with language disorders, discuss the major types of language disorders, and describe how practitioners treat language disorders.

KEY FEATURES OF THE TEXT

Each chapter bridges language-development theory and practice by providing students with a theoretical and scientific foundation to the study of language development. We emphasize the relevance of the material to students' current and future experiences in clinical, educational, and research settings.

Multicultural Considerations

Current perspectives emphasize the importance of taking into account multicultural considerations in understanding language development. This text promotes students' awareness of the way in which culture interacts with language development for children from diverse backgrounds within and beyond the many types of communities in the United States.

Research Foundations

Current initiatives in the educational, social science, and health communities emphasize the use of evidence-based practices. Such practices emphasize the importance of research results to making educational and clinical decisions. In keeping with this premise, we emphasize the research foundations of the study of language development, and use the most current empirical findings to describe children's language achievements.

Multidisciplinary Focus

The study of language development is constantly evolving and being influenced by many diverse disciplines; this multidimensional and multidisciplinary foundation attracts many students to the study of language development. We introduce exciting innovations in theory and practice from many diverse areas of research.

Easy-to-Read Format

Language Development from Theory to Practice is presented in a way that promotes student learning. First, the chapters are infused with figures, tables, and photographs to contextualize abstract and complex information. Second, important terms are highlighted for easy learning and reference. Third, discussion questions are integrated throughout to provide opportunities to pause and consider important information. All these features create opportunities for students to actively engage with the material in the text.

Pedagogical Elements

The text includes many pedagogical elements:

- Learning outcomes to organize each chapter
- Discussion questions interspersed throughout each chapter
- Video clips relevant to chapter material
- Chapter summaries
- Self-check, multiple-choice quizzes
- Activities that allow students to engage with language *Beyond the Book*
- Boxed inserts:
  - *Developmental Timeline*: We present milestones for language development, observable features of these milestones, and approximate ages for the milestones.
  - *Language Diversity and Differences*: We introduce cultural differences in language development and describe the observable features of these differences. We also discuss educational and clinical implications with regard to cultural differences.
  - *Research Paradigms*: We provide descriptions of various research paradigms used to inform our understanding of language development.
  - *Theory to Practice*: We discuss some implications of different theoretical perspectives for educational and clinical practice.

ACKNOWLEDGMENTS

We extend our thanks to our family members, friends, and colleagues who supported us throughout this revision. Among these persons are the Pence family, the Powell family, the Turnbull family, and the Justice and Mykel families. We are indebted to them for their interest in and support of this text.

We are grateful to a number of experts who reviewed this manuscript: Eileen Abrahamsen, Old Dominion University; Karin M. Boerger, University of Colorado–Boulder; Julie Dalmasso, Western Illinois University; Martin Fujiki, Brigham Young University; and Shannon Hall-Mills, Florida State University.

Brief Contents

Contents

5 Infancy: Let the Language Achievements Begin 122

6 Toddlerhood: Exploring the World and Experimenting with Language 158

7 Preschool: Building Literacy on Language   195

8 School-Age Years and Beyond: Developing Later Language   227

9   Language Diversity   262

10   Language Disorders in Children   290

1

Language Development

An Introduction

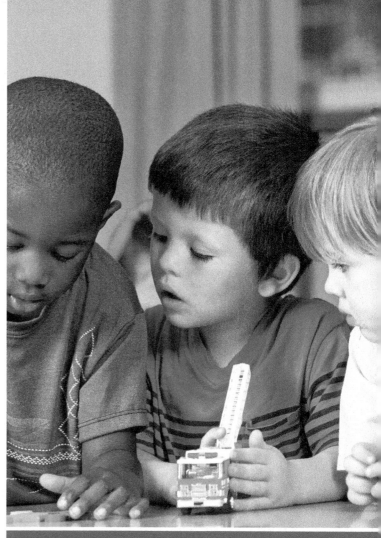

LEARNING OUTCOMES

After completion of this chapter, the reader will be able to:

1. Define the term *language*.

2. Describe how language relates to speech, hearing, and communication.

3. Describe the major domains of language.

4. Identify several remarkable features of language.

5. Discuss the distinction between language differences and language disorders.

Hundreds of scientists worldwide study the remarkable phenomenon of children's language acquisition. Each year, these scholars publish the results of numerous studies on children's language development in scientific journals, pursuing answers to such questions as:

- Does the language a child is learning (e.g., Chinese vs. English) influence the rate of language development?
- How do caregivers' interactions with their child affect the timing of their child's first word?
- Do children who show early delays in language development typically catch up with their peers?
- Do children learning a signed language develop language similarly to children learning a spoken language?
- Why do children with autism have such difficulties developing language skills?

These questions provide the student of language development a glimpse into many of the interesting topics language scientists focus on in their work around the world. These questions also suggest how important language research is to informing the everyday practices and activities of parents, teachers, psychologists, and other professionals invested in helping children achieve their fullest language development potential. That these questions have yet to be fully answered, shows that the study of language development is a constantly evolving and complex area of science in which practitioners have many more questions than answers.

In this chapter, we provide a general introduction to the study of language development and consider five major topics. In the first section, we answer the question "What is language?", and present a definition of *language* that we build on throughout this text. In the second section, we discuss differences among speech, hearing, and communication—three aspects of human development and behavior that are closely related but are nonetheless distinct capacities. In the third section, we address the five major domains of language, a topic we introduce here and discuss more fully in Chapter 2. In the fourth section, we examine several remarkable features of language, and in the fifth section, we describe differences in and disorders of language development—two topics we explore more comprehensively in Chapters 9 and 10.

WHAT IS LANGUAGE?

Language Defined

You probably have an intuitive sense of what language is because it is a human behavior you have acquired to a sophisticated level and use regularly for various purposes. In fact, you are using your language abilities as you read and analyze the content of this chapter. However, if you take a moment to define language more explicitly, you may find the task challenging. If you were to ask 10 classmates for a definition of language, each would likely respond differently. The same outcome would probably occur if you questioned 10 language researchers.

You are also most likely aware that language is a basic and essential human behavior that develops early in life. You probably recognize that language involves words and sentences and both expression (language production) and comprehension (language understanding). In addition, you know language is a process of the brain that helps people communicate their thoughts to other individuals, although you may be somewhat unclear about how language differs from speech and communication.

However, to be as specific as possible about what language is and is not, let's look at the official definition of the term *language* the American Speech-Language-Hearing Association (1982) uses:

The relationship between a word and its referent is arbitrary. English speakers use the word happy to represent an internal feeling of happiness, but any word would do.

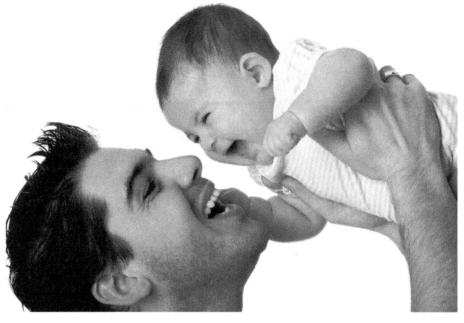

© Paul Hakimata/Fotolia

Language is a "complex and dynamic system of conventional symbols that is used in various modes for thought and communication."

Next, we delineate in more detail the specific characteristics of language identified in this definition:

1. *Language Is a System of Symbols.* The first characteristic of language warranting discussion is that it is a code, consisting of a system of symbols called morphemes. Morphemes are the smallest units of language that carry meaning; we combine them to create words. Some words consist of a single morpheme (e.g., *school*), but many words comprise two or more morphemes, such as *schools* (two morphemes—*school* + *-s*) and *preschools* (three morphemes—*pre-* + *school* + *-s*). These symbols can exist in spoken or written format, a point we'll return to shortly.

The term *code* refers to the translation of one type of information into another type of information; this involves the use of symbols. For humans to develop the capacity to use language thousands of years ago, perhaps the most important prerequisite was the human ability to use symbols, such as representing a specific concept with a specific sound (Christianson & Kirby, 2003). In language, we create words by using morphemes to represent myriad aspects of the world around our language community. For instance, as English speakers, we can represent an internal feeling of happiness by using the single word *happy*. When we use the word *happy* in a conversation with other people to describe our feelings, we use the word to translate our feelings. Although we can share feelings and ideas through other means—such as gesture, facial expression, and posture—words are much more specific and provide a uniquely powerful tool for communicating.

One important characteristic of language code is that the relationship between a word and its referent (the aspect of the world to which the word refers) is arbitrary. For example, although English speakers recognize that *happy* refers to a specific feeling, any other word (e.g., *sprit*, *nopic*, or *grendy*) would do. Likewise, one way English speakers can denote plurality is to attach the morpheme *-s* to words (e.g., *pens*, *dogs*). Because the relationship between the plural morpheme *-s* and its plural marking is arbitrary, English speakers could denote plurality in various other ways. In contrast, the code we use to organize words into sentences is not arbitrary; rather, we must follow specific rules for organizing thoughts into words and sentences, as we discuss next.

2.   *The System of Language Is Conventional.* The second characteristic of language is that the system of symbols is conventional, so the members of a community or culture can share it. The term *conventional* means users of a language abide by accepted rules. For instance, speakers of English agree to use the word *dog* (and related words and synonyms, such as *pup*, *puppy*, and *canine*) to refer to those companionable creatures, rather than other potential words, such as *boop* or *ming*. Speakers of Spanish use a different word to refer to this concept (*perro*), as do users of American Sign Language. Adhering to specific conventions allows all members of a language community to use language with one another as a tool for expression. A *language community* is a group of people who use a common language. In fact, somewhere in the history of the human species, a single language probably emerged within a social community of about 100 hominids (Cartwright, 2000). Some experts contend that language emerged within this community as a type of grooming behavior, essentially an efficient way to share socially useful information (Christiansen & Kirby, 2003). Accordingly, the numerous languages of the world emerged from this single community of language users.

Language communities emerge for many reasons. Some form as a result of geographic circumstances, as in the case of Ukrainian, the language people speak in Ukraine, a country in the western region of the former Soviet Union. Alternatively, a language community may emerge for sociological reasons, as in the case of Hebrew, which many persons of Jewish faith share, or American Sign Language, which persons in the U.S. Deaf community use. A language community can organize for economic reasons as well. For instance, the World Trade Organization (WTO), a global group that coordinates and regulates trade among 161 countries (as of April, 2015), conducts its activities in English, French, and Spanish.

3.   *The Language System Is Dynamic.* The third characteristic of language is that it is dynamic. This means language is in a state of activity and change, both within an individual who is acquiring language and within a community that uses a certain language. Let's consider first the case of the individual. As we discuss throughout this book, the acquisition of language begins at birth, or even before birth, in utero, and is in a state of change across the lifespan. Even as adults, our language skills are dynamic. As one example, we might seek to learn a second language. As another example, as we age, some aspects of our language skill decline. We might, for example, have increased difficulty finding the names for things (Capuron et al., 2011), which is a normal part of aging.

The language a community uses is also very dynamic. When the first edition of this book was published, in 2008, there was no such word as *selfie* (or *selfie stick*, for that matter). Sometime during the last eight years, this word entered the English language and is now in our vocabulary. In any language, words come and go and other changes happen as well, as we discuss more thoroughly in Chapter 9.

4.   *Language Is a Tool for Human Communication.* The final and perhaps most important characteristic of language requiring discussion is that it exists as a tool for communication. Communication is the process of sharing information, such as thoughts, feelings, and ideas, among two or more persons. Although other species are able to communicate, such as dogs, primates, birds, dolphins, and ants, the innate and specialized capacity of humans to use language as a tool to communicate is what makes the human species unique. For instance, although some primates may communicate alarms to one another using calls, these alarm calls seem to be general and do not symbolically represent a given predator (e.g., eagle) (Christiansen & Kirby, 2003). Experts therefore argue that "language is the most distinctive feature that distinguishes humans from other animals" (Wang & Minett, 2005, p. 263). Language itself is what supports the highly complex communication enjoyed by the human species, such as your ability to comprehend and learn from the complex matter contained within this text.

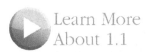

Learn More About 1.1

As you watch the video titled "What Is Language?" consider the different features of language and how language differs from other systems of communication. https://www.youtube.com/watch?v=GenkKxTk7bw

Language as a Module of Human Cognition

Beyond its role in supporting human communication, language is a cognitive tool that helps humans to develop the "picture of the world that we use for thinking" (Bickerton, 1995). This "picture of the world" includes not only symbolic representations of linguistic concepts (e.g., *big*, *fly*, *crazy*) that are organized in a vast network, but also the formal syntactic or grammatical rules that organize these concepts into orderly, surface-level representations. According to this proposition, first and foremost, language is a representational tool people use for thinking, and, second, this tool permits people to communicate their thoughts to other individuals.

Language probably emerged in the human species for the latter reason: to provide an efficient and effective means for communication within a community. In other words, language emerged as a cultural and social evolution, rather than a biological evolution: Our need and interest to communicate with others gave rise to the complexity of language over time (Christiansen & Kirby, 2003). Some experts suggest that language emerged in the human species because of increases in the size of human communities (e.g., from about 50 members in a group to more than 100 members), and therefore increases in the complexity of social dynamics (Dunbar & Aiello, 1993). With time, the neural circuitry of the human brain responded to the adaptive advantage of using language not only as a social tool but also as an inner representational tool, emerging as a specialized part of the human mind (Christiansen & Kirby, 2003).

The human brain uses language as a representational tool to store information and to carry out many cognitive processes such as reasoning, hypothesizing, memorizing, planning, and problem solving. These processes are sometimes called *higher-level* language skills to differentiate them from more basic-level language abilities. When applied to mathematical and scientific tasks, these higher-level abilities may be called *mathematical reasoning* and *scientific reasoning*; however, it is important to acknowledge the role of language in mathematical and scientific reasoning tasks. For instance, suppose you are asked to complete the following mathematical reasoning task:

> The average cost of a smart phone in the United States in 2015 is about $250. Assuming the prices of consumer goods decline about 3% per year, how much, on average, would a smart phone cost in 2020?

You would have difficultly generating an answer without using language as a tool. Although some persons may contend that they think in images and not in words, certain thoughts—such as "My trust in you has been shattered forever by your unfaithfulness"—are impossible to view as images and require language to be invoked as a representational tool (Bickerton, 1995, p. 22).

As we consider the definition of language, particularly its relation to cognition, we need to explore the concept of *modularity*. We introduce this concept here, and discuss it more thoroughly in Chapter 4. Modularity is a cognitive science theory about how the human mind is organized within the structures of the brain (Braisby & Gellatly, 2012). Questions about modularity concern whether the human brain contains a set of highly specific modules—regions of the brain developed to process specific types of information—or whether the human brain is itself a generalized module in which all parts work together to process information. A module is a specialized problem-solving device in the brain that responds to information of a restricted type. Because of the specificity of such modules, they are termed domain specific, meaning they can process only very specific types of information, such as depth perception within the visual system. Some cognitive theorists contend that the brain consists of very large domain-general modules, which carry out very general tasks like memory and reasoning, as well as domain-specific modules that execute very specific types of tasks.

? ! DISCUSSION POINT

Too many people in the world are without food. We need a solution to the global food-shortage problem. Try to reason through a solution to this problem without using language. Is it possible? Can an individual engage in complex reasoning without language?

With respect to language, some language theorists argue that the human brain contains a large number of language-specific modules, tightly clustered and highly interconnected, each of which processes specific types of linguistic information (see Curtiss, 2012). Such theorists contend that during human evolution, the neural circuitry of the brain became highly specialized in several regions to handle the task of developing and using language (Cartwright, 2000). In fact, researchers have long known that specific regions of the brain are associated with specific language abilities. For instance, people who sustain damage to certain areas of the left frontal lobe, such as during a stroke, often exhibit difficulty with basic grammar. These people may omit grammatical markers and speak with a "telegraphic" quality (e.g., "Tommy go store now"), which suggests this region of the brain governs aspects of grammar (Shapiro & Caramazza, 2003). The results of brain-imaging studies of the workings of undamaged brains also indicate that various regions of the brain correspond to highly specific aspects of language (Okada et al., 2013), a concept we elaborate on in Chapter 3.

Studies of children with language impairment (a group we discuss more thoroughly in Chapter 10) also provide some support for the notion of language modularity. Typically developing in all areas except for language, children with a condition called *specific language impairment* (SLI) exhibit problems in very precise aspects of grammar, such as marking verb tense. Verb tense marking includes, for instance, inflecting verbs with *-ed* to create the past tense, as in "Juan brushed his teeth." At ages 4 and 5 years, children with SLI have significant problems with past-tense marking (typically omitting it; Clahsen, Rothweiler, Sterner, & Chilla, 2014), even when other aspects of language development are proceeding normally. Across any number of languages, including English, German, and Swedish, this is a prominent marker of children with SLI (e.g., Clahsen et al., 2014). That verb structures are so clearly impaired in children with SLI suggests that, perhaps, there is a particular module of the brain that processes verb structures and that this is the site of disturbance in cases of SLI.

The concept of language modularity is not without its critics. Some theorists argue that language emerges in response to an individual's culture rather than in response to any specific internal architecture. Others argue that language is processed by a general neural network that operates on all aspects of language and that the hypothesized language modules lack "neurological reality" (Bickerton, 1995, p. 76). Bickerton, in a well-reasoned critique of modularity theory as it applies to language, showed that the results of research on disordered language due to developmental disability (e.g., cognitive impairment) and brain injury have failed to support the modularity concept. For instance, Bickerton reviewed studies of persons with damage to a specific area of the brain purportedly linked to grammar problems, noting that these individuals showed diverse patterns of syntactic impairment. Because the same module was likely damaged in these individuals, the expectation would be little variability in their impairment. At the same time, it is also important to recognize that, even if language processes are modular, this does not mean language functions specific to a given module (or area of the brain) cannot be subsumed by another area of the brain when injury occurs. We'll discuss the notion of brain plasticity in Chapter 3. Undoubtedly, researchers in the next several decades will better elucidate how language is represented in the neural architecture of the brain.

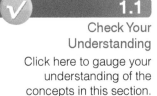

Check Your Understanding

Click here to gauge your understanding of the concepts in this section.

HOW DOES LANGUAGE RELATE TO SPEECH, HEARING, AND COMMUNICATION?

Language, speech, hearing, and communication together represent basic and interrelated human abilities. Although simple forms of communication such as gesturing do not necessarily require language, speech, and hearing, more advanced forms of communication—particularly speaking and listening—require them.

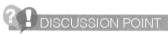

Often, the terms *language, speech, hearing,* and *communication* are used synonymously, but in fact they describe substantially different processes. We previously defined *language* as the rule-governed, code-based tool a person uses to represent thoughts and ideas. Once individuals formulate thoughts and ideas, they can communicate them to other people using speech or a manual sign system; otherwise, individuals can choose to keep thoughts and ideas to themselves (inner language) or can write them down (written language).

Speech describes the neuromuscular process by which humans turn language into a sound signal and transmit it through the air (or another medium such as a telephone line) to a receiver. Hearing is the sensory system that allows speech to enter into and be processed by the human brain. We described communication previously as the process of sharing information among individuals. Communication in the form of a spoken conversation between two persons involves language, hearing, and speech; in contrast, communication between two persons in an Internet chat room involves only language.

Speech

Speech is the voluntary neuromuscular behavior that allows humans to express language and is essential for spoken communication. In spoken communication, after people formulate ideas in the brain using language, they must then transmit the message by using speech. Speech involves the precise activation of muscles in four systems: respiration, phonation, resonance, and articulation. These four systems represent the remarkable coordination of a breath of air as it is inspired into and then expired from the lungs to travel up through the trachea, or windpipe (respiration). Within the trachea, the breath of air moves through the vocal cords, which are set into vibration to create one's voice (phonation). Then the breath of air proceeds into the oral and nasal cavities, where it resonates (resonation). Finally, the breath of air is manipulated by the oral articulators—including the tongue, teeth, lips, and jaw (articulation)—to emerge as a series of speech sounds that are combined into words, phrases, and sentences. Figure 1.1 illustrates these four systems.

When and how humans first began to use speech is the subject of considerable popular, philosophical, and scientific debate; estimates range from 2 million years ago with *Homo erectus* to only 35,000 years ago with *Homo sapiens* (Cartwright, 2000; Wang & Minett, 2005). Anatomically modern humans (based on remains

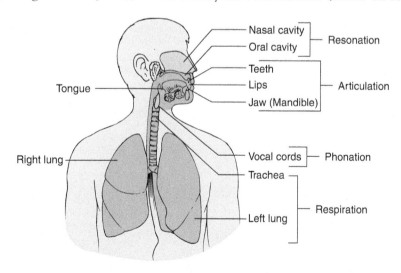

FIGURE 1.1

Systems involved with speech production.

Adapted from: Justice, Laura M., Communication Sciences & Disorders: An Introduction, 1st Ed., ©2006. Reprinted and Electronically reproduced by permission of Pearson Education, Inc., New York, NY.

found in Ethiopia) existed about 160,000 years ago, and it is believed that speech and language emerged sometime between 160,000 and 50,000 years ago when the human species experienced a "cultural explosion" (Wang & Minett, 2005). Although this continues to be debated, it is likely that speech became the mode for language expression because of its advantages over other modalities, such as gesturing or grunting (Christiansen & Kirby, 2003). Whereas gesturing requires a direct line of sight, speech enables communication in the dark, around corners, and from relatively far distances; speech also allows one to communicate when the hands are occupied, as when one is carrying an infant or working manually. In addition, speech allows an individual to communicate with a larger number of persons, which became necessary as the group size of early humans increased from small bands of hunter-gatherers of a dozen or so individuals, to larger organized communities of more than 100 members (Cartwright, 2000). Finally, and possibly most important, speech provides the medium for sharing language.

Model of Speech Production

We provide here a relatively basic model of speech production to show how speech moves from the brain to the articulators. A model is a way to represent an unknown event on the basis of the best current evidence governing the event. Models of speech production provide a theoretical description of how an individual can move from a cognitive representation ("I forgot to bring paper . . . I'll have to borrow a piece … I see she has an extra one in her notebook") to a clearly articulated spoken product ("May I borrow a piece of paper?").

Figure 1.2 presents a basic model of speech production involving three stages. The first stage is a perceptual event: The speech production process is initiated with a mental, abstract representation of the speech stream to be produced. This abstract representation is the language code, which provides a *perceptual target* of what is to be produced by speech. At the perceptual level, the code is represented by the phoneme. A phoneme is the smallest unit of sound that can signal a difference in meaning; we combine phonemes to produce syllables and words. For instance, the word *mama* comprises four phonemes, whereas the word *my* comprises two. In written form, phonemic representations are usually bounded by slashes; thus, the four phonemes in *mama* are /m/ /a/ /m/ /a/, and the two phonemes in *my* are /m/ /aɪ/. Conventionally, phonemes are represented by the symbols of the International

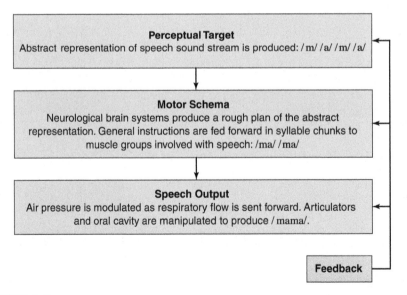

FIGURE 1.2

Model of speech production.

Source: Justice, Laura M., Communication Sciences & Disorders: An Introduction, 1st Ed., ©2006. Reprinted and Electronically reproduced by permission of Pearson Education, Inc., New York, NY.

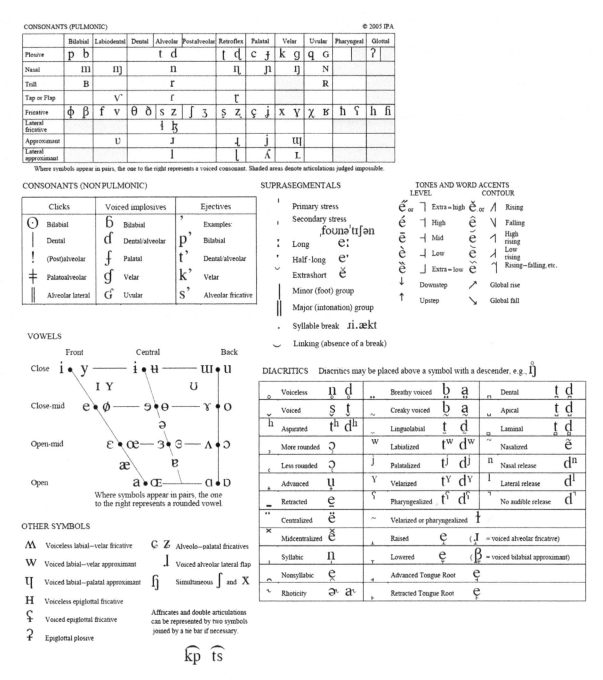

FIGURE 1.3

International Phonetic Alphabet.

Source: International Phonetic Association (updated 1993) copyright 1993 by International Phonetic Association.

Phonetic Alphabet (IPA), which is an international set of symbols that represents all of the phonemes of the world's languages. Figure 1.3 provides a reproduction of the IPA simply for illustrative purposes. (Shortly, we'll focus on the smaller subset of phonemes used in General American English; for a preview, turn to Table 1.2.)

The second stage of speech production is development of a *motor schema* to represent the perceptual language–based representation. This is a rough motor plan based on the abstract representation of the perceptual target. The rough plan organizes the phonemes into syllable chunks; for instance, for an infant who wants to call her mother, *mama* is represented as two syllables to be executed: /ma/ /ma/. The rough plan is sent forward to the major muscle groups involved with speech production. This stimulates the production of speech, or *speech output* in the

Humans can share language through many means, such as reading, writing, speaking, and communicating manually (e.g., sign language).

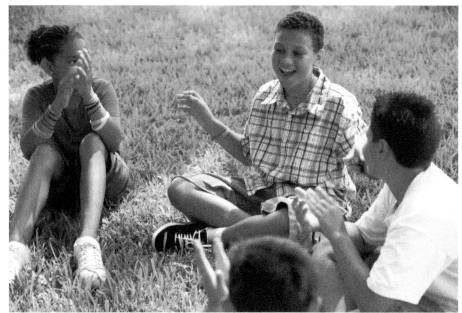

© Golden Pixels LLC/Alamy

third stage of speech production. The airflow, vocal fold vibration, and oral cavity movements are all finely manipulated to carry out the motor schema and to create speech. Ongoing feedback relays information about speech output back to the origination of the perceptual target and motor schema.

Relationship of Speech to Language

Speech is the voluntary and complex neuromotor behavior humans use to share language. Language does not depend on speech because people can share language by other means, such as writing, reading, and signing, or they can keep it to themselves as a tool for thinking. However, speech depends wholly on language because language gives speech its meaning. Without language, speech is just a series of meaningless noises. Persons with significant speech disorders, such as those occurring in some instances of cerebral palsy (a motor-based disorder present at birth), may be able to produce little or no speech, or they may produce unintelligible speech. These persons cannot use speech to transmit their thoughts to other people.

Speech and language are largely independent processes; thus, some persons can have no functional speech yet have excellent language skills. As an example, there is one relatively rare condition called *locked-in syndrome*, in which an individual has completely intact language and cognitive skills, but is unable to perform any voluntary movements (i.e., has complete paralysis) with the exception of eye movement. Persons with locked-in syndrome can learn to communicate with others through eye movements, such as blinking. However, it is also the unfortunate case that many persons with locked-in syndrome don't receive the opportunity to communicate because their consciousness is unrecognized by everyone *except* the person with the condition (Chisholm & Gillett, 2005). Nick Chisholm, who as a 23-year-old New Zealander who was injured while playing rugby, describes his experience after having locked-in syndrome for 5 years this way: "When you're like this (despite having 24 hour care) it's an incredibly lonely existence at times. It's amazing how much time I have to think about things now since the accident. There's heaps of thoughts that I don't bother even expressing" (Chisholm & Gillett, 2005, p. 96).

Hearing

When people produce speech to share language for communication, not only a sender (the speaker) but also a receiver (the listener) is necessary. The receiver's task is to receive and comprehend the information the speaker conveys, and hearing

? ! DISCUSSION POINT

Speech and language are independent processes, as the case of locked-in syndrome illustrates. Can you think of other illustrations of the independence of speech and language?

is essential to both *reception* and *comprehension* of spoken language. Hearing, or audition, is the perception of sound, and it includes both general auditory perception and speech perception.

Sound Fundamentals

So that you understand hearing and how it relates to language and speech, we will provide a brief overview of acoustics, or the study of sound. The transmission and reception of speech involve four acoustic events: creation of a sound source, vibration of air particles, reception by the ear, and comprehension by the brain (Champlin, 2011):

1. *Creation of a Sound Source.* A sound source sets in motion a series of events. The sound source creates a disturbance—or set of vibrations—in the surrounding air particles. When you bring your hands together to clap, doing so sets the air particles near the sound source into a complex vibratory pattern. Likewise, when you produce the word *coffee*, it sets the air particles near the sound source (in this case, just in front of your mouth) into a complex pattern of vibration.

2. *Vibration of Air Particles.* Fundamentally, sound is the movement or vibration of air particles. The air particles, set in motion by the sound source, move back and forth through the air (or another medium, such as water). How *fast* the particles move back and forth is the sound frequency, or pitch. How *far apart* the particles move when they move back and forth creates intensity, or the loudness of the sound. When you clap your hands or say a word, you set the air particles around the sound source into a vibratory pattern, and how the particles move carries information about frequency (pitch) and intensity (loudness). This information is represented in the movements of air particles between the sender and the receiver.

3. *Reception by the Ear.* The ear is specially designed to channel information carried by the air-particle vibrations into the human body. The ear is a complex structure with three chambers. The outer chamber (the outer ear) captures the sound and channels it to the middle chamber (the middle ear). The middle chamber then forwards the acoustic information to the inner chamber (the inner ear), which contains the cochlea. From the cochlea, the auditory information travels up the auditory nerve to the auditory regions of the brain.

4. *Comprehension by the Brain.* The auditory centers of the brain—located in the left hemisphere—translate the auditory information sent through the ear and along the auditory nerve. If the information that arrives at the brain involves speech sounds, the speech and language centers of the brain facilitate the comprehension process. If the information that arrives at the brain is not a speech sound (e.g., a clap of the hands or the hum of a fan), the speech and language centers are not involved. The human brain differentiates sound information as speech and nonspeech; in fact, the human ear and the brain are designed to be "remarkably responsive" to processing the sounds of speech (Borden et al., 1994, p. 176).

Speech Perception

Speech perception refers to how the brain processes speech and language. Speech perception is different from auditory perception, which is a more general term describing how the brain processes any type of auditory information. Processing a clap of the hands or the hum of a fan involves auditory perception, but processing the word *coffee* requires speech perception. The brain differentiates between general auditory information and speech sounds, processing speech differently than other auditory stimuli.

Speech perception involves specialized processors in the brain that have evolved specifically to respond to human speech and language. Infants enter the world with biologically endowed processing mechanisms geared to the perception of speech, and with exposure to a specific language (or languages), the perceptual mechanism

Learn More About 1.2

As you watch the video titled "Auditory Transduction (2002)," consider how the physiological process of hearing can impact a person's speech and communication skills. https:// www.youtube.com/ watch?v=PeTriGTENoc

is calibrated to reflect this language. Calibration of the speech perception mechanism is aided by a few capacities of the young child. First, young children show a preference for auditory rather than visual information; this phenomenon is called *auditory overshadowing* (Sloutsky & Napolitano, 2003), a principle of early development suggesting that young children have a bias toward attending to auditory information in their environment. Second, young children—mostly infants—show a striking ability to process and analyze speech as a particular type of auditory stimulus. From an early age, infants "engage in a detailed analysis of the distributional properties of sounds contained in the language they hear," which helps calibrate their speech perception abilities for their native language or languages (Tsao, Liu, & Kuhl, 2004, p. 1068).

In fact, this detailed analysis appears to involve the infant's use of statistical learning (Hay, Pelucchi, Estes, & Saffran, 2011). Believe it or not, infants appear to assess statistical regularities among the sounds they hear in the speech stream around them and use these regularities to identify and learn the words of their native language. To learn new words, infants need to be able to isolate words within running speech so as to recognize that the three sounds in *cup*, blended together, represent the entity "cup." Infants calculate statistics on the durations between phonemes, for instance, to identify whether the phonemes are likely to mark word boundaries, as in *my#cup*, in which the # marks the word boundary (Hay et al., 2011).

At the most basic level, speech perception involves processing phonemic information, such as the four phonemes in the word *coffee* (/k/ /a/ /f/ /i/) or the three phonemes in the word *cup* (/k/ /ʌ/ /p/). Sometimes, analogies are made between how the brain processes a series of phonemes in a spoken word, and how a reader reads a series of letters in a written word, as if speech perception involves the sequential one-on-one processing of individual speech sounds. This analogy is incorrect. When humans produce phonemes, the phonemes overlap with one another in a process called coarticulation. For instance, the initial /k/ in *coffee* and the initial /k/ in *coop* are produced differently because the initial /k/ in each word carries information about the subsequent vowels, which differ. The /k/ in *coffee* is influenced by the subsequent *ah* sound, whereas the /k/ in *coop* is influenced by the subsequent *oo* sound. As a result, the /k/ in *coop* is produced with rounded lips in anticipation of the *oo* sound. *Coarticulation* is the term that describes this "smearing," or overlapping, of phonemes in the production of strings of speech sounds. The articulators (lips, tongue, etc.) coarticulate speech sounds because doing so is much more efficient than producing just one sound at a time, and the speech-processing mechanisms of the brain have evolved to process the rapidly occurring and coarticulated speech sounds.

Communication

We defined communication previously as the process of sharing information among two or more persons, usually differentiated as the sender (speaker) and the receiver(s) (listeners). Typically in communication, only one person is the sender, although this is not always the case, such as when students coauthor a paper. In addition, although communication may at times involve only one receiver, it can also involve numerous receivers, such as when the re-elected president, Barack Obama, gave his second inaugural speech to an estimated audience of more than 1 million on Washington, D.C.'s National Mall.

Regardless of the number of senders and receivers, communication involves four basic processes: formulation, transmission, reception, and comprehension. The sender formulates and then transmits the information he or she would like to convey, and the receiver takes in and then comprehends the information. *Formulation* is the process of pulling together your thoughts or ideas for sharing with another person. *Transmission* is the process of conveying these ideas to another person, often by speaking, but alternatively by signing, gesturing, or writing. *Reception* is the process of receiving the information from another person, and *comprehension* is the process of making sense of the message.

Symbolic communication, also called referential communication, occurs when an individual communicates about a specific entity (an object or event), and the relationship between the entity and its referent (e.g., a word) is arbitrary (Leavens, Russell, & Hopkins, 2005). For instance, the 1-year-old who says "bottle" to request something to drink is communicating symbolically because the relationship between the word *bottle* and its referent is arbitrary. Symbolic communication also "knows no limitations of space or time" (Bickerton, 1995, p. 15).

However, some communication is not symbolic and is thus constrained to a particular space and time. Preintentional communication is communication in which other people assume the relationship between a communicative behavior and its referent. For example, a cat's purr and an infant's cry are types of preintentional communication. The cat and the baby are communicating, but the communicative partner must infer the actual referent or goal of the communication. The infant's cry could mean "I am really hungry" or "This blanket is too hot." In contrast, intentional communication is relatively precise in its intent and the relationship between the communicative behavior and its referent is not arbitrary. Some forms of intentional communication are very transparent (called iconic communication) because of the clear relationship between the message and its referent (Bickerton, 1995). For instance, when an infant points to a bottle, or a chimpanzee gestures toward a banana, the act is intentional, iconic communication.

Whether communicating intentionally or symbolically, people share information for three basic purposes: to request ("May I have some cake?"), to reject ("I don't want this cake"), and to comment ("This cake is delicious"). Requesting, rejecting, and commenting need not use language, as any adult interacting with an 8-month-old infant can attest. Infants at this age can request, reject, and comment using an array of nonlinguistic yet intentional means, including crying, laughing, gesturing, smiling, and cooing. However, as infants develop as language users, they begin to use language and speech as a means to disseminate their needs and wants more precisely. By 1 year of age, toddlers use language for all three purposes, even if their vocabulary is not yet well developed ("Bottle?" "Bottle!" "Bottle.").

The combination of speaking and listening is a common mode of communication called oral communication. However, communication need not involve speaking or listening. A person can reject by turning away, a baby can comment by smiling, and a dog can request by panting at the door. What is unique about *human* communication though, is the use of *language* and *speech* in the communication process. In much of this text, we emphasize the development and use of language as a tool for uniquely human, sophisticated communication.

Model of Communication

Figure 1.4 provides a model of communication that includes three essential components: (a) a sender to formulate and transmit a message, (b) a receiver to receive and comprehend the message, and (c) a shared symbolic means for communication. Figure 1.5 shows the roles of language, speech, and hearing in formulation, transmission, reception, and comprehension during communication.

In addition to these basic processes is another aspect of communication: *feedback* (see Figure 1.4). Feedback is information the receiver provides to the sender. In effective communication, the receiver provides continual feedback, and the sender responds to this feedback to maintain the ongoing effectiveness of the communication process. The feedback system is what makes communication *active* and

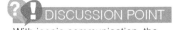

DISCUSSION POINT

With iconic communication, the relationship between the symbol used for communication and the referent is transparent. Provide some other examples of iconic communication common in the life of a university student.

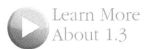

Learn More About 1.3

As you watch the video titled "Brain Highways: Speech and Language," consider how speech and hearing processes are related in a child's language comprehension and how this can impact a child's development. https://www.youtube.com/watch?v=1jiFNqKF7gA

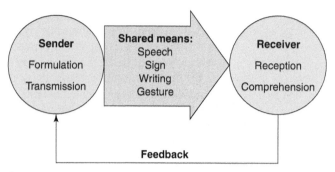

FIGURE 1.4

Model of communication.

Source: Justice, Laura M., Communication Sciences & Disorders: An Introduction, 1st Ed., ©2006. Reprinted and Electronically reproduced by permission of Pearson Education, Inc., New York, NY.

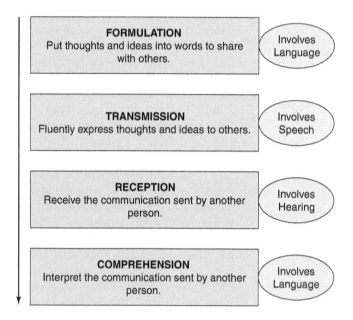

FIGURE 1.5

Roles of language, speech, and hearing in communication.

Source: Justice, Laura M., Communication Sciences & Disorders: An Introduction, 1st Ed., ©2006. Reprinted and Electronically reproduced by permission of Pearson Education, Inc., New York, NY.

dynamic. It is active because both sender and receiver must be fully engaged. It is dynamic because the receiver is constantly sending feedback that the sender interprets and uses to modulate the flow of communication.

A receiver can provide feedback in numerous ways. Linguistic feedback includes speaking, such as saying "I totally agree," "I hear what you are saying," or "Wait; I don't get it." It also includes vocalizing, such as saying "mm-hmm" or "uh-oh." Nonlinguistic feedback, or extralinguistic feedback, refers to the use of eye contact, facial expression, posture, and proximity. This type of feedback may supplement linguistic feedback or it may stand alone. Paralinguistic feedback refers to the use of pitch, loudness, and pausing, all of which are superimposed over the linguistic feedback. These linguistic and nonlinguistic forms of feedback keep the communication flowing, and provide the speaker with valuable information concerning the receiver's comprehension.

When communicating, people often supplement their speech and language with nonlinguistic, or extralinguistic feedback, such as eye contact, facial expressions, posture, and proximity.

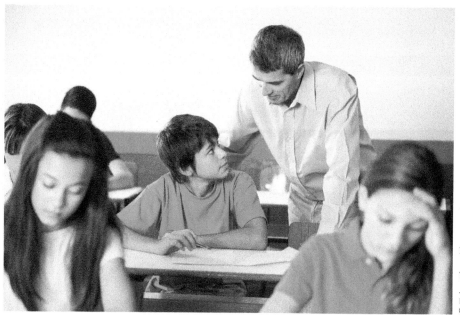

© Tyler Olson/Shutterstock

For communication to be effective, the receiver's feedback is just as important as the information the sender provides. The sender and the receiver use feedback to prevent communication breakdowns from occurring:

CHILD: I need that one.

FATHER: This one?

CHILD: No, that one.

FATHER: This here?

CHILD: No. (starts crying)

FATHER: Maybe it's this one?

CHILD: Yeah, I said that one.

If you look closely at this snippet of conversation, you should be able to find a communication breakdown that seems to occur because of inadequacies of both the sender and the receiver. The child appears not to have the language abilities to produce sufficiently explicit information about what he or she desires, and the father does not provide adequate feedback to clarify the lack of specificity. Eventually the father repairs the breakdown, which is called a conversational repair. Minor communication breakdowns occur in every conversation but are easily recognized and repaired if the sender is closely monitoring the receiver's feedback and the receiver is providing ongoing feedback. More serious communication breakdowns occur when receivers do not provide appropriate types or amounts of feedback or when senders do not attend to the feedback.

Purpose of Communication

The primary purpose of communication is to provide and solicit information. Humans communicate to provide information about their feelings and to obtain information from other people. Individuals communicate to share information about trivial and exciting events and to describe their needs and desires. Table 1.1 provides one system of differentiating the major purposes of communication. All of these purposes are vitally important for developing and maintaining social relationships with other people, as well as for meeting personal basic needs and satisfying desires.

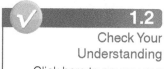

1.2

Check Your Understanding

Click here to gauge your understanding of the concepts in this section.

TABLE 1.1
Seven purposes of communication

PURPOSE	DESCRIPTION	EXAMPLE
Instrumental	Used to ask for something	"Will you pass me the butter, please?"
Regulatory	Used to give directions and to direct others	"Go ahead and sit down over there."
Interactional	Used to interact and converse with others in a social way	"How was the game last night?"
Personal	Used to express a state of mind or feelings about something	"There is no way I passed that test!"
Heuristic	Used to find out information and to inquire	"Do you know how much this book is?"
Imaginative	Used to tell stories and to role-play	"Okay, let's practice what you're going to say when you call her."
Informative	Used to provide an organized description of an event or object	"So, we got to the hotel, and they had no record of our reservation. Then, they tell me they have no rooms left at all. . . ."

Source: Based on *Learning How to Mean: Explorations in the Development of Language Development* by M. A. Halliday, 1975, London: Arnold; and "Presentation of Communication Evaluation Information" by C. Simon and C. L. Holway, in *Communication Skills and Classroom Success* (pp. 151–199), edited by C. Simon, 1991, Eau Claire, WI: Thinking Publications.

WHAT ARE THE MAJOR DOMAINS OF LANGUAGE?

Form, Content, and Use

Language is a single dimension of human behavior that consists of several distinct domains. In Chapter 2 we discuss these domains more deeply; however, we introduce them here as their understanding will be useful in Chapter 4, when we discuss prominent theories of language development.

A classic representation of the domains comprising language distinguishes among content, form, and use (Lahey, 1988). Consider the following utterances by 3-year-old Adelaide: "I beating you up the stairs." "I wonned!" "I am so fast." These utterances provide an array of analytical possibilities for characterizing Adelaide's language. First, you can consider the *form* of Adelaide's utterances. Form is how words, sentences, and sounds are organized and arranged to convey content. When you consider form, you examine such things as sentence structure, clause and phrase usage, parts of speech, verb and noun structures, word prefixes and suffixes, and the organization of sounds into words. For instance, in examining the form of Adelaide's utterances, note that she uses three simple sentences, the first of which contains a prepositional phrase (*up the stairs*). She uses various parts of speech, including nouns (*stairs*), pronouns (*I*), articles (*the*), prepositions (*up*), verbs (*running*), and adverbs (*so*). Adelaide also uses a number of speech sounds, including a variety of vocalic sounds (i.e., vowels) and several consonantal sounds (i.e., consonants; e.g., /b/, /w/, /f/).

In considering form, you must take a closer look at how sentences are structured. Examination of Adelaide's sentence structures reveals that each sentence contains a subject, which, in all cases, is the personal pronoun *I*. Each sentence also contains a predicate, or verb, structure. In her three short utterances, Adelaide uses three different verb structures. In the first sentence, *I beating you up the stairs*, she uses the transitive verb *beating*, which requires an object (i.e., you). Note that although she has inflected the verb *beat* with the present progressive marker *-ing* to show that the actions are occurring continuously in the present, she has also omitted the auxiliary verb *am*. In the

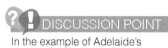
DISCUSSION POINT

In the example of Adelaide's language, she said the word *wonned*. What are some possible explanations for this error?

second sentence, Adelaide uses the verb *wonned*. In this case, she has produced the irregular past tense form of *win* but has added the past tense marker for regular verbs, *-ed*. This verb is an intransitive verb, which does not require an object, and none is provided. In the third sentence, the verb structure comprises a *be* verb (*am*) that serves as the main verb in the sentence and requires a subject complement (*so fast*).

Second, you can consider content, which refers to the meaning of language—the words used and the meaning behind them. We humans convey content through our vocabulary system, or lexicon, as we select and organize words to express our ideas or to understand what other individuals are saying. You can consider the content of Adelaide's utterances in a variety of ways: She uses 12 words; of these, she repeats one word (*I*) several times, for a total of 10 different words. The words *beating*, *wonned*, and *fast* create lexical ties across the utterances because conceptually they work together to denote that a race of some type is occurring. The words she uses and the concepts she expresses through these words are fairly concrete. She does not use figurative or idiomatic words, nor does she use abstract language. The focus is clearly on the here and now. Language that focuses on the immediate context is contextualized, and typically the content of highly contextualized language is concrete and supported by cues within the environment (e.g., gestures, facial expressions). Thus, in this particular example, the context in which Adelaide speaks provides important information that supplements the content of the language. In contrast, imagine that Adelaide was telling the story of this race over the telephone to her grandmother. She would need to be much more precise to convey the content. When we share language with little reliance on the context for conveying content, it is decontextualized.

Third, you can consider the language *use*. Use pertains to how people draw on language functionally to meet personal and social needs. When you examine this domain of language, you are asking about the intentions behind the utterances and how well the utterances achieve these intentions. Thus, you examine individual utterances to consider their intent. One possible scheme is Halliday's seven communication functions (see Table 1.1). For the analysis of Adelaide's language use, you can conclude that the intentions behind her utterances are primarily interactional (language used to interact socially) and personal (language used to express a state of mind).

Examination of use also involves consideration of how well language achieves these intentions—for example, whether an individual can maintain a topic through several turns in a conversation, can regulate the participation of other people (e.g., through eye contact, facial expressions, pausing), and can adjust language given the particular demands of the communicative situation and the listener's needs. Because analysis of use requires understanding the context in which language is occurring, it may be difficult to evaluate one's language use by reading a transcript. For example, you would have no way to know from the transcript of Adelaide's utterances whether she is meeting the contextual needs of the situation, and whether she is regulating her language use effectively to achieve her intentions.

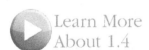

Learn More About 1.4

As you watch the video titled "Language Domains," consider how each domain allows for detailed specificity in communication. https://www.youtube.com/watch?v=WrNi7VrumJU

Components of Form, Content, and Use

Form, content, and use represent a three-domain system used to represent and organize the major dimensions of language. A five-component system is also often used, which provides a slightly more refined description of the components of each of the three domains. The five components are phonology, morphology, syntax, semantics, and pragmatics. The first three—phonology, morphology, and syntax—are three components of form, whereas the components of semantics and pragmatics are synonymous with the domains of content and use, respectively. Following is a brief description of each component; these topics are considered in more depth in Chapter 2:

1. Phonology (form) refers to the rules of language governing the sounds that make syllables and words. Every language has a relatively small number of meaningful sounds, or *phonemes*.General American English (GAE; also called *Standard American*

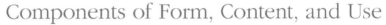

TABLE 1.2

Vowels and consonants of General American English

CONSONANT SYMBOL	EXAMPLE	CONSONANT SYMBOL	EXAMPLE
b	_b_at	r or ɹ	_r_ose
p	_p_at	s	_s_un
d	_d_ip	ʃ	_sh_ine
t	_t_ip	f	_f_it
g	_g_ive	tʃ	_ch_urch
h	_h_ot	θ	_th_ink
j	_y_es	ð	_th_at
k	_c_at	v	_v_et
l	_l_ot	w	_w_ash
m	_m_ine	z	_z_ag
n	_n_ose	ʒ	trea_s_ure
ŋ	ri_ng_	ʤ	_j_ail

VOWEL SYMBOL	EXAMPLE	ARTICULATORY FEATURES
i	f_ee_t	high, front, unrounded
ɪ	f_i_t	high, front, unrounded
e	m_a_ke	mid, front, unrounded
ɛ	b_e_t	mid, front, unrounded
æ	c_a_t	low, front, unrounded
u	bl_ue_	high, back, rounded
ʊ	p_u_ll	high, back, rounded
ɔ	b_ough_t	mid, back, rounded
o	g_o_	mid, back, rounded
a	b_o_x	low, back, unrounded
ʌ	b_u_g	mid, central, unrounded
ə	_a_round	mid, central, unrounded
ɝ	b_ir_d	mid, central, unrounded
ɚ	fath_er_	mid, central, unrounded

Source: Justice, Laura M., Communication Sciences & Disorders: An Introduction, 1st Ed., ©2006. Reprinted and Electronically reproduced by permission of Pearson Education, Inc., New York, NY.

English) has about 39 phonemes (give or take a few, depending on the dialect), as shown in Table 1.2. GAE relies on the combination of 15 vowels and 24 consonants to create about 100,000 words. Some languages use more phonemes; others use fewer.

Allophones are the subtle variations of phonemes that occur as a result of contextual influences on how phonemes are produced in different words. For instance, the two /p/ phonemes in *pop* are produced differently, given the position of each in the word. The initial /p/ is aspirated, meaning that it is produced with a small puff of air. In contrast, the final /p/ is unaspirated. (The final /p/ can be aspirated but typically is not.) The two /p/ sounds in *pop* are allophonic variations of a single phoneme, and many phonemes have several allophones. In addition, each language has rules governing how sounds are organized in words, called phonotactics. For instance, in English the phoneme /g/ never directly follows /s/ or /l/ at the beginning of a syllable.

2. Morphology (form) pertains to the rules of language governing the internal organization of words. Previously, we defined *morpheme* as the smallest unit of language that carries meaning; many words contain two or more morphemes. We can "morph" (manipulate) words in a variety of ways to change their meaning. For instance, we can add prefixes to words to change their meaning—such as by adding the morpheme *pre-* to words to create *preschool*, *predisposition*, *preview*, and *pretest*. Also, we can use suffixes to add grammatical information to words (i.e., to indicate basic grammatical information such as tense or plurality). These types of suffixes are called *grammatical morphemes*. Grammatical morphemes include the plural *-s* (*cat–cats*), the possessive *'s* (*mom–mom's*), the past tense *-ed* (*walk–walked*), and the present progressive *-ing* (*do–doing*), to name a few. Morphology is an important linguistic tool that not only allows us to add precision to language (e.g., "Tamika walk" vs. "Tamika had walked"), but also to expand vocabulary exponentially using a relatively small core of words (base vocabulary) and morphing them into a much larger pool of word families (e.g., *school, schools, schooling, schooled, preschool*).

3. Syntax (form) refers to the rules of language governing the internal organization of sentences. Knowledge of the rules governing syntax enables us to readily turn the simple statement *He did it* into the question *Did he do it?*, and to embed one simple sentence (e.g., *Andre is angry*) in another (e.g., *Andre is not coming*) to produce a complex sentence (e.g., *Andre, who is angry, is not coming*). Syntax is what permits a child to produce a seemingly endless sentence by linking a series of simple sentences: *This is Thomas and he is so mad at Lady and Lady goes off the siding and here comes Percy and Thomas gets out of the way and Percy is coming so fast*. In short, whereas semantics provides the meaning to utterances, syntax provides the structure. Noam Chomsky's well-known proposition that *Colorless green ideas sleep furiously* illustrates the difference between semantics and syntax, in which a sentence is devoid of meaning but conforms to sophisticated syntactic rules.

4. Semantics (content) refers to the rules of language governing the meaning of individual words and word combinations. When people produce a given word (e.g., *cat*) or phrase (*black cat*), they express a certain meaning. Semantics thus involves consideration of the meaning of various words and phrases. For instance, you know that a *culprit* is someone who has done something wrong; the word *run* has many meanings, whereas the word *stapler* has only one meaning; the phrase *bent over backwards* has both a figurative and a literal meaning; and the words *papaya*, *banana*, and *kiwi* go together conceptually. If you ask a person to produce the first word that comes to mind when he or she hears the word "vehicle," the semantic relationship among words might provoke the person to respond "car" (or, alternatively, "truck" or "tractor"). Knowledge of semantics tells you something is wrong with the sentence linguist, Noam Chomsky produced, *Colorless green ideas sleep furiously*, and differentiates the meaning the words express (semantics) from the grammar that organizes them into a sentence (syntax) (Pinker, 1994).

5. Pragmatics (use) pertains to the rules governing language use for social purposes, and is a synonym for the term *social communication*. Pragmatics com-

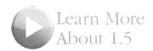

Learn More About 1.5

As you watch the video titled "Fantastic Feature We Don't Have In the English Language," consider how English creates form, content, and use and how other languages do the same but with different features. https://www.youtube.com/watch?v=QYlVJlmjLEc

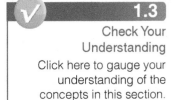

1.3

Check Your
Understanding

Click here to gauge your
understanding of the
concepts in this section.

prises the set of rules that govern three important aspects of the social use of language: (a) using language for different functions or intentions (communication intentions); (b) organizing language for discourse, including conversation; and (c) knowing what to say and when and how to say it (social conventions). In using language for social purposes, pragmatic rules govern linguistic, extralinguistic, and paralinguistic aspects of communication, such as word choice, turn taking, posture, gestures, facial expression, eye contact, proximity, pitch, loudness, and pauses.

WHAT ARE SOME REMARKABLE FEATURES OF LANGUAGE?

Language is one of the most extraordinary capacities of the human species, and young children's extremely rapid language acquisition is one of the most remarkable aspects of early development. Given the thousands of scientific studies exploring the extraordinariness of language, including how children go about learning the languages of their communities, you might assume nothing is left to learn about language development. Such an assumption could not be further from the truth. There are many mysteries that remain regarding how children develop their language abilities and, indeed, how humans acquired language in the first place.

Why is language such a mystery? In part, its mysteriousness relates to several remarkable features of language that work together to make it a particularly complicated area of study, albeit one that continues to capture the attention of numerous scholars around the world. In this section, we consider five of these remarkable features of language: acquisition rate, universality, species specificity, semanticity, and productivity.

Acquisition Rate

Faced with the task of explaining how children develop their remarkable language skills, scholars have often noted that the sheer acquisition rate of language makes it difficult to study. For instance, consider the following interaction between a mother and her 30-month-old daughter:

TAJIKA: Thomas the very useful engine is in the siding.

MOTHER: He's in the what?

TAJIKA: The siding. This is the siding.

MOTHER: Oh, that's the siding?

This brief interaction shows the extraordinary capacity of young children to learn and use new words at a stunning rate. *Siding* is a part of a train track that runs off the main course. In this vignette, Tajika has placed her miniature Thomas the Tank Engine on the siding. Her mother did not know the meaning of *siding*, but Tajika clearly did.

Erica Hoff, a scientist who studies early language development, stated that language development reveals the genius in all children (Hoff, 2013), whereas others have referred to infants and young children as "scientists in cribs" (Gopnik, Meltzoff, & Kuhl, 2009). The reference to children as geniuses and young scientists is based on the fact that children acquire the complexities of language at a seemingly miraculous rate: Although at birth children understand and use no words, within a year, they begin to understand and use several words, and by about 24 months, they have a vocabulary of several hundred words and can combine them into short sentences. Whereas the 1-year-old can say only "mama" to request something to drink, the 3-year-old can say, "Mom, Daddy said I could have some chocolate milk and I think I'll have it in the pink sippy cup."

The years of early language acquisition, from birth to about puberty, are often called a critical period (or sometimes a *sensitive period*) for language development, meaning that a window of opportunity exists during which language develops most rapidly and with the greatest ease. (We will discuss the concept of a critical period in more depth in Chapter 3.) A critical period for language development also implies periods of time in which the environment has particularly important impacts on language growth.

One important study of the critical period, as it applies to language development, involved research on institutionalization of infants in Romania (Nelson et al., 2007). Institutionalized care in Romania, at least until the early 2000s, typically featured very limited stimulation of infants, in part due to the very high child-to-caregiver ratio in such settings (Smyke et al., 2007). In this study, institutionalized infants were randomly assigned to remain in institutionalized care or to be placed in foster homes, in which presumably, stimulation would be greater because of a decrease in the child-to-caregiver ratio. An important part of this study, in addition to assessing the benefits of foster-care placements, was testing the critical-age hypothesis; the researchers did this by varying the time when children were moved into foster care: 14 children were placed in foster care before 18 months, 16 children between 18 and 24 months, 22 between 24 and 30 months, and 9 after 30 months (Nelson et al., 2007). If a critical period is operating, within which language development is most readily influenced by features of the environment, we might expect that children placed earlier in foster care would exhibit better language skills than children placed later. In fact, this is exactly what researchers found when they measured the language abilities of the foster-care children at 3.5 years of age. On standardized measures of language ability, those placed earlier had the highest scores, and those placed later had the lowest scores, with a gap of about 15 points separating those with the earliest versus the latest placements.

The critical period in the human species for language development is similar to the critical periods in other species for acquisition of behaviors considered essential for survival. For instance, songbirds show a critical period for song learning, although considerable differences in the ways in which songbirds acquire songs occur among the more than 4,000 songbird species (e.g., some songbirds require early exposure to songs for song learning, whereas others can develop song in isolation; Brenowitz & Beecher, 2005). Because only one species of *Homo sapiens* exists, the critical period of language development applies to all children everywhere.

DISCUSSION POINT

In this section, we consider the concept of critical period as it applies to language development. To what other areas of development does the concept of critical period apply?

Universality

Language is ubiquitous among the communities of the world. Every human culture has one language, and sometimes many languages, and all are equally complex. The universality of language, as Steven Pinker wrote in *The Language Instinct* (1994),

> fills linguists with awe, and is the first reason to suspect that language is not just any cultural invention but the product of a special human instinct. . . . Cultural inventions vary widely in their sophistication from society to society. . . . [L]anguage, however, ruins this correlation. There are Stone Age societies, but there is no such thing as a Stone Age language. (p. 26)

The universality concept, as applied to language, suggests all persons around the world apply the same cognitive infrastructure to the task of learning language, and that this cognitive infrastructure is particularly suited to the task of developing symbolic representations for objects and actions (Christiansen & Kirby, 2003). Although world languages clearly vary in their syntactic organization (e.g., some languages do not have auxiliary verbs, whereas others do; see Tomasello, 2005), the cognitive infrastructure is the same for all languages. Therefore, the way in which children learn language, and the time points at which they achieve certain milestones appear to be fairly invariant among global language communities.

Species Specificity

Language is strictly a human capacity. No other animals share this aptitude; thus, human language shows species specificity. Although many nonhuman species can communicate, their communication abilities tend to be relatively iconic, such that there is a transparent relationship between *what* is being communicated and *how* it is being communicated. One study of the communication skills of domestic dogs (Border Collies, for those interested in the details) revealed they were able to fetch an object when shown a miniature version of the object (Kaminksi, Tempelman, Call, & Tomasello, 2009). (They did less well when asked to fetch objects shown in a photograph.) The study found domestic dogs could comprehend human communication that featured iconic signs. Although this is an interesting feat, it pales in comparison to what even very young children can do, as little is iconic about human language. For instance, a 2-year-old would have little difficulty comprehending the phrase "Mommy will be home soon" even though it is not iconic at all.

Animal communication systems differ in another important way from human communication systems, specific to its hierarchical properties. Human language provides a syntactic framework that permits the combination of ideas into larger hierarchical propositions; in fact, humans can produce an endless array of novel constructions with the tool of syntax. Although animals can learn sequences of complex actions, the hierarchical complexity of human language far exceeds the capabilities of even the most sophisticated of nonhuman primates (Conway & Christiansen, 2001). No other animal has a communication system that provides the means for combining symbols in the way syntax allows humans to use language.

Semanticity

Human language allows people to represent events that are decontextualized, or removed from the present—to share what happened before this moment or what may happen after this moment. This concept is called semanticity or, alternatively, displacement. As mentioned previously, human language has no time or space boundaries because the relationship between a referent and the language used to describe it is completely arbitrary. For instance, the word *cup* has no relationship to that to which it refers; the relationship is completely arbitrary. As such, a person can say the word *cup* without having a cup present, and other people will know to what the person is referring. Semanticity (or displacement) is the aspect of language that allows people to represent the world to others, a remarkable capacity shared by no other species.

Productivity

Productivity describes the principle of combination—specifically, the combination of a small number of discrete units into seemingly infinite novel creations. Productivity is a phenomenon that applies to other human activities—such as mathematics and music—as well as to language. With a relatively small set of rules governing language, humans can produce an endless number of ideas and new constructions. For instance, humans use only a small set of sounds (speakers of GAE use about 39) and can combine these small units—according to a set of rules they know intuitively (e.g., /g/ cannot follow /l/ in English at the beginning of a syllable)—into an infinite number of words. Likewise, humans use a relatively small number of words and with them, can create an infinite variety of new sentences, most of which no one has ever heard. Because of the remarkable principle of productivity, you could, right now, produce a sentence that no other person has ever uttered.

Although many nonhuman species can communicate, their communication is iconic in that a transparent relationship exists between what is being communicated and how it is being communicated.

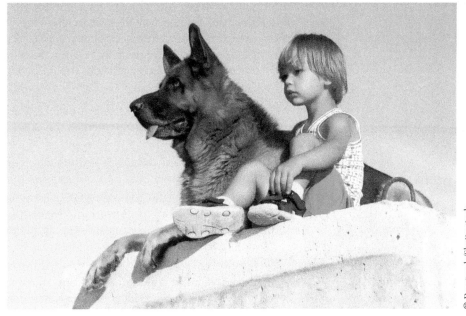

© Berezandr/Shutterstock

√ **1.4**
Check Your Understanding
Click here to gauge your understanding of the concepts in this section.

The principle of productivity is inherent in language in its earliest stages of acquisition: Children who are 18 months old and have about 50 words in their vocabulary can combine and recombine this small set of words to produce sentences that neither they nor others have ever heard. This feature of language is unique to humans because the units of nonhuman communication systems cannot be recombined to make new meanings. For instance, night monkeys have 16 communication units. These units cannot be recombined to make more than 16 possible ways to communicate because the principle of productivity does not apply (Bickerton, 1995).

WHAT ARE LANGUAGE DIFFERENCES AND LANGUAGE DISORDERS?

For most children, language development follows a fairly invariant path. Children around the world typically begin to communicate using words around the same time (12 months), and they often begin to combine words to form two-word combinations (e.g., *daddy shoe, mommy go*) by around 18 months. From that point, they accrue thousands of words in their productive vocabulary by age 5 years and achieve an adultlike grammar well before puberty. However, although this general developmental trajectory characterizes most children, it does not describe them all. In fact, a comparison of any two children of about the same age will reveal considerable differences in the form, content, and use of their language. Such differences relate to the language being learned, gender and temperament, and the language-learning environment. In addition, some children show mild to severe disorders in language acquisition as a result of innate genetic predispositions, developmental disability, or injury or illness. In Chapter 10, we provide a more in-depth examination of these topics.

Language Differences

Language difference is a general term that describes the variability among language users. Two children of exactly the same age will likely show a range of differences if their language abilities are compared. For example, they may differ in the number of words they understand, the length of their sentences, the types of words they use, and the way they share language with other people during conversation. Sometimes the differences between two individuals are subtle. However, in other instances the differences may be more significant and may even compromise communication. For instance, consider the following descriptions of young children in the United States:

- Lamika, a 5-year-old girl, speaks a dialect of African American English. She attends a child care center in which all the other children and her teachers speak GAE.

- Angela, a 3-year-old child with hearing loss, communicates by using Signed Exact English. She attends a special preschool for children with hearing loss, and most of her peers sign with American Sign Language.

- Jack, a 2-year-old child, is learning Spanish and English simultaneously. His family speaks both languages at home. In his preschool, which includes mostly monolingual Spanish-speaking children, he speaks primarily Spanish but sometimes uses the grammar of English.

- Mimi, a 3-year-old child adopted from China at age 18 months, uses fewer vocabulary words and produces shorter sentences than other children in her child care center.

These examples reveal how children (as well as adults) who live in culturally and linguistically diverse communities show variability in their language. In this section, we discuss several major factors that help explain differences among individuals—specifically, dialect, bilingualism, gender, genetic predisposition, and language-learning environment.

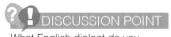

DISCUSSION POINT
What English dialect do you speak? What dialects do your friends speak? To what extent do these differences affect your communication with one another?

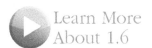

Learn More About 1.6

As you watch the video titled "The Psychology of Accents," consider your own perception of accents and how these perceptions may influence how you interact with others.
https://www.youtube.com/watch?v=CSp9ghRymgk

Dialect

Dialects are the natural variations of a language that evolve within specific cultural or geographic boundaries. These variations affect form, content, and use. Given the many speakers of English around the world, the fact that numerous English dialects exist is not surprising. In the United States, common dialects include Appalachian English, African American English, and Spanish-Influenced English. Each of these dialects may show subtle to more significant variations in form, content, and use from those of the GAE dialect. This finding is also true of the dialects of English spoken around the world, including those of Great Britain, Australia, and New Zealand.

Every language includes a range of dialectal variations, and the number of dialects for a given language increases when users of a language are spread across a large geographic region, when significant geographic barriers isolate one community from other communities, or when social barriers are present within a language community. Language Diversity and Differences: *African American English* provides an in-depth look at the African American English dialect. We provide a more thorough discussion of language diversity and differences, including dialects, in Chapter 9.

Bilingualism

Although many children in the United States learn a single language (monolingualism), others acquire two or more languages (bilingualism). Hawaii is the only officially bilingual state (English and Hawaiian), although a number of states are unofficially bilingual, providing services in multiple languages. This is particularly the case in cities, like the international hub of Miami, Florida, in which the population is very culturally and linguistically diverse. With such diversity increasing across the United States, it is not surprising that today, about one-fifth of Americans speak a language other than English at home (U.S. Census Bureau, 2013).

Bilingualism is the norm in many countries, such as Belgium, where many citizens speak both French and Dutch. (There are in fact three official languages in Belgium, as some persons also speak German.) Canada is officially bilingual (English and French), and the constitution requires that services be available in both languages. India has a staggering 23 official languages, and most persons are trilingual, speaking Hindi, English, and the language of their community. Children who are raised bilingually often show language differences not seen in children who are raised monolingually, such as interchanges between the syntax and the vocabulary of the two languages they are learning. This phenomenon is called code switching (Muñoz, Gillam, Peña, & Gulley-Faehnle, 2003). For instance, a child who is bilingual in Spanish and English may produce a sentence in Spanish that includes an English phrase or an English sentence that reflects Spanish syntax.

Children who learn multiple languages can do so simultaneously or sequentially. With *simultaneous bilingualism*, children acquire their two languages concurrently. With *sequential bilingualism*, children develop one language initially, then acquire a second language later. Sequential bilingualism is relatively common for Hispanic children in the United States who learn Spanish at home but then develop English in preschool or elementary school. The English skills of a sequential

LANGUAGE DIVERSITY AND DIFFERENCES

African American English

The English language has many dialects. The term *dialect* refers to natural variations in form, content, and use within a single language. In the United States, African American English (AAE) is a prominent dialect used not only by some African American individuals, but also by persons of various other ethnicities and races. An individual's use of AAE is typically influenced by the amount of contact that person has with AAE-speaking peers rather than by his or her ethnic or racial heritage, a point that holds true for any English dialect.

Sociolinguists, who study variability in languages as a function of social influences, have provided rich descriptions of some of the most prominent features of AAE that distinguish it from GAE (e.g., Labov, 1972). Some features of AAE involve language form, including phonology (e.g., reduction of final consonant clusters, such as /mos/ in AAE vs. /most/ in GAE) and grammar (e.g., omission of the copula verb, such as "that hers" in AAE vs. "that is hers" in GAE; Charity, Scarborough, & Griffin, 2004). Additional features of AAE involve language content and use.

Like all other English dialects, AAE is a systematic, rule-governed system with its own rules and conventions that influence form, content, and use. In every way, AAE is equivalent in its complexity to any other English dialect (Goldstein & Iglesias, 2013). This point is important because some scholars in the past suggested that AAE is an "impoverished" version of English, a perspective that shows a clear lack of understanding of dialectal variations, including the fact that all languages (and their dialects) are equivalent in complexity. Still, in many language communities around the world, people value and assign greater prestige to some dialects than others.

In the United States, some experts contend that speakers of AAE face risks in educational achievement because their dialect differs from the one used most commonly in schools, sometimes called *School English* (*SE*; Charity et al., 2004). One reason for this risk may be a mismatch between the AAE speaker's representation of linguistic features and the features prominent in the dialect of his or her teachers, which often (but not always) is GAE (Charity et al., 2004). Another possibility is that some teachers, particularly those who speak the GAE dialect, may have a negative bias toward pupils who speak AAE, holding lower expectations and providing less effective instruction to these pupils. However, because some research shows that the level of familiarity with SE among pupils who speak AAE is associated positively with their reading achievement (Charity et al., 2004), practitioners must improve their understanding of how dialectal variations both aid and inhibit children's success in school.

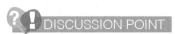

DISCUSSION POINT

Fewer children are raised bilingually in the United States than in a number of other countries. Why? Why might this trend change in the future?

Spanish–English child who is bilingual in the early stages of development will differ from those of a child who learned both Spanish and English from birth, and both children may show some differences in language form, content, and use from those of monolingual English-speaking children.

Although the language a child learns has clear influences on his or her language development—for instance, the stories Chinese-speaking children produce differ in their organizational structure from those of English-speaking children (Wang & Leichtman, 2000)—all languages are approximately equal in complexity. In other words, although some differences can be seen among children as a function of the language (or languages) they are learning, all languages use the same infrastructure of the human brain and thus are similar in complexity (Bickerton, 1995).

Gender

One relatively well-known fact is that girls have an advantage over boys in language development. Girls usually begin talking earlier than boys do (Karmiloff & Karmiloff-Smith, 2001) and develop their vocabulary at a faster rate than boys do in the early years of life (Rowe, Raudenbush, & Goldin-Meadow, 2012). Also, boys are more likely to have significant difficulties with language development, or language impairment; in fact, prevalence estimates show a ratio of about 2 or 3 boys to 1 girl (Dale, Price, Bishop, & Plomin, 2003; Spinath, Price, Dale, & Plomin, 2004). Despite these apparent differences between the genders, Kovas and colleagues (2005) pointed out that gender differences in language development are relatively minor, particularly as children move beyond toddlerhood into the preschool years.

Why such gender differences in language development occur is unclear. Experts point to the possibility of both biological and environmental influences (Kovas et al., 2005). For example, parents may talk more often to girls than to boys, which would help speed language development. Alternatively, hormonal factors may contribute to these differences.

Genetic Predisposition

Any preschool teacher is well aware that young children of about the same age show incredible variability in their language development. Some of this variability relates to genetic predisposition. As a complex human trait, language ability is unlikely to reside on a single gene. However, evidence points to the influence of different alleles from a set of genes on all aspects of language development, including syntax, vocabulary, and phonology (Stromswold, 2001). Twin studies are one method researchers use to estimate the contribution of genetics to language development, as well as the heritability of language disorders (see Research Paradigms: *Twin Studies*). In twin studies, researchers compare the language abilities of identical (*monozygotic*, or *MZ*) and fraternal (*dizygotic*, or *DZ*) twins; MZ twins are genetically identical, whereas DZ twins share 50% of their genetic material. Twin studies allow researchers to identify the exact contributions of genetic and environmental influences to language development.

How much of human language ability is inherited? The results of one study involving 787 pairs of twins revealed that about 16% of the variability in language ability in 4-year-old children could be attributed to heritability (Kovas et al., 2005). However, language disorders among twins seem to be more strongly influenced by genetic factors than do language disorders among children in the typical population; in fact, about 49% of variability in language ability can be attributed to heritability (Spinath et al., 2004). If one MZ twin has a language impairment, the other twin has about an 85% likelihood of also having the impairment.

Language-Learning Environment

The language-learning environment in which children are reared exerts considerable influence on their language development. Although children bring biologically

RESEARCH **PARADIGMS**

Twin Studies

Both genetic and environmental influences play significant roles in language development. However, identifying the exact contributions of genetic influences relative to environmental influences can be difficult. One way to estimate the unique influences of genetics versus environment is *twin studies*, or the *twin method* (Kovas et al., 2005). When monozygotic (MZ) or dizygotic (DZ) twins grow up in the same household, they are assumed to share 100% of their environmental influences, both prenatally (in the womb) and postnatally (in the home environment; Kovas et al., 2005). Researchers interested in estimating the influence of genetic versus environmental influences on language development collect measures of language from sets of twins, often repeatedly across time. These researchers use a number of sophisticated statistical techniques to determine the genetic heritability of certain language skills by comparing MZ and DZ twins. They also can isolate environmental influences on language by carefully controlling the amount of variability in language skill that can be attributed to genetic influences.

One of the largest twin studies to date is the Twins Early Development Study (TEDS), conducted in the United Kingdom, and supported financially by the United Kingdom's Medical Research Council (Trouton, Spinath, & Plomin, 2002). This study involved 6,963 sets of twins; 2,351 were MZ twins, 2,322 were same-gender DZ twins, and 2,290 were opposite-gender DZ twins. All the twins were born in the United Kingdom between 1994 and 1996, and their language development was studied at ages 2, 3, and 4 years by using parent questionnaires. Twins born with severe medical or genetic problems or perinatal complications were not included in the sample, nor were twins whose zygosity could not be determined and those whose parents did not speak English at home (Spinath et al., 2004). Various studies have been conducted by using the data from these twins not only to examine genetic and environmental influences on language development, but also to compare language development for boys versus girls, and to estimate the heritability of language impairment. As a result of TEDS, researchers will be able to answer numerous questions in the next decade by using data from these nearly 14,000 children.

endowed abilities and propensities to the language-learning task, the neural architecture that supports language acquisition is an "open genetic program" (Cartwright, 2000, p. 195). This term means the neural architecture is calibrated on the basis of input from the environment, or the "actual evidence" children receive from the environment, concerning the form, content, and use of the language or languages to which they are exposed (Cartwright, 2000). In short, everything the child experiences in his or her environment will help calibrate his or her language-learning apparatus.

The environmental aspects that seem to figure most prominently in the young child's language development are the quantity and quality of language experienced. *Quantity* refers to the sheer amount of language a child experiences. *Quality* refers to the characteristics of the language spoken in the child's caregiving environment: the types of words (e.g., nouns, verbs, adverbs), the construction of sentences (e.g., simple, complex, compound), the intention of sentences (e.g., directives, declaratives, interrogatives), and the organization and specificity of stories (e.g., emotional expression, situational details). How often toddlers and preschoolers participate in conversations with their caregivers is significantly associated with language growth in the first few years of life, indicating that sheer volume of talk is important (Zimmerman et al., 2009). However, children who are exposed to an array of complex sentence forms (e.g., sentences with subordinate clauses, such as *That boy who hit me is not my friend*), in addition to simple sentence forms, (e.g., *That boy is not my friend*) will use more complex sentence forms than those used by children not exposed to such syntax (Huttenlocher, Vasilyeva, Cymerman, & Levine, 2002). In short, characteristics of the language to which children are exposed in their prominent caregiving environments (home, preschool, etc.) contribute to the variability in children's language development.

DISCUSSION POINT

Young children who participate in many conversations at home have better language skills than children who participate in few conversations. Explain why there are differences in the conversational opportunities children experience in American homes.

Studies of infants reared in mainstream United States communities have revealed one particularly important aspect of the language-learning environment: caregiver responsiveness. This term refers to the promptness, contingency, and appropriateness of caregiver responses to children's bids for communication through words or other means (Tamis-LeMonda, Bornstein, & Baumwell, 2001). Experts contend responsiveness provides a significant aid to children's language development because it reflects the child's current topic of interest, and provides sensitive input that promotes semantic and syntactic learning. Higher degrees of caregiver responsiveness during infancy and early toddlerhood are associated with accelerated rates of language development in children. For instance, the results of one study revealed children of highly responsive mothers achieved the 50-word milestone, on average, at age 15 months, whereas children of less responsive mothers were more likely to achieve this milestone at about age 21 months (Tamis-LeMonda et al., 2001). The contribution of caregivers' responsive and sensitive language input to children's language development indicates quality of language input is just as important as quantity. See Theory to Practice: *Children Who Are Linguistically Reticent in the Classroom* for a description of how the relation between temperament and language has influenced practice in the area of promoting linguistic interactions with children who are reticent.

Language Disorders

Like any complex human trait, the ability to develop language in a timely and effortless manner can be adversely influenced by heritable weaknesses in the language mechanism, as well as by the presence of certain developmental disabilities and brain injuries. Children with language impairment show significant difficulties in the development of language, typically achieving language milestones more slowly than other children, and exhibiting long-standing difficulties with various aspects of language form, content, and use. Next, we provide a brief overview of childhood language impairment, a topic we address in more detail in Chapter 10.

Heritable Language Impairment

Children with a heritable language impairment exhibit depressed language abilities, typically with no other concomitant impairment of intellect. Because of its specificity to the functioning of language, this condition is often called specific language impairment (SLI), and it affects about 7%–10% of children (Beitchman et al., 1989; Tomblin et al., 1997). SLI is the most common type of communication impairment affecting children. It is the most frequent reason for administering early intervention and special education services to toddlers through fourth graders.

Evidence suggests SLI is a heritable condition, as indicated by both twin studies and family pedigree studies (Lai, Fisher, Hurst, Vargha-Khadem, & Monaco, 2001; Spinath et al., 2004). The results of twin studies reveal a strong likelihood for an MZ twin to have SLI if his or her twin is affected. Family pedigree studies show a strong likelihood for a child to have SLI if a parent is affected.

Developmental Disability

Language impairment often co-occurs with certain developmental disabilities. In such cases, language impairment is considered a secondary disorder because it results secondary to a primary cause. Common causes of a secondary language impairment include intellectual disability and autism spectrum disorder. Intellectual disability is a "condition of arrested or incomplete development of the mind, which is especially characterized by impairment of skills manifested during the developmental period" (American Association on Mental Retardation [AAMR], 2002, p. 103). For intellectual disability to be diagnosed, an individual must also exhibit limitations in adaptive behavior, and the activities of daily living, such as difficulties with conceptual skills

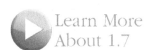

Learn More About 1.7

As you watch the video titled "What is SLI?" consider how a language disorder may go undetected in an individual for a long period of time. https://www.youtube.com/watch?v=Pqu7w6t3Rmo

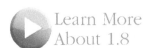

Learn More About 1.8

As you watch the video titled "Speech & Language Therapy: Helping Michael," consider how all the areas of form, content, and use can be impacted by speech and language therapy. https://www.youtube.com/watch?v=MpdjP0zHeBc

(communication, functional academics, self-direction, health and safety), social skills (social relationships, leisure), or practical skills (self-care, home living, community participation, work; AAMR, 2002). One cause of intellectual disability is Down syndrome, which is due to a chromosomal anomaly during the initial stages of fetal development. Whether intellectual disability occurs because of Down syndrome or other causes, it is often accompanied by significant language impairment.

Another type of secondary language impairment is *autism spectrum disorder* (ASD). *ASD* is an umbrella term describing a variety of developmental conditions characterized by significant difficulties in social relationships and communication with others, and restricted and repetitive behaviors. These difficulties are apparent within early childhood, but may become more apparent over time, as the demands to engage in complex communication with others increase (American Psychiatric Association, 2013). The number of children affected by ASD has increased over the last several decades, with current estimates indicating that about 1 in 68 children have ASD (Centers for Disease Control and Prevention, 2014). Children with autism spectrum disorder usually exhibit mild to profound secondary language impairment, and some children with this disability never develop productive use of language. A condition related to ASD is

THEORY TO PRACTICE

Children Who Are Linguistically Reticent in the Classroom

The frequency with which children use language as a tool to communicate with other people varies substantially among individual children. To some extent, frequency relates to a child's facility with his or her language, but it also relates to temperament. *Temperament* describes an individual's "innate way of approaching and experiencing the world" (Kristal, 2005, p. 5), and it is a theoretical construct of human behavior that helps researchers understand why some children are bold and energetic, others are sensitive and timid, and some are inflexible (Kristal, 2005). Given that language development requires a child to experience input from the environment to "calibrate" his or her language-learning mechanisms, a reasonable conclusion is that a child's temperament might influence the amount of language input he or she experiences. For instance, a child who is bold may solicit more language from parents and teachers, whereas the child who is reticent and shy may solicit less language.

Theoretical perspectives on the potential interaction of language development and temperament suggest that an *interaction* occurs between these two constructs or that they influence one another. The results of studies on the possible interaction of language and temperament provide support for this theory. For example, Evans (1996) found that 18 kindergartners characterized by teachers as very reticent (e.g., rarely asking for assistance when it was needed, seldom participating in class discussions) performed more poorly than their more talkative

peers on a variety of language ability measures in first grade. What remains unclear is whether some children are less talkative because they have less developed language skills, or whether children with less developed language skills are less talkative.

Theory and research on the possibility of a temperament–language interaction have important implications for instruction in the preschool and kindergarten classroom, in which several important goals include fostering children's language skills, promoting socialization among children, and promoting children's ability to use language for a variety of purposes. Teachers may have difficulty helping children who are verbally reticent achieve these goals. One approach that has been tested for increasing children's language use and complexity in the preschool classroom is training teachers to use interaction-promoting responses (Cabell et al., 2011). Examples of interaction-promoting responses include (a) using a variety of questions, (b) inviting children to take turns, and (c) scanning the classroom and inviting uninvolved children to participate. Evidence shows that when teachers use these and other language-promoting techniques in the preschool classroom, the children talk more and use more complex vocabulary and grammar. Although the effects of these techniques have not been determined specifically for children who are verbally reticent, they provide a promising way to translate theory and research on the temperament–language interaction to inform practice.

social communication disorder (SCD), also called *pragmatic communication disorder* (American Psychiatric Association, 2013). Individuals with SCD have particular difficulty in the use of social communication, such as following the rules of conversation (e.g., taking turns, using eye contact) and comprehending more complex and abstract language (e.g., understanding a joke or idiom). SCD is distinctive from ASD in that individuals typically have higher levels of language skill and do not show the restrictive and repetitive behaviors characteristic of ASD. Historically, persons with SCD may have been referred to as having "high-functioning ASD," but in more recent years, it is recognized that SCD is best conceptualized as a particular type of disability that is distinct from that of autism.

Brain Injury

Language impairment can also occur as a function of damage or injury to the mechanisms of the brain involved with language functions. Brain injuries can occur in utero (before birth) and perinatally (during the birthing process), but they can also occur after birth; these injuries are called acquired brain injuries. Acquired brain injuries are a leading cause of death and disability among young children. Brain damage resulting from physical trauma, particularly blunt trauma to the head, is referred to as traumatic brain injury (TBI). Annually, about 500,000 children (0 to 14 years of age) in the United States experience TBI, with the highest rate among infants and toddlers (Langlois, Rutland-Brown, & Thomas, 2007). Causes of TBI in children include abuse (e.g., shaken baby syndrome), intentional harm (e.g., being hit or shot in the head), accidental poisoning through ingestion of toxic substances (e.g., prescription medications, pesticides), car accidents, and falls. Injuries may be *diffuse*, affecting large areas of the brain, or *focal*, affecting only one specific brain region. The frontal and temporal lobes of the brain, which house the centers for most executive functions (e.g., reasoning, planning, hypothesizing) and language functions, are often damaged in head injuries (Eden & Stevens, 2006).

Even though it is popularly believed that the brain of the young child can readily heal following brain injury (because of plasticity), this does not seem to be the case (Catroppa & Anderson, 2009). One possible reason for this misperception is that some young children may have delayed onset of impairment; problems sustained during a brain injury may not be evident until years later, when damaged areas of the brain are applied to complex skills and activities.

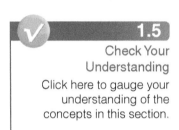

1.5

Check Your Understanding

Click here to gauge your understanding of the concepts in this section.

SUMMARY

Language is a complex and dynamic system of conventional symbols used in various modes for thought and communication. The human brain uses language as a representational tool to store information and to carry out many cognitive processes, such as reasoning, hypothesizing, and planning. As a communication tool, language provides a productive and efficient means for sharing information with other people. Some researchers consider the human capacity for language to reside in a particular module of the brain; others contend that a more general neural network serves language processes.

Language, speech, hearing, and communication are different albeit interrelated processes. Speech is the voluntary neuromuscular behavior that allows humans to express language and is essential for spoken communication. Hearing is the perception of sound, which includes both general auditory perception and speech perception. Speech perception involves specialized processors in the brain that have evolved specifically to respond to human speech and language. Communication is the act of sharing information among two or more people. Although communication need not involve speech, language, and hearing, the capacity for humans to use these processes to share information makes human communication the most sophisticated among all species.

Language comprises three major domains: form, content, and use. *Form* is how words, sentences, and sounds are organized and arranged to convey content. Form includes phonology (rules governing the sounds used to make syllables and words), morphology (rules governing the internal organization of words and syllables), and syntax (rules governing the internal organization of sentences). *Content* is the meaning of language, including the specific words people use and the concepts words and groups of words represent. *Use* describes the functions language serves, or how people draw on language functionally to meet personal and social needs.

Five remarkable features of language make it particularly fascinating to both researchers and practitioners. First is the acquisition rate of language; young children exhibit a striking capacity for developing language rapidly and efficiently. Second is the universality of language. Language is ubiquitous among world communities, and every human culture has one or more languages that its members share. The third feature is species specificity. Language is a uniquely human capacity; no other animal species shares this aptitude. The fourth feature is semanticity. Human language allows people to represent events that are decontextualized,

or removed from the present, including not only real events of the past or future, but also events and concepts that are wholly imaginary and abstract. The fifth feature is productivity—or the principle of combination—which is how the rule-governed code of language provides its users with a generative code by which they can combine a small number of discrete units (e.g., phonemes, morphemes) into seemingly infinite novel creations.

Comparing the language achievements of any two persons, whether children or adults, will reveal considerable individual differences in the content, form, and use of language. *Language differences* and *language disorders* are terms that describe this variability in language achievements among individuals. Language differences occur because of the natural variability in language achievement that results from different dialects, bilingualism, gender differences, genetic predisposition, and varied language-learning environments. A language disorder occurs when an individual shows significant difficulties in language achievement; such disorders result from heritable language impairment, developmental disability, and brain injury.

 Apply Your Knowledge

Click here to apply your knowledge to practical scenarios.

BEYOND THE BOOK

1. Search http://www.youtube.com for a video of a toddler in a conversation with his or her parent. Prepare a transcript of all utterances the toddler produces. Classify each utterance according to its primary purpose (see Table 1.1). What purposes occur most often? Least often?

2. With a classmate, discuss the pros and cons of adopting an official language or languages in the United States. (Currently, there is no official language.)

3. Watch a video or live feed of a person being interviewed by a popular television personality During the interview, assess the types of linguistic,

nonlinguistic, and paralinguistic feedback the person provides. What types of feedback seem to characterize this person?

4. Language is a rule-governed system. Communicating with friends via text-based systems, such as text messaging, seem to have their own set of rules. What are some of these rules? How did these rules come about and how do they spread?

5. In small groups, discuss the benefits of teaching a very young child to use sign language (e.g., to learn "baby signs.") Also discuss why so many parents seem interested in helping their children to sign before they can talk.

 Check Your Understanding

Gauge your understanding of the chapter concepts by taking this self-check quiz.

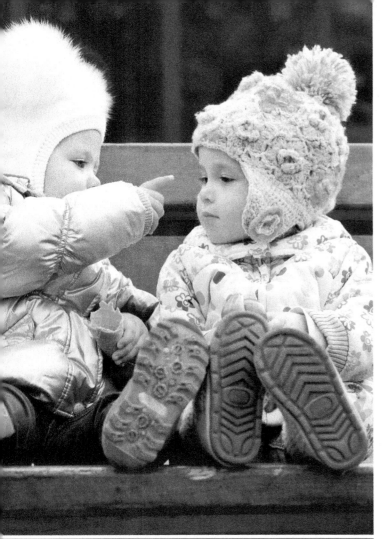

2

Building Blocks of Language

LEARNING OUTCOMES

After completion of this chapter, the reader will be able to:

1. Discuss important concepts related to early phonological development.

2. Discuss important concepts related to early morphological development.

3. Define the term *syntactic development*.

4. Identify major building blocks in early semantic development.

5. Explain important concepts related to early pragmatic development.

In Chapter 1, we discussed how language is a single dimension of human behavior that comprises three interrelated domains: form, content, and use. Children's language development involves achieving competency in each of these domains, and, subsequently in this book, we discuss major accomplishments in each domain for infants (Chapter 5), toddlers (Chapter 6), preschoolers (Chapter 7), and school-age children (Chapter 8). In this chapter, we present these three domains in more detail to prepare you for the in-depth discussions in Chapters 5–8, and for the various theories related to language development in Chapter 4.

As children develop their language from infancy forward, their achievements in each language domain grow by leaps and bounds as they master, and then expand on the basic building blocks of form, content, and use. Recall from Chapter 1 that the five components of the three domains are as follows: phonology, morphology, syntax, semantics, and pragmatics. Phonology, morphology, and syntax are components of form, whereas semantics and pragmatics are components of content and use, respectively. In this chapter, we identify and discuss the basic building blocks for each component of the three domains. We start by describing three *phonological development* building blocks: becoming sensitive to prosodic and phonotactic cues in streams of speech, developing internal representations of the phonemes of the native language, and becoming phonologically aware. We then turn to the building blocks of *morphological development*—acquiring grammatical (inflectional) and derivational morphemes—and *syntactic development*—increasing utterance length, using different sentence modalities, and developing complex syntax. We then discuss the building blocks of *semantic development*, which include developing a lexicon, learning new words, and organizing the lexicon for efficient retrieval. Finally, we describe the *pragmatic development* building blocks: acquiring communication functions, learning conversational skills, and gaining sensitivity to extralinguistic cues. As we discuss each building block, we briefly examine important influences—such as gender, socioeconomic status, and language impairment—on children's achievements.

WHAT IS PHONOLOGICAL DEVELOPMENT?

Phonological development involves acquiring the rules of language that govern the sound structure of syllables and words. We discuss in Chapter 1 how every language has a relatively small number of meaningful sounds, or *phonemes*. Phonemes are the individual speech sounds in a language that signal a contrast in meaning. In General American English, for instance, /r/ and /l/ are two different phonemes because exchanging one sound for the other creates a different meaning (e.g., *low* vs. *row*; *liver* vs. *river*). Words that differ by only one phoneme, such as *low* and *row*, are called minimal pairs. As children develop their phonological system, they develop an internal representation of each phoneme in their native language, which is important to differentiate minimal pairs. In essence, a phonological representation is a neurological imprint of a phoneme that differentiates it from other phonemes. Having this imprint (internal representation) does not necessarily correspond to being able to produce a phoneme, as we can see here in this exchange between the second author and her 3-year-old son, Griffin:

GRIFFIN: We need to "sine" the mirror.

LJ: Sign the mirror?

GRIFFIN: No, we need to "sign" it. (emphasizes the initial /s/)

This exchange implies that Griffin has an internal representation of the "sh" sound (the initial phoneme in *shine*), and perceives the meaningful difference in the minimal pairs *shine* and *sign*; however, his production does not match that internal representation. This is not an uncommon sort of exchange with children in this age range, whose internal phonological representations seem to be more sophisticated than their expressive capabilities (at least for certain sounds, such as "sh" and "th").

Phonological development also involves developing sensitivity to the phonotactic rules of a person's native language; these rules specify "legal" (i.e., acceptable) orders of sounds in syllables and words and the places where specific phonemes can and cannot occur. Early in development, children become sensitive to both. For example, they recognize that /l/ + /h/ is an illegal combination of sounds in English, and that /t/ + /s/ is legal in the final position of a syllable (e.g., *pots*) but illegal in the initial position.

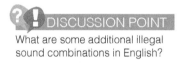

DISCUSSION POINT

What are some additional illegal sound combinations in English?

Phonological Building Blocks

Phonological development begins immediately after birth (if not before) as the infant experiences speech in the environment. Here, we describe three key building blocks in phonological development, and provide more detail in subsequent chapters: (a) using cues to segment streams of speech, (b) developing a phonemic inventory, and (c) becoming phonologically aware.

Cues to Segment Streams of Speech

One of the earliest phonological tasks infants face is parsing the streams of speech occurring in the world around them. Early in development, infants exhibit the capacity to use specific cues within the speech stream to parse it into smaller units (e.g., words) and to separate simultaneously occurring speech streams (e.g., the speech on the television vs. the mother's speech; Hollich, Newman, & Jusczyk, 2005). One strategy infants use to parse speech streams is to draw on prosodic and phonotactic cues (Estes, 2014; Gerken & Aslin, 2005).

When using prosodic cues, infants draw on their familiarity with word and syllable stress patterns, or the rhythm of language, to break into the speech stream. For example, infants exposed to English rapidly become sensitive to prevalent stress patterns in English words, including the strong–weak stress pattern in such words as *little* and *grammar* (Thiessen & Saffran, 2003). During the first year of life, infants use their knowledge of predominant word-stress patterns to locate boundaries between words in running streams of speech. For example, they presume that a word boundary occurs following two syllables of a strong–weak stress pattern, given the prevalence of this word-stress pattern in English. For the infant who hears "little boy," this cueing strategy helps him to isolate *little* and *boy* as separate words. Infants also recognize relatively early that pauses often occur at the boundaries between clauses and phrases (Gerken & Aslin, 2005; Hawthorne & Gerken, 2014). Infants' sensitivity to the way in which pausing marks linguistic boundaries within speech streams, such as clause segments, may support their syntactic development because it provides the opportunity to analyze how smaller syntactic units combine to form larger units of speech (Hawthorne & Gerken, 2014).

Infants also use phonotactic cues to parse the speech stream. Early in development, infants become sensitive to the probability that certain sounds will occur both in general and in specific positions of syllables and words (Jusczyk, Luce, & Charles-Luce, 1994). Thus, when encountering a speech stream containing the phoneme sequence /gz/, the English-learning infant recognizes the improbability that this sequence starts a word. In contrast, this sequence is both legal and probable in the final position of a word (*dogs, eggs*), and he or she uses knowledge of these probabilities to segment a likely word boundary following the sequence. Knowledge of phonotactic probabilities and improbabilities is an important tool for the infant to use to segment novel words from a continuous speech stream (Estes, 2014).

Phonemic Inventory

Another major building block in phonological development is the child's acquisition of internal representations of the phonemes composing his or her native language—termed phonological knowledge—and his or her expression of these phonemes to produce syllables and words—termed phonological production or *expression*. Children develop a full phonemic inventory gradually as they make more and more fine-tuned distinctions among phonemes. When their inventory is relatively small, children use a single phoneme (e.g., /d/) to express multiple phonemes (e.g., /t/, /d/, /k/, and /g/). This means a 2-year-old might say both "take" and "cake" as "dake." Children gradually add more phonemes until their inventory is complete and adultlike.

The child's phonemic inventory includes both vowels and consonants. Vowels develop prior to consonants, typically in the first year of life. In contrast, not all consonants are acquired or expressed at the same time; some emerge early in development (early consonants) and others emerge later (late consonants). Several factors influence the timing of development for specific phonemes, including the phoneme's frequency of occurrence in spoken language, the number of words a child uses that contain a given phoneme, and, to some extent, the articulatory complexity of producing the phoneme (Amayreh, 2003; To, Cheung, & McLeod, 2013). Because of these influences, the order of consonantal acquisition varies among languages; for example, English-speaking children master /z/ earlier than Arabic-speaking children because this phoneme occurs more frequently in English than in Arabic (Amayreh, 2003).

In general, children's phonological knowledge and production are sufficiently well developed by age 3–4 years to provide for fully intelligible speech. Although some consonantal phonemes will elude mastery for several more years, the child's inventory is large enough to allow reasonable substitutions of mastered phonemes for those yet to be mastered (e.g., /d/ for the initial sound in *that*). Figure 2.1 provides a summary of the order of mastery for the English consonantal phonemes. Examining this figure, note that an early-emerging phoneme is /m/ and a later-emerging phoneme is /v/. Why do you think /m/ would emerge early and /v/ later among English-speaking children?

Phonological Awareness

Phonological awareness is an individual's ability to attend to the phonological units of speech through implicit or explicit analysis. We can examine an individual's phonological awareness using a variety of simple oral tasks (so the individual completing the tasks must *listen* to the phonological units and not *read* them):

1. *Syllable counting:* How many syllables are in the word *psychologist*? (Answer: four)

2. *Rhyme detection:* Of these four words, which two rhyme: *four, boat, hat, door*? (Answer: *four, door*)

3. *Initial sound identification:* What is the first sound in the word *boat*? (Answer: /b/)

4. *Initial sound elision:* Say the word *boat* without the /b/. (Answer: *oat*)

5. *Phoneme counting:* How many sounds are in the word *justice*? (Answer: six)

All of these tasks require an individual to attend to the phonological units of words, ranging from fairly large units (syllables, item 1) to the smallest units (each individual phoneme, item 5). Of the five tasks, the latter three are the most challenging because one has to attend to the smallest units of phonology by identifying or eliding the first sounds in words (items 3, 4, and 5), or by counting all of the phonemes in a word (item 5). When an individual is able to attend explicitly to the individual phonemes in words, as is necessary for task 5, he or she is said

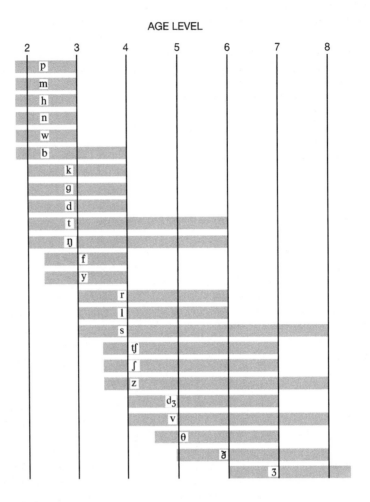

FIGURE 2.1

Order of acquisition for English consonantal phonemes.

Source: Reprinted with permission from "When Are Speech Sounds Learned?" by E.K. Sander, 1972. Journal of Speech and Hearing Disorders, 37,p. 62. Copyright 1972 by American Speech Language Hearing Association. All rights reserved.

to have phonemic awareness (awareness of the individual phonemes of a language). Although young children demonstrate phonological awareness as early as 2 years, which is apparent in their ability to produce rhyming patterns and engage in word play (e.g., "Lily-Lily-bo-Billy . . ."), children typically do not exhibit phonemic awareness until several years later (Anthony et al., 2011).

Phonological awareness provides an important bridge between language development and reading achievement (Melby-Lervåg, Lyster, & Hulme, 2012). This is particularly true for alphabetic languages, such as English, in which the written script represents phonemes using letter-to-sound pairings for individual letters (*B* = /b/) and letter sequences (e.g., *OUGH* = /o/). Phonics instruction teaches children the relationships between letters and sounds, and children who are "phonologically aware" can better profit from phonics instruction than children who are unaware (see Metsala & Ehri, 2013). Many children in the United States struggle to develop basic word-reading skills, and for many of these children, a contributor to this struggle is underdeveloped phonological awareness (Fuchs et al., 2012). Systematically teaching children to attend to the phonological structure of language, through the use of games and other similar activities, is an important aspect of early-reading instruction that can have long-term, positive effects on future reading achievement (Suggate, 2014).

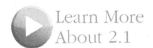

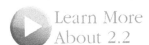

Influences on Phonological Development

Some children develop their phonological skills much more slowly than other children, which may signal a phonological disorder if the delay is significant. As we address in Chapter 10, such a disorder compromises the child's achievement of the building blocks discussed in the previous sections. In this section, we discuss two additional, well-established influences on phonological development.

Native Language

Infants' phonological development is influenced significantly by the phonemic composition of the language (or languages) to which the infants are exposed. Speech sounds that are phonemic in one language may not be phonemic in another. Thus, children learning Arabic acquire representations of the phonemic inventory of Arabic and not the inventory of English (or any other language); for this reason, Arabic-speaking children will not develop a phonemic representation of /p/ because it is not phonemic in their language.

Even when a given speech sound is phonemic in two languages, children may acquire it at different times, depending on the frequency with which it appears in words and its similarity to other phonemes in the language inventory. In other words, the functional load of a phoneme can vary among languages. *Functional load* refers essentially to the importance of a phoneme in the phonemic inventory of the language, which corresponds to the volume of words that are distinguishable by that phoneme (Wedel, Kaplan, & Jackson, 2013). If we draw again on the comparison of English and Arabic, English-speaking children master /z/ by about age 4 years (Grunwell, 1997), whereas Arabic-speaking children do not master this phoneme until after age 6 years (Amayreh, 2003). In English, the phoneme /z/ has a high functional load, in part because it is used for pluralization (e.g., *vans, dogs*), whereas in Arabic it has a low functional load (Amayreh, 2003).

Linguistic Experience

Even among children who are learning the same language, differences exist in the timing of their establishment of phonological representations and in their production of different phonemes (McCune & Vihman, 2001). Children develop phonological representations through their exposure to phonemic contrasts in their

Infants use various tactics to break into the streams of speech they hear around them. For instance, early in life, infants use their implicit knowledge of sound patterns in their native language to identify boundaries between words in the speech stream.

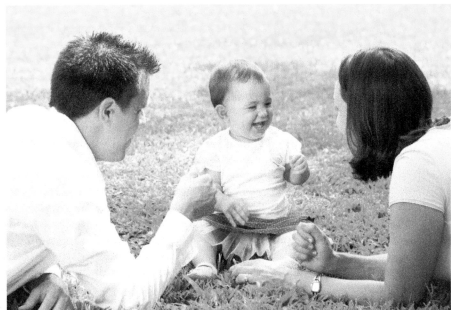

© michaeljung/Shutterstock

language; thus, differences in the timing of phonological development occur, at least in part, because of variability in children's phonological exposure. The internal phonological representations of children reared in lower-income homes can be less mature and distinct than those of children of the same age reared in higher-income homes, probably because of variations in the children's exposure to language (McDowell, Lonigan, & Goldstein, 2007). The same holds true for children with a history of chronic ear infections, whose phonological representations are less mature than those of children without such a history (Haapala et al., 2014). This is because children with chronic ear infections experience periods in which linguistic exposure is compromised.

2.1

Check Your Understanding

Click here to gauge your understanding of the concepts in this section.

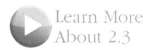

Learn More About 2.3

As you watch the video titled "An Introduction to Morphology," notice how morphology influences other areas of language (specifically syntax and semantics).

https://www.youtube.com/watch?v=syjbhT45J14

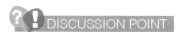

DISCUSSION POINT

Using the word *school*, identify all the morphemes that can be added to it to inflect it. Classify each morpheme as grammatical or derivational.

WHAT IS MORPHOLOGICAL DEVELOPMENT?

Children's *morphological development* is their internalization of the rules of language that govern word structure. Morphemes are the smallest meaningful units of language, and many words include several morphemes. Morphemes allow the grammatical inflection of words, as in adding *-ed* to *walk* to create the past tense verb *walked*, and they can change the syntactic class of words, as in adding *-like* to the noun *child* to create the adjective *childlike*. Morphological development thus provides children with the tools for grammatical inflection, as well as a means for expanding their vocabulary from a smaller set of root words (e.g., *child*) to an exponentially larger set of derived forms (e.g., *childless*, *childlike*, *childish*).

Morphological Building Blocks

Morphological development involves acquiring two types of morphemes: grammatical morphemes (also called *inflectional morphemes*) and derivational morphemes. As discussed in Chapter 1, grammatical morphemes include the plural *-s* (*cat–cats*), the possessive *'s* (*mom–mom's*), the past tense *-ed* (*walk–walked*), and the present progressive *-ing* (*do–doing*), to name a few. Derivational morphemes change a word's syntactic class and semantic meaning. For example, taking the word *like*, we can add both prefixes (*dislike*, *unlike*) and suffixes (*liken*, *likeable*, *likeness*) to vary its meaning and syntactic role in a sentence.

Grammatical Morphemes

Children's earliest words and sentences contain few grammatical morphemes, but only for the first year or two. At about age 2 years, children begin to use the first-appearing grammatical morpheme, the present progressive *-ing*. Whereas before then, the child might ask, "Where Mommy go?", he or she now asks, "Where Mommy going?" In subsequent chapters, we discuss in more detail the child's timing and course of acquisition for learning the major grammatical morphemes, which include not only the present progressive *-ing*, but also the plural *-s*, the possessive *'s*, and the past tense *-ed*, as shown in Table 2.1. Note that the grammatical morphemes in Table 2.1 include not only suffixes, but also several free morphemes. Suffixes (and prefixes) are called bound morphemes because they must be bound or attached to other morphemes. In contrast, free morphemes can stand alone; they include both words with clear semantic referents (e.g., *dream*, *dog*, *walk*), and words that serve primarily grammatical purposes (e.g., *his*, *the*, *that*). Children's early achievements in grammatical morphology include acquiring not only bound morphemes but also several free morphemes that serve purely grammatical purposes, including the prepositions *in* and *on*, and the articles *the*, *a*, and *an*.

The child's acquisition of the major grammatical morphemes, which follows a fairly invariant course in both the order and the timing of acquisition, is a subtle, but important achievement in early childhood. Although parents do not often

TABLE 2.1

Grammatical morphemes acquired in early childhood

GRAMMATICAL MORPHEME	AGE (IN MONTHS)	EXAMPLE
Present progressive -ing	19–28	"Baby eating"
Plural -s	27–30	"Doggies"
Preposition in	27–30	"Toy in there"
Preposition on	31–34	"Food on table"
Possessive 's	31–34	"Mommy's book"
Regular past tense -ed	43–46	"We painted."
Irregular past tense	43–46	"I ate lunch."
Regular third-person singular -s	43–46	"He runs fast."
Articles a, the, an	43–46	"I want the blocks"
Contractible copula be	43–46	"She's my friend."
Contractible auxiliary	47–50	"He's playing."
Uncontractible copula be	47–50	"He was sick."
Uncontractible auxiliary	47–50	"He was playing."
Irregular third person	47–50	"She has one."

Source: Information from *A First Language: The Early Stages*, by R. Brown, 1973, Cambridge, MA: Harvard University Press.

applaud (or possibly even notice) when their children first begin to inflect verbs for past tense, grammatical morphology enables the child to move from speaking with a "telegraphic quality" (e.g., "Baby no eat"), to a more adultlike quality ("The baby's not eating"). And, although parents often seem to coach their children to use new important words (as in "Say 'bottle'!" and "Say 'mama'!"), they don't seem to do the same for grammatical morphemes ("Add *s* to 'bottle'!"). However, and perhaps thankfully so, parents don't need to coach their children to use grammatical morphemes at all, as children figure out the rules for when to use them, even at very young ages (Zapf & Smith, 2007).

When researchers study children's grammatical morphology, they often examine obligatory contexts of use, and determine whether the child has omitted or included the obligatory morpheme. An obligatory context occurs when a mature grammar specifies the use of a grammatical marker; for instance, in the phrase *The girl's house*, the possessive *'s* is considered obligatory. Thus, if a child says "The girl house," he or she is omitting the possessive (*'s*) morpheme in an obligatory context. As another example, if a child says "two baby," he or she is omitting the plural (*s*) in an obligatory context. When children include a grammatical morpheme in 75% or more of obligatory contexts, they are said to have mastered the morpheme.

Derivational Morphemes

We add derivational morphemes to root words to create derived words. The corpus of words derived from a common root word (e.g., *friend, friendless, friendliness, befriend*) share derivational relations. We can create derived words by attaching morphemes, both prefixes and suffixes, to root words to yield *polysyllabic words* (words containing more than one syllable). Table 2.2 presents some common

TABLE 2.2

Common derivational prefixes and suffixes

PREFIX	EXAMPLES	SUFFIX	EXAMPLES
un-	unease	-y	guilty
dis-	disappear	-ly	happily
re-	rerun	-like	adultlike
pre-	preview	-tion	adoption
uni-	unitard	-ful	bountiful
tri-	tricycle	-less	tactless
inter-	intergalactic	-er	bigger
fore-	forecast	-est	hardest
post-	postdate	-ness	gentleness
co-	cohabitate	-ish	selfish
im-	immodest	-able	amicable
anti-	antipathy	-ician	pediatrician
sub-	subarctic	-ism	organism
in-	ineffective	-logy	anthropology
un-	unplug	-phobia	arachnophobia

Source: Information from *Word Study for Phonics, Vocabulary, and Spelling Instruction* by D. R. Bear, M. Invernizzi, S. Templeton, and F. Johnston, 2004, Upper Saddle River, NJ: Merrill/Prentice Hall.

prefixes and suffixes used for derivational purposes. Because each prefix and suffix can be combined with many root words, derivational morphology is a powerful tool for adding precision to a person's lexical base.

Influences on Morphological Development

One of the seminal works of child language research is Roger Brown's (1973) book, *A First Language.* In this key work, Brown carefully described children's development of 14 grammatical morphemes, showing how a core of grammatical morphemes emerged in a uniform order among children (see Research Paradigms: *Longitudinal Studies*). These morphemes appear in Table 2.1. Brown's work had a tremendous influence on the field of child language research, prompting many researchers to focus on describing other such universalities in child language development.

Since then, researchers have begun to appreciate the importance of studying individual differences in language acquisition, and identifying specific influences that do and do not affect the normal course of language acquisition. For example, researchers have questioned whether a child's native language influences his or her development of grammatical morphology. Contrary to what you might expect, children learning languages that are richly inflected (e.g., Spanish) do not acquire novel morphemes at faster rates than those of children learning less richly inflected languages (e.g., English).

Second Language Acquisition

Persons learning a second language that differs considerably in its grammatical morphology from their native language may never master the grammatical morphology of the second language (Bialystok & Miller, 1999; Jia, Aaronson, & Wu, 2002). For instance, native Chinese speakers who learn English as a second language find the plural marker difficult to master because plurality is not inflected morphologically in the Chinese language (Jia, 2003). This is particularly true when persons learn a second language at an older age rather than at a younger age, or when a specific morpheme is not inflected in a person's native language. However, even for younger children, learning the grammatical morphology of a second language can be challenging. Jia's (2003) longitudinal study of 10 Chinese-speaking children during a 5-year period focused on the acquisition of the plural -s, which is not grammatically inflected in Chinese. Three of the 10 children, even after 5 years' immersion in English, never mastered the plural morpheme, and those who did so were usually younger at their initial immersion in English. The three children who

RESEARCH **PARADIGMS**

Longitudinal Studies

Longitudinal studies are a type of research that involves following individuals over time. Some of these studies may last for only several weeks or months, whereas others follow individuals for many years. The National Institute of Child Health and Human Development (NICHD), for instance, supported a network of 10 research teams across the United States (the Early Child Care Research Network [ECCRN]) to follow 1,364 children, all born within a 24-hour period in 1991, for 15 years into adolescence. The children were tested repeatedly over time, and the data they provided have answered numerous questions about many developmental phenomena, including language (e.g., NICHD ECCRN, 2005). An overview of the study is available online (https://www.nichd.nih.gov/research/supported/Pages/seccyd.aspx).

In language-development research, longitudinal studies have a particularly rich tradition, providing important insights to very nuanced aspects of children's earliest language acquisitions, such as the emergence of grammatical morphemes (Brown, 1973). Roger Brown's documentation of three children—whom he called Adam, Eve, and Sarah—is one of the most well-known longitudinal studies of language development. Then a professor at Harvard, Brown and his students visited the homes of the three children weekly for several years. The team audio-recorded the children's language and then transcribed it in the university's research lab; these transcripts (and what could be learned from them) were the topic of regular seminars among the research team (Pinker, 1999). This work was groundbreaking in documenting the systematic and ordered progression of grammatical morpheme emergence, such as the use of verb tense markers

(e.g., present progressive -ing and past tense -ed). Brown's work also resulted in new conceptualizations regarding how children's language growth can be monitored over time by using the mean length of utterance (MLU) as a metric. The longitudinal transcripts of Adam, Eve, and Sarah are still available for the research community to use.

Because children today are different than the children enrolled in longitudinal studies that have ended, such as the NICHD ECCRN study and the Brown study, newly launched longitudinal studies continue to inform our understanding of language development. For instance, an increasing number of children in the United States are bilingual, speaking Spanish at home in the early years and transitioning to English for formal schooling. Our understanding of language development among these youngsters is only now emerging. To contribute to this effort, the Language and Reading Research Consortium (LARRC) longitudinal study was launched in 2010 to conduct a 5-year investigation of children's development of language and reading skills from age 4 to 9 years (see Language and Reading Research Consortium, 2015). The study follows a cohort of English-speaking children as well as a cohort of bilingual English/Spanish-speaking children. Children in this study completed a 7-hour battery of assessments each year for 5 years, with assessments transcending all five dimensions of language. As researchers examine the language and reading development of LARRC participants, we stand to learn a great deal more about the role of language skills in future reading achievement, for both English-speaking and English/Spanish bilingual children.

did not master the plural morpheme used it in fewer than 80% of obligatory contexts, typically omitting the plural marker.

Dialect

Dialects are the variants of a single language. The dialects of a language vary in a number of important ways from the "general dialect," including their morphology. Even among speakers of a single language (e.g., English), achievement of specific morphological building blocks can vary substantially as a function of the morphological features of the dialect the speakers are acquiring. In the United States, one dialect many speakers share is African American English (AAE). Some morphological features of AAE differ from those of General American English (GAE), including the use of copulative, or *be*, auxiliary verbs; verb tense inflections; and possessive and plural inflections (Charity, Scarborough, & Griffin, 2004). For instance, a GAE speaker may say, "Tom's aunt," whereas an AAE speaker may say, "Tom aunt," omitting the possessive marker. Some children learn only the AAE dialect, whereas others learn the AAE dialect before, while, or after learning the GAE dialect. AAE-speaking students who have more knowledge of GAE tend to perform better in reading development, possibly because less of a mismatch occurs between the written form of language they encounter in school (which uses GAE) and the dialect they speak (Charity et al., 2004). At least in part, the mismatch between AAE and GAE involves differences in morphology, particularly grammatical inflections. Alternatively, it may also be that AAE-speaking students who have more knowledge of GAE have a strong capability to code-switch; that is, to switch between their two dialects (Connor & Craig, 2006; Craig, Zhang, Hensel, & Quinn, 2009). Children who can readily switch between dialects may have a heightened meta-linguistic awareness, which can support reading development. In this regard, there may be benefits to helping children acquire the ability to switch between dialects, with a focus on helping children understand the value of their own dialect and the value of learning the dialect used in schooling.

Language Impairment

Language impairment affects morphological development, often in significant ways. In fact, one hallmark of specific language impairment (SLI), a developmental language disorder we mentioned in Chapter 1 and discuss more thoroughly in Chapter 10, is difficulty with grammatical morphology. For instance, whereas typically developing

✓ 2.2
Check Your Understanding
Click here to gauge your understanding of the concepts in this section.

Many English dialects are spoken in the United States. One common dialect is African American English (AAE), which varies from other dialects in some aspects of semantics, morphology, phonology, and syntax.

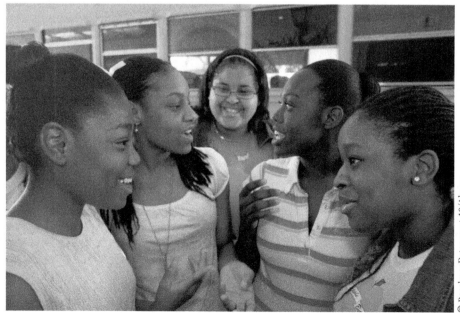
© RosaIreneBetancourt 10/Alamy

children use the present progressive -ing with more than 80% accuracy, children with SLI use it with only 25% accuracy (Conti-Ramsden & Jones, 1997). In general, children with SLI seem to have very specific difficulties with verb tense markings, such as the past tense inflection and the third-person singular inflection (e.g., He runs.).

WHAT IS SYNTACTIC DEVELOPMENT?

Syntactic development is children's internalization of the rules of language that govern how words are organized into sentences. As Pinker (1994) stated in his seminal work on language acquisition, *The Language Instinct*,

> When a dog bites a man that is not news, but when a man bites a dog that is news. . . . The streams of words called "sentences" . . . tell you who in fact did what to whom. (p. 83)

As children progress from single-word users to conveyers of complex thoughts and ideas that involve stringing many words together, they develop a fine-tuned understanding of how to organize words into sentences that carefully specify "who did what to whom", as well as what they want ("May I please watch the Thomas video?"), remember ("Mommy, Daddy told me we couldn't go to the toy store"), and imagine ("I think if we go to the toy store I'll get to buy a new movie"). Children develop this sophisticated ability to organize words into larger propositions by gradually internalizing the grammatical system of their language. Essentially, *grammar* refers to the rules and principles that speakers of a language use to structure sentences. An example of such a rule is the use of the nominative pronoun form (e.g., *I, he, she*) rather than the objective form (e.g., *me, him, her*) when a personal pronoun follows a *be* verb; thus, "It is he" is considered grammatically correct; "It is him" is considered incorrect. These rules and principles are in the minds of native speakers, a mental grammar that allows people to produce and comprehend the syntactic rules of their language with remarkable rapidity and ease.

Syntactic Building Blocks

The grammatical system a child acquires from birth onward is a "discrete combinatorial system" consisting of a *finite* number of discrete elements that allow the child to produce an *infinite* number of sentences (Pinker, 1994). As children internalize this combinatorial system, they exhibit three major syntactic achievements: (a) an increase in utterance length, (b) use of different sentence modalities, and (c) the development of complex syntax.

Utterance Length

A major accomplishment that most children achieve with relative ease by their sixth birthday is the production of utterances that are, on average, nearly as long as those of adults. Contrast these two utterances produced by Tahim:

18 MONTHS: Daddy no.

60 MONTHS: No, put that one over there, there on the blocks I set up.

At 18 months, Tahim's utterance length averages 1.3 morphemes, whereas at 60 months his average utterance length exceeds 8 morphemes. Like Tahim, most children show a gradual increase in utterance length from ages 1 to 6 years, and these increases reflect the children's ability to chain together morphemes to produce an infinite variety of sentences.

Calculating the mean number of morphemes per utterance—referred to as mean length of utterance (MLU)—provides a simple proxy for estimating the syntactic complexity of children's utterances, at least in the first 5 years of development.

To calculate an MLU for a child, one makes a transcript of consecutive utterances the child speaks (ideally at least 50 different utterances), calculates the number of morphemes per each utterance, and divides this by the total number of utterances. Children with an average MLU of two morphemes speak with a telegraphic quality in which grammatical markers (e.g., articles, conjunctions, auxiliary verbs) are omitted, as in Tahim's "Daddy no." In contrast, children with an average MLU of four morphemes use a variety of grammatical markers to organize their sentences, including articles, conjunctions, and auxiliary verbs. In other words, when children produce longer utterances, they do not simply string words together haphazardly (e.g., "Daddy no go up"), but they use various grammatical structures to organize sentences in precise and adultlike ways ("Daddy, I really don't think we should go up there").

Sentence Modalities

Once children begin to combine morphemes to create longer and longer utterances, they begin to produce sentences of various types, or modalities. During the early years of syntactic development, children become increasingly skilled at producing different sentence types that vary not only in their pragmatic intent, but also in their syntactic organization. In large part, the differences among sentence types reside in how words are grammatically organized at a surface level.

Declaratives.   Declarative sentences make a statement, and simple declaratives often use these six organizational schemes (Eastwood & Mackin, 1982):

1. Subject + Verb: *I bake.*
2. Subject + Verb + Object: *I bake bread.*
3. Subject + Verb + Complement: *I feel good.*
4. Subject + Verb + Adverbial phrase: *I feel good today.*
5. Subject + Verb + Indirect object + Direct object: *She gave Tommy the hammer.*
6. Subject + Verb + Direct object + Indirect object: *She gave the hammer to Tommy.*

Three-year-old children have commonly mastered most of these basic declarative patterns, and even use coordinating and subordinating conjunctions (like *and, but,* and *so*) to link several of them, as in "I am working and she is too!" An important point is that during the early years of language acquisition, children are never taught explicitly *how* to produce these and other types of declarative sentences; rather, they intuit the rules from the language they experience around them and gradually become capable of producing an infinite variety of declaratives on the basis of these internalized rules.

Negatives.   Any adult who has spent much time with children recognizes that many of them master the use of the negative sentence fairly early in development. Following are a few examples:

"No, I not going!"

"I don't want to!"

"I'm not eating that!"

"Don't do that!"

Negative sentences express negation and rely on such words as *no, not, can't, don't,* and *won't.* The child's development of the art of negation involves learning where to insert these negative markers into sentences. Bellugi's (1967) extensive research on the language development of three children showed that the syntactic structure of negative sentences emerges in a predictable order. Children's first use of the negative sentence modality typically has a pattern in which the word *no* is placed at the beginning of the sentence, as in "No eat that." Soon afterward, the negative word moves inside the sentence next to the main verb, as in "I not eat that" and "You no do that." By age 4 years, many children use the auxiliary forms of verbs that approximate adultlike negation, as in "You can't do that" and "I don't want to go." However, other and more nuanced negative sentences may not emerge until several years later, such as passive sentences containing the modal verb *won't* ("She won't be getting a prize"), and negative sentences that involve probability estimates ("I'm not sure if she'll get the prize").

Interrogatives. Interrogative sentences involve the act of questioning. Children become amazingly sophisticated at organizing sentences to obtain information from other people:

> "Why is that light green?"
>
> "What happened?"
>
> "Who did it?"
>
> "Where are you going?"
>
> "Is it snowing?"
>
> "He's sad; isn't he?"

Although individuals can pose questions using declarative sentences by raising the intonation at the end ("He's going?"), syntax provides an important vehicle for question asking that children discover early in life. Children's development of the interrogative sentence modality includes two major question types: *wh-* questions and yes–no questions. Many children's earliest interrogatives include *wh-* words, such as *what, where,* and *why,* as in "What that?", "Where Daddy go?", and "Why he not here?" Children's repertoire of question words expands during the preschool years to include *who, whose, when, which,* and *how. Wh-* questions seek specific information about time, place, manner, reason, and quantity (Jacobs, 1995), whereas yes–no questions seek a yes or no response, as in "Are we going?" and "Can you see me?"

In producing interrogatives, children draw on specific syntactic rules to organize sentences for questioning purposes. Consider the syntactic differences between this declarative sentence and its interrogative counterpart:

> *Declarative:* He is sleeping.
>
> *Interrogative:* Is he sleeping?

In forming the yes–no interrogative, children must move the auxiliary verb *is* from its place following the subject *he* and preceding its main verb, *sleeping* so it appears before the subject. As simple as yes–no questions may seem, they require a sophisticated syntactic maneuver that children master at relatively young ages.

Children acquire the ability to draw on specific syntactic rules to pose *wh*-questions as well. For example, to ask the question, "What do you like?", the child must generate the *wh*-word corresponding to the missing information in the declarative version of the sentence (in this case, the word *what*, corresponds to the missing information in the declarative sentence "You like X", so the sentence becomes "You like what"). The child must also place the *wh-* word in the initial noun phrase slot, and "empty" the object slot (so the sentence "You like what" becomes "What you like"), and insert an auxiliary verb before the subject (in this case *do*, so "What you like" becomes "What do you like?"). There are a number of other ways to produce *wh*-questions, depending on whether you are asking about the subject or predicate of the sentence. However, for the purposes of this chapter, it is most important to recognize that children acquire and implement a set of complex syntactic rules to form questions without having anyone teach them how to do so.

Complex Syntax: Linking Phrases and Clauses

The syntactic development of young children is often monitored by calculating their MLU. Though MLU is a handy tool for estimating children's syntactic development, it does not provide much detail concerning more nuanced achievements in syntax, particularly the child's use of phrase and clause structures. A *phrase* is a cluster of words organized around a *head*. Types of phrases include noun phrases (*the tall, angry <u>boy</u>*), prepositional phrases (*in the <u>bucket</u>*), adjectival phrases (*very <u>happy</u>*), and verb phrases (*was <u>saddened</u>*; in each example, the head of the phrase is underscored). With phrasal development, sentences become increasingly elaborate, as shown in Figure 2.2. As children begin to use more elaborate phrase structures, they develop skill in phrasal coordination, which allows them to connect phrases, as in this sentence in which *and* links two noun phrases: *I'm putting on my coat and my hat.*

A *clause* is a syntactic structure containing a verb or a verb phrase; when we produce sentences, we often join a number of clauses by using specific rules. For instance, the sentence, *I'll go and you stay* contains two independent clauses (*I'll go; you stay*) conjoined with the coordinating conjunction *and.* The sentence, *That boy who hit me is in time-out* contains a dependent clause (*who hit me*) embedded within an independent clause (*That boy is in time-out*).

From age 3 years on, children begin to master the art of conjoining and embedding clauses to create sentences of not only increasing length, but also increasing syntactic complexity. Table 2.3 presents information about R. Brown's (1973) stages of grammatical development; as the table shows, when children's utterances average 3.5 morphemes in length, the art of sentence embedding emerges. At this stage (Stage IV), children begin to use complex sentences featuring embedded subordinate clauses (*That's mine <u>because Mommy gave it to me</u>*), embedded *wh-* questions (*I don't know* why he did it), and relative clauses (*That boy <u>who hit me</u> took the crayons*). At this point in development, children move from using simple syntax to complex syntax, which refers to the use of phrase and clause structures, as well as conjunctive devices for organizing internal structures of sentences. Table 2.4 presents some examples of complex syntax. Analyses of complex syntax examine children's use of different types of phrases and clauses, such as relative and infinitive clauses, as well as ways in which children embed and conjoin phrases and clauses by using coordinating and subordinating conjunctions.

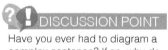
DISCUSSION POINT

Have you ever had to diagram a complex sentence? If so, why do so many students find this activity such a challenge when they have been able to produce complex sentences since early childhood?

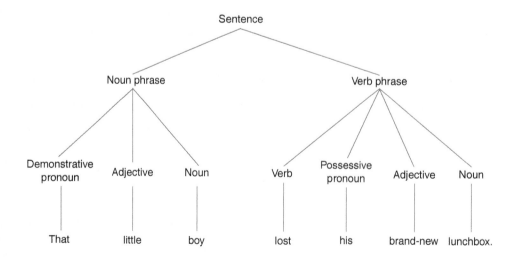

FIGURE 2.2

Example of the phrase structure of a sentence.

TABLE 2.3
Stages of grammatical development

STAGE	MLU RANGE (MIDPOINT)	STAGE DESCRIPTION
I	1.0–1.99 (1.75)	Single-word utterances predominate. Grammatical inflections not used.
II	2.0–2.49 (2.25)	Two- and three-word utterances predominate. Grammatical inflections emerge (e.g., present progressive marker, plural marker). Emergence of grammar as child follows basic word-order patterns (e.g., Agent + Action: "*Mommy go*"; Agent + Action + Object: "*DeeDee ate bone*").
III	2.5–2.99 (2.75)	Emergence of different sentence modalities: yes–no questions, *wh-* questions, imperatives (e.g., "Fasten your seat belt"), and negatives.
IV	3.0–3.99 (3.5)	Complex sentences emerge to feature multiclause sentences, such as object–noun phrase complements ("I think I'm tired"), embedded *wh-* questions ("That's why she went outside"), and embedded relative clauses ("Clifford, who was so good, is still waiting").
V	4.01	Emergence of coordinating conjunctions and adverbial conjuncts ("I am tired because I didn't take a nap"; "I'm helping Daddy do the dishes and make dinner").

MLU = mean length of utterance.
Source: Based on *A First Language: The Early Stages* (1–59) by R. Brown, 1973, Cambridge, MA: Harvard University Press.

TABLE 2.4
Examples of complex syntax

SYNTACTIC FEATURE	EXAMPLE
Double embedding	"I'm not going to think about what happened."
Infinitive clause with differing subject	"Bobby wants Mommy to go too."
Object relative clause	"That's the train I lost."
Subject relative clause	"The girls who signed up didn't pay."
Wh- infinitive clause	"Tell her what to do."
Complex sentence with subordinating conjunction	"I can't go when she wants me to."
Compound sentence with coordinating conjunction	"The kids are sleeping but the teacher's about to leave."
Subject complement clause	"The kids signing up didn't know it cost money."
Perfect aspect verb	"The dog had caught it already."
Passive voice sentence	"The doll was found after we looked everywhere."
Postnoun elaboration	"Other colors like green and yellow might work too."
Multiclause sentence	"Because she didn't call first, we didn't know to wait and left without her."

Source: Based on "Grammar: How Can I Say That Better" by S. Eisenberg in *Contextualized Language Intervention* (pp. 145–194), edited by T. Ukrainetz, 2006, Eau Claire, WI: Thinking Publications.

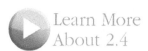

Learn More About 2.4

As you watch the video titled "'Syntactic Trees and X' Theory – Linguistics Topic 10," notice that syntax comprises multiple language components and these components combine to create a language's grammar.
https://www.youtube.com/watch?v=7UOcoQr0hvg

Influences on Syntactic Development

Syntactic development is considered a relatively resilient aspect of language, proceeding in a mostly uniform pattern in both the type and the timing of development. Resilient aspects of language are those that seem to be impervious to change in conditions (Goldin-Meadow, 2014), as appears to be the case for syntax. Evidence for the resilience of syntax is evident in the case of "homesigners," which refers to children born profoundly deaf to hearing parents who do not have exposure to any conventional sign language (Goldin-Meadow, 2014). When this occurs, children will develop their own manual communication system to communicate with others. When homesigners have the opportunity to congregate, they have the opportunity to grow their own language absent of the influence of any other language. Studies of homesigner languages, such as Al-Sayyid Bedouin Sign Language, which emerged over several generations in a small isolated community in southern Israel, reveal complex and systematic syntactic properties govern them (Sandler, Meir, Padden, & Aronoff, 2015), thereby suggesting the resilience of syntax as an important aspect of language.

Given the perspective that syntactic development is relatively resilient, historically, researchers have tended to emphasize the similarities in syntactic development among children, as in Brown's research (see Research Paradigms: *Longitudinal Studies*). Consequently, relatively little research has focused on individual differences among children and the factors that give rise to these differences. Researchers are increasingly focusing on identifying and understanding factors that affect syntactic development. We consider two of them next.

Child-Directed Speech

Child-directed speech (CDS) refers to the talk directed to children by others, including parents and other caregivers (Saxton, 2008). The speech to which children are exposed can vary with respect to its syntactic complexity. For instance, one child might be exposed primarily to short, simple sentences, whereas another might frequently hear long, complex sentences. That such variability in children's language-learning environments exists, allows us to examine whether and how much this variability is associated with children's syntactic development (Goldin-Meadow, 2014).

In fact, a large body of work shows that the syntax to which children are exposed in CDS relates to their syntactic development. For instance, young children often make pronoun case errors in which they use the subjective case *me* in place of the nominative case *I*, as in "me do it" and "me cook it." Interestingly, children whose caregivers use a larger number of "me + verb" sequences in their CDS—as in "Let me do it" and "Did you see me doing it?"—produce a larger number of me-for-I errors (Kirjavainen, Theakston, & Lieven, 2009). This is not to say that caregivers cause their children's language errors, but rather that children's linguistic experiences contribute to their language acquisition.

The utterances children experience in their linguistic environments typically contain numerous exemplars of simple syntax—grammatically well-formed utterances containing simple noun phrases and verb structures (Huttenlocher, Waterfall, Vasilyeva, Vevea, & Hedges, 2010). However, what seems more variable is children's exposure to exemplars of more complex syntax, such as embedded relative clauses, auxiliary-fronted yes–no questions, and *wh-* questions (Huttenlocher, Vasilyeva, Cymerman, & Levine, 2002). Importantly, children who hear complex syntax more often in their environment produce greater amounts of complex syntax at an earlier age than do children who hear complex syntax less frequently (Kirjavainen et al., 2009). Hoff (2003) explained this phenomenon by using the *learning-from-input hypothesis*, which emphasizes that the grammatical properties of children's language use depend on exposure to the properties in CDS. The results of two studies by Huttenlocher et al. (2002) substantiate this point. In these studies, researchers examined the syntactic properties of mothers' language at home and preschool teachers' language in the classroom. The researchers studied the relationship between complex syntax contained in parents' and teachers' language and children's syntactic development. The results of these studies revealed differences in maternal use of complex syntax between lower socioeconomic status (SES) and middle SES parents (see Figure 2.3). The results also showed a strong linear relationship between children's exposure to complex syntax and their development of complex syntactic forms, as depicted in Figure 2.4. Considering how such findings may translate into practice, Theory to Practice: *Language-Focused Curricula* describes efforts to increase teachers' use of complex syntax in preschool classrooms.

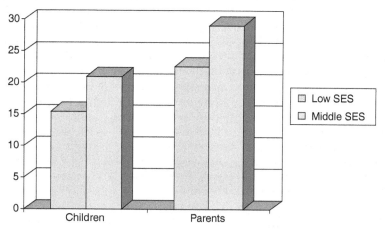

FIGURE 2.3

Percentage of mothers' and children's sentences containing complex syntax.

SES—socioeconomic status.

Source: Adapted from *Cognitive Psychology*, Vol. 45, J. Huttenlocher, M. Vasilyeva, E. Cymerman, and S. Levine, "Language Input and Child Syntax," p. 348. Copyright 2002.

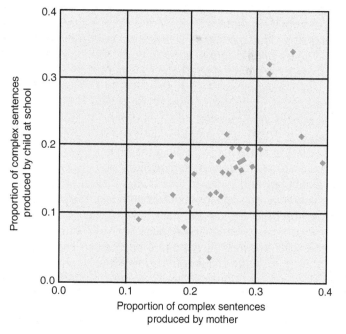

FIGURE 2.4

Relationship between mothers' and children's production of complex syntax.

Republished with permission of Elsevier Science and Technology Journals, from "Language Input and Child Syntax," J. Huttenlocher, M. Vasilyeva, E. Cymerman, and S. Levine in Cognitive Psychology, Vol. 45 p. 337-374. permission conveyed through Copyright Clearance Center, Inc.

Language Impairment

Although exposure is important to supporting children's developments in syntax, the environment is not all that matters. Both developmental and acquired language disorders often disrupt syntactic comprehension and production. We discuss this topic more deeply in Chapter 10, yet provide a preview here.

Developmental language disorders are present at birth. Language disorders that affect *only* language (and no other aspect of development, such as cognition) are viewed as "specific"—hence, the term *specific language impairment* (SLI). Children with SLI have significant problems with language, but no other disabilities. However, some language disorders are secondary, resulting from or occurring concomitantly with other disabilities, such as cognitive impairment. Both specific and secondary language impairments often affect syntactic development, sometimes profoundly. For example, children with SLI produce shorter sentences than their nonimpaired peers (Laws & Bishop, 2003), and have particular difficulty with verbs. For this reason, children with SLI may use other words to "fill in" holes in sentences created by verb omissions, such as "Colin lady ticket," "Lights on my camera," and

---

THEORY TO PRACTICE

Language-Focused Curricula

In this chapter, we've discussed how the linguistic environment children experience relates to their development of linguistic form, content, and use. *Child-directed speech* (CDS) is the term researchers use to describe an important aspect of children's linguistic environment (Saxton, 2008). In recent years, researchers have become increasingly interested in studying CDS in preschool classrooms (Huttenlocher et al., 2002), recognizing that the majority of children in the United States today participate in preschool education in the years prior to formal schooling. At the same time, researchers have also begun to explore how the linguistic environments—including CDS—of preschool classrooms might be improved through implementation of language-focused curricula (Pence, Justice, & Wiggins, 2008). Language-focused curricula are designed to improve the linguistic environment of preschool classrooms by increasing teachers' use of complex vocabulary and syntax in their CDS.

An early exemplar of language-focused curricula was developed by Betty Bunce and her colleagues at the University of Kansas Language Acquisition Preschool (Bunce, 1995). Bunce developed a comprehensive curriculum for early childhood teachers that involved embedding specific language-facilitation strategies in a variety of classroom activities, such as dramatic play, group reading, and art. Strategies included modeling advanced vocabulary and syntax (e.g., verb tense markings), asking open-ended questions to engage children in extended conversations, and prompting children to initiate dialogues with others. The two authors of this text conducted a large-scale evaluation of Betty Bunce's curriculum, involving 14 teachers and nearly 200 preschool children enrolled in their classrooms (Justice, Mashburn, Pence, & Wiggins, 2008; Pence et al., 2008). Seven of the teachers implemented Bunce's language-focused curriculum for an academic year, whereas the other seven teachers implemented their typical classroom curriculum. The results of this study indicated children who made the greatest gains in expressive language over the academic year were those whose teachers used the language-facilitation strategies at the highest levels (Justice et al., 2008). Efforts to develop language-focused curricula and evaluate them for their impacts when used in everyday classrooms are important in using developmental research to improve children's educational experiences.

"Not that the horse, where a big horse?" (Conti-Ramsden & Jones, 1997, p. 1307). Children with language impairment secondary to Down syndrome (DS) also show significant difficulties with syntactic development. Adolescents with DS produce sentences averaging only four morphemes long, shorter than those produced by typically developing 6-year-olds (Laws & Bishop, 2003).

Acquired language disorders occur as a result of injury or illness that damages the language centers of the brain. Strokes, for instance, occur when the blood

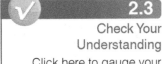

2.3
Check Your
Understanding
Click here to gauge your
understanding of the
concepts in this section.

supply to the brain is stalled; this can cause a language disorder if parts of the brain involved with language processes are damaged. In some instances of stroke, the damage affects the part of the brain involved with syntax; this can cause an individual to lose the ability to produce syntactically complex language. One study of four adults with this type of acquired language disorder revealed their utterances averaged about four morphemes in length; complex sentences composed only 5% of all their sentences, and less than one-third of their sentences were grammatically correct (Thompson, Shapiro, Kiran, & Sobecks, 2003).

WHAT IS SEMANTIC DEVELOPMENT?

We now turn to the topic of *semantic development*, which refers to an individual's learning and storage of the meanings of words. Given that we have just discussed the topic of syntax, it is helpful to understand that children's semantic and syntactic development is highly interrelated, potentially emerging synchronously (Dixon & Marchman, 2007). For instance, children's acquisition of grammatical morphemes, such as the plural marker, is closely related to their acquisition of count nouns (e.g., *dog, bottle, toy*). Now, to dig more deeply into the topic of semantics, let's consider the following conversations between the second author and her daughter at age 3:

Friday, at home in the kitchen:

ADELAIDE: Mommy, what's this? (points to a vent on the baseboard)

LJ: That's a vent. A vent lets air come into the room.

ADELAIDE: It's a vent.

Saturday, at the children's museum:

ADELAIDE: There's another went, Mommy. (*points to a speaker embedded in the wall*)

LJ: A went? What's a went?

ADELAIDE: A went puts air into the room.

LJ: Oh! You mean *vent*. That's a speaker; it looks like a vent, but that makes noise. People speak through it.

These two conversational snippets are useful to understanding the processes by which children learn and store new words. When encountering a new word, the child must develop an internal representation of the word that includes its phonological form (the specific sounds in it and their order), its grammatical role (e.g., verb, pronoun, noun), and its conceptual meaning. In this example, notice how readily Adelaide incorporated a new word—*vent*—into her vocabulary. These excerpts also show how knowledge of a specific word matures with time and that a child's early knowledge and use of a word may be incomplete. With additional exposure to the word in various contexts, Adelaide's initial representation will develop from a relatively immature state, to a more flexible, adultlike representation.

Semantic Building Blocks

Semantic development involves three major tasks for the language learner: (a) acquiring a *mental lexicon* of about 60,000 words between infancy and adulthood, (b) learning *new words* rapidly, and (c) organizing the mental lexicon in an efficient *semantic network*.

Mental Lexicon

A person's mental lexicon (or simply the *lexicon*) is the volume of words he or she understands (receptive lexicon) and uses (expressive lexicon). Typically, the receptive lexicon is larger because an individual usually understands many more words than he or she actually uses. Estimates of the size of a child's lexicon show that its volume increases remarkably quickly during the first several years of life—from only several words at age 12 months, to 300 words at age 24 months, to 60,000 words by early adulthood (Fenson, Dale, Reznick, Bates, & Thal, 1994). A typical child acquires about 860 words per year between ages 1 and 7 years, averaging about 2 new words per day during this period (Biemiller, 2005).

One long-standing belief in the field of child language acquisition is that children undergo a vocabulary spurt, or word spurt, that begins near the end of the second year and continues for several years. The term *spurt* implies that children transition from a slow stage of development to a rapid stage of development, with an inflection point differentiating the stages (Ganger & Brent, 2004), as illustrated in Figure 2.5A. This inflection point implies that there is a sudden burst in lexical growth at a given point. However, some researchers contend relatively few children (25% in one study of toddlers' lexical growth) experience a vocabulary spurt (Ganger & Brent, 2004). Rather, most show a continuous, linear increase in their vocabulary size (Figure 2.5B), suggesting the concept of a vocabulary spurt is not a universal principle but applies to only some children. Thus, although the lexicon undergoes remarkable growth, whether lexical growth is appropriately represented

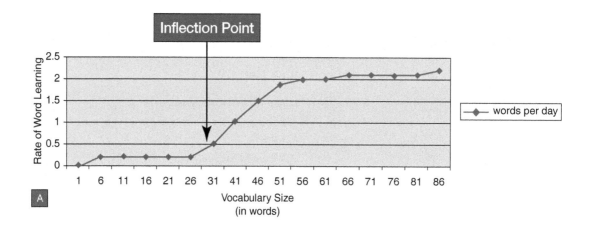

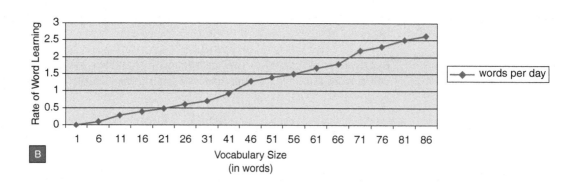

FIGURE 2.5

Lexical development featuring a vocabulary spurt (Graph A) compared with gradual linear growth (Graph B).

Source: Based on "Reexamining the Vocabulary Spurt" by J. Ganger and M. R. Brent, 2004, *Developmental Psychology, 40,* 621–632.

as a spurtlike phenomenon rather than as a more continuous, linear trajectory is unclear.

When practitioners think about the size of a child's lexicon, they consider not only its volume, but also the individual lexical items it contains. A *semantic taxonomy* differentiates words on the basis of their semantic roles (Ingram, 1989). One classic semantic taxonomy differentiates children's lexical items into five categories (Ingram, 1989):

1. *Specific nominals* refer to a specific object (e.g., *Daddy, Fluffy*)
2. *General nominals* refer to all members of a category (e.g., *those, cats*)
3. *Action words* describe specific actions (e.g., *up*), social-action games (e.g., *peekaboo*), and action inhibitors (e.g., *no*)
4. *Modifiers* describe properties and qualities (e.g., *big, mine*)
5. *Personal–social words* describe affective states and relationships (e.g., *yes, bye-bye*)

Children's early lexicons, comprising the first 50 or so words, typically contain at least one word in each semantic category. K. Nelson's (1973) classic longitudinal study of 18 children's early lexical development revealed that general nominals predominated, corresponding to 51% of all words in the lexicon, and specific nominals and action words composed an additional 14% and 13%, respectively, of lexical entries. Modifiers (9% of words) and personal–social words (8% of words) composed a relatively small number of children's early lexical items. (An additional 4% of the words did not fit any of these categories.) Of these general and specific nominals, most refer to tangible, concrete items, such as *shoe* and *cup*; infants' understanding of more abstract nominals develop along a more protracted timeline (Bergelson & Swingley, 2013).

New Words

When a child encounters a word for the first time, his or her knowledge of the word is incomplete; in fact, the child's knowledge of the word is just beginning. Take the word *umbrella*, for instance. Following initial exposure to this novel word, a child may have a general understanding of its meaning and may even begin to express the word, albeit not always correctly (Brackenbury & Fey, 2003). For instance, a child might see a hanger on the floor of her parents' closet and call it an "umbrella." Between the initial exposure to a word and achieving a deepened flexible understanding of it, word knowledge is in a "fragile" state, meaning the child will likely make errors in understanding and using words (McGregor, Friedman, Reilly, & Newman, 2002). It will take a bit of time for the child to learn the fairly constrained meaning of the word *umbrella*, and to learn a hanger has its own name.

A number of factors influence the rapidity with which a child develops an adultlike understanding of a word. We consider three of them next:

1. *Concept represented by the word.* As children engage in learning a new word, some words are clearly easier to learn than others because of the concepts the words express. For instance, children acquiring English learn the words *go* and *hit*, which refer to concrete actions, more easily than *think* and *know*, which represent abstract concepts (Gleitman, Cassidy, Nappa, Papafragou, & Trueswell, 2005). Words referring to abstractions are considered "hard words" (Gleitman et al., 2005) because they are relatively difficult for children to learn compared with other words. Words are hard when the concept to which they refer is not accessible to the child. Consequently, children often do not acquire words that describe beliefs and mental states—such as *think* and *know*—until age 3 or 4 years, whereas they learn words such as *see* and *walk* earlier (Gopnik & Meltzoff, 1997). A related concept is the notion of imageability, which concerns how readily an individual can generate a mental image of a word (Ma, Golinkoff, Hirsh-Pasek, McDonough, & Tardif, 2009).

Apple and *cup* have very high imageability, whereas *tomorrow* and *believe* have low imageability (Ma et al., 2009). Young children learn words with high imageability earlier than words with low imageability (Ma et al., 2009).

2. *Phonological form of the word.* When an individual learns a new word, he or she must acquire not only knowledge of the conceptual referent of the word, but also its phonological form (Nash & Donaldson, 2005). Two substantial differences exist among the phonological features of words. First, the relationship between the phonological form of a word and the concept to which it refers is most often arbitrary, but this is not true in all cases. Exceptions include onomatopoeic words, such as *boom* and *crash*, in which a more transparent relationship exists between the phonological form of the word and the concept it represents. Not surprisingly, many young children use onomatopoeic words first to refer to objects (e.g., calling a cow a *moo* or a cat a *meow*) instead of their more conventional labels. Second, some words contain sounds and sound sequences that occur relatively often in spoken language, called *common sound sequences* (e.g., the first two sounds in *sit*), whereas other words contain sounds and sound sequences that occur infrequently, called *rare sound sequences* (e.g., the first two sounds in *these*; Storkel, 2003). Children learn words containing common sound sequences more readily than words containing rare sound sequences (Storkel, 2003).

3. *Contextual conditions at initial exposure.* Children's initial and subsequent exposures to a new word vary considerably according to the contextual conditions in which the word is embedded. Children draw on many sources of contextual information to develop and refine their internal representations of novel words (Gleitman et al., 2005). They draw on information from the linguistic context, such as the grammar of the utterance containing a new word (e.g., "This is a vent" vs. "I dropped my ring into the vent"), and the extent to which semantic features of the word are described (e.g., "A vent blows air into a room" vs. "I think the vent isn't working"). One important source of variation in young children's learning of new words is whether, in fact, the child is attending to the word's referent when exposed to its label. By way of illustration, consider these two scenarios, both of which take place when a father is bathing his 11-month-old infant. For the purpose at hand, consider the word *shovel* as novel to Jonas:

> Scenario 1: The infant is inspecting a yellow plastic duck in his hand. The dad is holding a green plastic shovel. The dad says, "Jonas, look here. I have a shovel."
>
> Scenario 2: The infant is inspecting a green plastic shovel in his hand. The dad is holding a yellow plastic duck. The dad says, "Jonas, look at that. You have a shovel."

These two scenarios are strikingly similar, yet they exemplify two distinct ways in which children may be exposed to novel words. Scenario 1 illustrates a lead-in, in which an adult labels an object or event that is outside of the child's attentional focus; Scenario 2 illustrates a follow-in, in which an adult labels an object or event that is currently the child's attentional focus (Shimpi & Huttenlocher, 2007). Researchers have long contended that the follow-in is more influential to children's vocabulary growth than the lead-in; this is because the child does not have to shift his or her attention, and thus has greater resources to allocate to the task of learning a new word. However, it also seems that lead-ins that are successful in shifting the child's attention to the novel focus can also support children's word learning (Shimpi & Huttenlocher, 2007).

Children also draw on information from the extralinguistic context, seeking overt cues from the environment that clearly label or define the referent of a new word, such as the eye gaze and gestures of their conversational partners (Jaswal & Markman, 2001a, 2001b). In ostensive word-learning contexts, a great deal of contextual information is provided about a novel word either linguistically

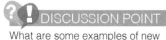

DISCUSSION POINT
What are some examples of new or novel words you have heard recently?

Children refine their knowledge of the meaning of a new word through repeated exposure to the word in different contexts.

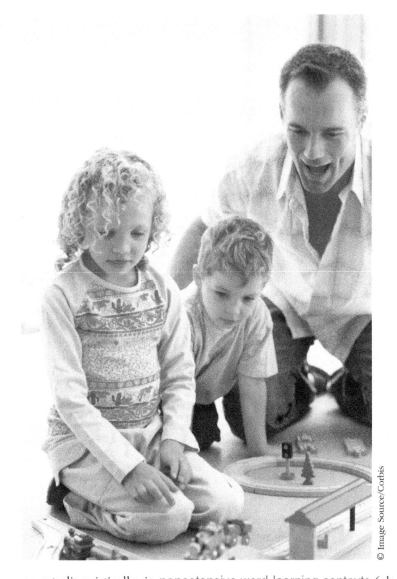

© Image Source/Corbis

or extralinguistically; in nonostensive word-learning contexts (also called *inferential contexts*), little contextual information is provided to help a person derive the meaning of a new word. In general, children's word learning is better in ostensive than nonostensive word-learning contexts. For example, when extralinguistic cues—such as pointing—are combined with a variety of linguistic cues—such as juxtaposing a novel word (*beak*) against a known word (*bird*): "See the bird? Look, a beak!"—children's word learning is superior to that when only one type of information is provided (Saylor & Sabbagh, 2004). In short, to develop a representation of a new word, children use various tools to draw on information from the linguistic and extralinguistic contexts in which the word is embedded.

Semantic Network

A person's mental lexicon, comprising the store of words he or she understands and uses, is not organized randomly; rather, as the human brain acquires new words, they are stored in a semantic network in which its entries are organized according to connective ties among them. The connections among words vary in strength from strong to weak according to the extent to which they share syntactic, phonological, or semantic features. For instance, the association between the pronouns *him* and *her* is fairly strong because of similarities in syntactic roles; so is the association between *pin* and *pit* because of shared phonological features, and between *whale* and *dolphin* because of semantic similarities. Thus, a person's mental lexicon contains a vast network of lexical entries linked by connective ties that vary in relative strength. Sometimes slips of the tongue provide evidence of the connective ties within one's lexicon, such as saying, "I slammed my finger, I mean toe."

An important point is that in a semantic network, the entries themselves do not carry meaning; the links between the entries do (De Deyne, Navarro, & Storms, 2013). Theories on how an individual accesses specific entries in the semantic network emphasize a process called spreading activation, in which activation of specific entries spreads across the network according to the strength of connections among entries. For instance, if the word *bird* is activated, a number of additional entries in the semantic network are also activated because of semantic similarities (e.g., *wings, robin, canary*; Harley, 2001).

As a child learns new words, they are stored in his or her semantic network. Young children often make a number of naming errors (McGregor et al., 2002); such errors are particularly prominent in the second year of life (Dapretto & Bjork, 2000). For instance, a child may call a *kangaroo* a *mouse*, or a *saddle* a *chair* (McGregor et al., 2002). These types of errors provide an interesting glimpse into the organization of a child's semantic network; calling a *kangaroo* a *mouse* suggests that these two entries are stored closely and that the lexical representation of *mouse* may be stronger (i.e., more robust) than that of *kangaroo*. The strength of the word *mouse* interferes with the child's lexical access to the *kangaroo* entry, which may be relatively fragile (McGregor et al., 2002). As the child's lexical representation of *kangaroo* strengthens, naming accuracy improves, and this entry becomes "less vulnerable to retrieval failure" (McGregor et al., 2002, p. 343).

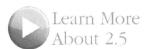

Learn More About 2.5

As you watch the video titled "Developing Semantics in Your Preschooler | Getit Young Moms," observe the various avenues by which parents can foster their children's semantic growth and how these strategies can influence other language skills as well. https://www.youtube.com/watch?v=2R0tC1FKNMY

Influences on Semantic Development

Several factors influence not only the rate and ease with which children build their lexicon, but also their efficiency in retrieving words from the lexicon.

Gender

In the first several years of language acquisition, girls usually have larger vocabularies and learn words more easily than boys (Bornstein, Hahn, & Haynes, 2004), a phenomenon apparent in a variety of cultures (Eriksson et al., 2012). In fact, one study of 2-year-olds' expressive vocabularies revealed girls know an average of 363 words versus 227 words for boys (Bornstein et al., 2004). However, these early differences often attenuate, if not disappear, by age 6–7 years (Bornstein et al., 2004). Most likely, these early differences in semantic development result from a combination of biological, psychological, and social variables (Bornstein et al., 2004). Biologically, there are some distinctions between the brain organization of girls and boys, which may have some bearing on developmental differences between the two genders with respect to early language growth, as well as other skills (Tomasi & Volkow, 2012). Psychologically and socially, gender-typed interests likely also have large influence on the types of interactions children experience (Hines, 2011). For instance, research results suggest that girls in child care receive more attention from teachers than boys (NICHD Early Child Care Research Network, 1997), which raises the possibility that early gender differences in semantic development result not only from biological differences, but also from opportunities to learn language from adults.

Language Impairment

Children who exhibit a developmental disorder of language (SLI) typically have significantly smaller vocabularies than those of their peers without SLI (Nash & Donaldson, 2005). Difficulties in learning new words and poorly organized semantic networks contribute to these differences in lexical size. In a study of the rate at which 4- to 5-year-old children learned new words, Gray (2003) determined the number of learning trials children needed to learn a new word. During each learning

A significant relationship exists between the number and types of words children hear in their environment and the size of their vocabulary.

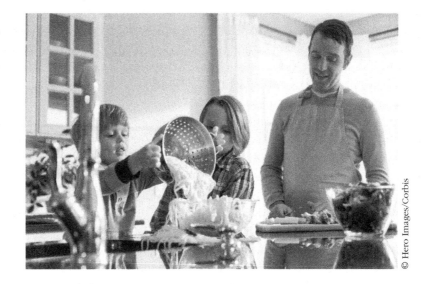

© Hero Images/Corbis

trial, children were exposed to a novel word during play activities in which the adult modeled the word and prompted the child to produce it. Typically developing children required an average of 11.6 trials to produce a new word, compared with nearly 14 trials for children with SLI. In addition to learning new words more slowly, many children with SLI exhibit word-finding errors and slower retrieval of items from the semantic network (Friedmann, Biran, & Dotan, 2013). This likely contributes to the slower pace of vocabulary development in children with SLI.

Language Exposure

Numerous studies have revealed a significant relationship between the number and types of words children hear in their environment and the size of their vocabulary (Hoff, 2003; Hurtado, Marchman, & Fernald, 2008). Children reared in orphanages who experience relatively little language input typically show depressed vocabularies (Glennen, 2002). The same finding is true for children reared in low-SES households compared with children living in higher-SES households (Rowe, 2009), presumably because children in low-SES households are exposed to fewer words. As Neuman (2006) pointed out, one explanation for this substantial variability in children's exposure to words as a function of SES is the striking effect of poverty on parents' emotional resources, which compromises the quality and frequency of parents' conversational interactions with their children. Given that 14 million children in the United States live in poverty, of whom 6 million live in extreme poverty (Wright, Chau, & Aratani, 2010), this early vocabulary achievement gap is a significant educational problem in the United States. Language Diversity and Differences: *Language Development and Children Living in Poverty* covers this topic in more detail.

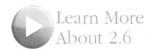

Learn More About 2.6

As you watch the video titled "An Introduction to Colourful Semantics," notice how semantics and speech–language therapy for semantics can impact multiple areas of language (specifically syntax). https://www.youtube.com/ watch?v=17smjL8Y21s

2.4
Check Your Understanding

Click here to gauge your understanding of the concepts in this section.

WHAT IS PRAGMATIC DEVELOPMENT?

Pragmatic development involves acquiring the rules of language that govern how language is used as a social tool. Such development involves using language for different purposes, being able to enter and hold conversations, and taking into account the circumstances and goals of the participants in a conversation.

Pragmatic Building Blocks

Three important aspects of pragmatic development are (a) using language for different communication functions, (b) developing conversational skills, and (c) gaining sensitivity to extralinguistic cues. These areas of pragmatic development are key

LANGUAGE DIVERSITY AND DIFFERENCES

Language Development and Children Living in Poverty

Often the term *diversity* brings to mind the cultural differences that arise from religion, race, ethnicity, country of origin, and ability or disability. However, in many countries, substantial cultural differences exist between people who are economically advantaged and those who are economically disadvantaged. In the United States, children living in poverty comprise a singularly large cultural group: Twenty percent of all children younger than age 18 years (14 million) reside in households with annual incomes below the poverty threshold ($19,157 for a family of four), and 50% live in low-income homes (twice the annual poverty threshold; Wright et al., 2010). African American and Hispanic children in the United States are about three times as likely to live in poverty as their White counterparts.

You might wonder what poverty has to do with language development, particularly the building blocks discussed in this chapter. Unfortunately, a strong negative relationship exists between poverty and language achievement. Children raised in poverty and in low-income households consistently know fewer words, produce shorter utterances, use a smaller variety of words, and have less developed phonological skills than peers raised in more advantageous circumstances (see Hoff, 2013). Beyond language, poverty affects many other areas of child development, including cognition and learning, motor development, socioemotional functioning, and general health.

When considering how poverty most affects language, researchers point to two major influences: parental socioemotional resources and parental access to material resources. Concerning the first, poverty takes an immense toll on parents' socioemotional resources; significantly higher rates of maternal depression occur when financial resources are stressed (Mistry, Biesanz, Taylor, Burchinal, & Cox, 2004). Compared with higher-income mothers, mothers living in poverty show lower levels of warmth, responsiveness, and sensitivity when interacting with their young children (Wallace, Roberts, & Lodder, 1998). High levels of maternal sensitivity and responsiveness directly support children's language development. Parents who reside in poverty often do not have the socioemotional resources to provide the levels of sensitivity and responsiveness to promote their children's early development (Goodman et al., 2011).

Poverty also undermines a family's material and financial resources. Families living in poverty do not have access to the same level of medical care as advantaged families, so their children often have more handicapping illnesses and injuries that may affect language development (e.g., chronic middle ear infections). Likewise, these families cannot take advantage of the "lessons, summer camps, stimulating learning materials and activities, and better quality early childhood care" available to children from advantaged backgrounds (Neuman, 2006, p. 30). Not surprisingly, hundreds of researchers have documented the deleterious effects of poverty on the building blocks of language and the "dramatic, linear, negative relationships between poverty and children's cognitive-developmental outcomes" (Neuman, 2006, p. 30).

building blocks that emerge during early childhood and are then gradually refined during later childhood, adolescence, and adulthood.

Communication Functions

When people use language in social contexts, behind every utterance is an intention, or communication function. For instance, the following three utterances produced by 2-year-old Eva vary in their function:

"Give me that."

"Mommy going outside?"

"I love my doggie."

Likewise, consider these three utterances by 4-year-old Zachary:

"No, put that one up on top of the digger."

"Addie, did you bring Thomas the Train to school today?"

"I actually think my mom is coming after nap."

TABLE 2.5

Basic communication functions (purposes of communication)

FUNCTION	DESCRIPTION
Instrumental	Used to ask for something
Regulatory	Used to give directions and to direct others
Interactional	Used to interact and converse with others in a social way
Personal	Used to express a state of mind or feelings about something
Heuristic	Used to find out information and to inquire
Imaginative	Used to tell stories and to role-play
Informative	Used to provide an organized description of an event or object

Source: Based on *Learning How to Mean: Explorations in the Development of Language Development* by M. A. Halliday, 1975, London: Arnold; and "Presentation of Communication Evaluation Information," by C. Simon and C. L. Holway, in *Communication Skills and Classroom Success* (pp. 151–199), edited by C. Simon, 1991, Eau Claire, WI: Thinking Publications.

Take a moment to study each of Eva's and Zachary's utterances and consider the intention behind it. The intentions you identify for each utterance reflect the children's mental states, beliefs, desires, and feelings. These examples also reveal how children must learn to use language "differently in different situations according to the circumstances and communication goals of the participants" (Bloom & Tinker, 2001, p. 14).

Early in life, children acquire a basic range of functions, and across their life spans they become increasingly sophisticated in expressing these functions. For instance, consider the communication function of regulation, in which an individual uses communication to control other people's behavior. Consider differences in how this function might be expressed at 1, 5, 13, and 21 years. Table 2.5 (which appeared in Chapter 1) defines this function and several other basic communication functions.

Although many basic communication functions emerge in the first several years of life, children gain increasing competence in their ability to use these functions successfully. Consider again, as an example, the use of regulation, in which a person uses language to direct or control other people's behaviors. Although toddlers typically use direct requests to obtain objects from other people ("Give me that"), preschoolers use direct requests with peers but indirect requests ("May I have that, please?") with adults and more dominant peers (Becker Bryant, 2005).

Developing a range of communication functions is an important aspect of language development that emerges in infancy and continues through adolescence and adulthood. As important as these functions are for children's use of language for self-expression, they may also propel other aspects of language development forward, such as vocabulary and grammar. The intentionality hypothesis proposes that children's experiences using language to engage with other people fosters their development of form and content; such experiences motivate the child to "express and articulate increasingly elaborate . . . representations" (Bloom & Tinker, 2001, p. 79).

Therefore, mastering of a range of communication functions allows a person to use language as an instrument to convey his or her mental state to other people and to use language as a social-interactional tool. To accurately express a communication function to another person, children draw on their language abilities in other domains, including vocabulary, morphology, syntax, and phonology (Bloom & Tinker, 2001). When skills are uneven across domains, communication breakdowns may occur. For example, consider 3-year-old Hakuta, who wants his mother to read him a story. Hakuta's phonological skills are underdeveloped, which renders his request completely unintelligible. Thus, expressing communication functions depends on achievements in a number of language domains.

Conversational Skills

When children express communication functions, they do so in exchanges with other people, called conversations. One key aspect of pragmatic development is developing understanding of conversational schema (Siegel, 2013). Schema are the building blocks of cognition and, in essence, are internalized representations of the organizational structures of various events (Atherton & Nutbrown, 2013). When children have a robust representation of a particular schema, their cognitive resources are freed from navigating the organizational structure of the event so that they can acquire new information within the event. For example, consider your first visit to the university library. The organizational schema of the library was unfamiliar; thus, during your first visit, you focused considerable cognitive effort on developing a schematic representation of the library, including how information was cataloged and where materials were located. After internalizing this schema, you could, during future visits, devote more cognitive energy to looking for and assimilating the information you were seeking (see Neuman, 2006).

Conversations have a schema as well: initiation and establishment of a topic, navigation of a series of contingent turns that maintain or shift the topic, and resolution and closure (see Figure 2.6). This macrostructural schema provides a broad organizational framework in which many additional microstructural schemata are embedded. Microstructural schemata a child must acquire include navigating topic shifts, negotiating conversational breakdowns, and knowing how much information to provide according to whether listeners share background information. Children must learn how to enter a conversation in which they were not previously involved. To do so, they must identify the frame of reference for

Initiation and establishment of topic	A: So, I meant to ask you, what did you think about the test? B: Boy, that was rough, wasn't it?
Navigation of a series of contingent turns that maintain or shift topic	A: Yeah, I definitely didn't study enough. I was really surprised by the essay. B: I know. I thought it was going to be on pragmatics. I didn't even study the semantic stuff. A: Well, I did, but obviously not enough. B: I went into that test with an A; it's probably shot now. A: Yeah, I feel the same way.
Resolution and closure	A: Well, we ought to go back in. B: Yeah, I definitely can't afford to miss anything. Talk to ya later. A: See ya.

FIGURE 2.6

Macrostructural schema of a conversation.

the conversation and then establish themselves as sharing that frame of reference (Liiva & Cleave, 2005).

Development of a conversational schematic begins soon after birth as infants engage in increasingly sustained periods of joint attention with their caregivers. *Joint attention* describes instances in which infants and caregivers focus attention on a mutual object; in such exchanges, the infant must coordinate his or her attention between the social partner and the object of interest (Moore & Dunham, 2014). Periods of joint attention, which systematically increase in duration and frequency during the first 18 months of life, provide the child with early schematic representations of conversational organization; like conversation, periods of joint attention feature a communication bid or conversational initiation, a period of sustained turn taking on a single topic, and then a resolution. Caregivers naturally assume the most control during these early *protoconversations*, often interpreting children's vocal or gestural contributions to "fill in the gaps" and using various techniques to redirect children's attention to the conversation (Tomasello, 1988).

Experiences participating in the protoconversations of infancy and toddlerhood help children develop schematic representations of mature conversations in which both participants maintain topics across turns. This is particularly true when young children participate in protoconversations embedded in highly scripted routines focused on concrete objects, such as play with a familiar toy (Tomasello, 1988). In these scripted and familiar routines, children usually assume more active conversational roles and produce longer turns than in less structured and unfamiliar routines.

As children increase their range of conversational partners beyond their immediate caregivers, they show gradual improvements in their ability to initiate and sustain conversations. Studies of preschoolers' conversations during snack time in their classrooms provide an interesting snapshot of what young children like to talk about. Can you guess? If you said "themselves," you are right! Nearly 80% of what 3- and 4-year-olds converse about over snacks involves people—themselves (as in "I can count to ten," "I got a Batman shirt like that") and their listeners ("You always spill," "I see you have slippers on"; O'Neill, Main, & Ziemski, 2009).

An interesting avenue of pragmatic growth is learning how to enter conversations with others. By first grade, children can successfully enter peer conversations, contributing a turn in the ongoing conversation within 1 minute of entering a conversation. Once in a conversation, first graders' verbal contributions are significant, averaging 61 utterances during only 10 minutes (Liiva & Cleave, 2005). Thus, in a relatively short period, children move from being fairly passive participants in caregiver-mediated protoconversations to active participants in extended conversations with peers.

Sensitivity to Extralinguistic Cues

When individuals use language for social-interactional purposes, they draw on a variety of extralinguistic devices to aid communication, such as posture, gesture, facial expression, eye contact, proximity, pitch, loudness, and pausing. Consequently, pragmatic development also involves developing sensitivity to these extralinguistic cues, such as how, during a conversation, a person's facial expression conveys additional content beyond the words themselves.

Previously in this chapter, we discussed how children must use a variety of tactics to "break into" the streams of speech occurring around them. Attending to extralinguistic cues surrounding the speech stream is an important tool children use early in life to make sense of the language directed at them; for instance, 6-month-olds can follow the gaze of their adult conversational partners to map adult words onto objects in the environment (Morales, Mundy, & Rojas, 1998). Infants also attend to prosodic elements of caregivers' speech to make probabilistic estimates of where word boundaries occur in the speech stream (Shukla, White, & Aslin, 2011).

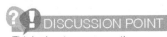

DISCUSSION POINT

Think about a conversation you had recently that did not go smoothly. What are some specific features of a less-than-optimal conversation?

Beyond infancy, children become increasingly attuned to drawing on extralinguistic information to comprehend and produce language in social-interactional contexts. They learn how to use facial expressions, gestures, stress, and loudness to convey their intentions more precisely, and they attend to these elements in conversations with other people to derive meaning beyond that contained in words alone. Studies examining children's register variations provide interesting data concerning children's developing skills in this area of pragmatic development. The term register refers to stylistic variations in language that occur in different situational contexts; for instance, consider how you vary your language form, content, and use when making a request of a best friend versus your college professor.

During the preschool years, children show varying registers during their dramatic play, assuming different speaking styles, for example, when playing house or school (Anderson, 2014). In a study of 4- to 8-year-old children, researchers observed them while they enacted a family situation, a classroom situation, and a doctor situation. The study results showed that boys and girls at all ages varied their pitch, loudness, and speaking rate as they performed different roles; for instance, the children used higher pitches for mothers, louder voices for fathers, and the highest pitches for other children (Anderson, 2000). Even the youngest children in the study showed clear stylistic variations when taking on different speaker roles. Compared with the older children, the youngest relied mostly on prosodic variations for register changes, whereas the older children varied the words and syntax of utterances and were able to "stay in role" for longer periods of play. Given the importance of facial expression, posture, eye contact, and other extralinguistic cues to the success (or failure) of children's communication with other people, the fact that children acquire sensitivity to these aspects of language early in development is not surprising.

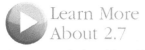

Learn More
About 2.7

As you watch the video titled "Steven Pinker on Language Pragmatics," observe how pragmatics impacts our understanding of language and communication. Also consider how human communication would be different if we did not have pragmatics. https://www.youtube.com/watch?v=VKbp4hEHV-s

Influences on Pragmatic Development

As children become competent language users, they show differences in a range of pragmatic aspects of language. Some of these differences arise from personal disposition, particularly temperament, whereas others relate to social and cultural contexts of development. We next discuss these two influences on pragmatic development.

Temperament

Temperament is the way in which an individual approaches a situation, particularly one that is unfamiliar; put simply, *temperament* describes a person's behavioral style or personality type (Kagan & Snidman, 2004). Some individuals are uninhibited, or bold, whereas others are inhibited, or shy. When placed in unfamiliar situations, inhibited children appear wary and fearful, have problems sustaining attention, and are verbally reticent. In contrast, uninhibited children seem eager to explore the situation, are interactive with and responsive to other people, and adjust quickly. These individual differences in behavioral style reflect biologically based heritable variations in neurochemistry (Kagan & Snidman, 2004).

Children's temperament may be apparent in their pragmatic style. For instance, children who are shy and inhibited talk less and smile less often during communications with other people than bold, uninhibited children (Kagan & Snidman, 2004). In elementary classrooms, bold children interact more with teachers and peers. Such differences in temperament may give rise to individual differences in language development because bold children initiate and engage in conversations with other people more frequently than shy children, which provides more opportunities for bold children to practice and refine their conversational abilities (Evans, 1996).

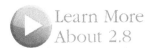

Learn More About 2.8

As you watch the video titled "What Is Pragmatic Language Impairment?" think about what type of intervention a child would need in this situation. https://www.youtube.com/ watch?v=Dk9kULgUkSQ

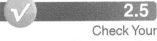

2.5

Check Your Understanding

Click here to gauge your understanding of the concepts in this section.

Social and Cultural Contexts of Development

Social and cultural communities have distinct rules about how language should be used during social interactions. These rules govern, for instance, how conversations are organized and how speakers address one another. When we (the authors of this book) were children, we addressed our friends' parents as "Mr. _____" and "Mrs. _____." Modern-day children often call friends' parents by their first names, which shows how this pragmatic rule has changed in one generation.

As members of specific social and cultural communities, children exhibit pragmatic development that reflects the pragmatic rules of the larger community. In one cultural community, adults may socialize children to never initiate conversations with adults, but rather to "speak when spoken to." Conversely, in another community, children may be socialized to initiate conversations with adults often, and their success in doing so may be hailed as evidence of linguistic precocity. Likewise, children in one community may be socialized to limit eye contact during conversations with other people, whereas in another community children may be socialized to view maintenance of eye contact as a gesture of respect. When practitioners consider a child's achievement of specific pragmatic building blocks—including his or her development of communication functions, conversational skills, and sensitivity to extralinguistic cues—they must recognize these skills are not developed in a vacuum. Instead, achievements in each area reflect the socialization practices children experience at home, at school, and in the community.

SUMMARY

As children's language develops, they achieve competence in form (phonology, morphology, syntax), content (semantics), and use (pragmatics). In this chapter, we discuss the basic building blocks corresponding to each of these areas.

Phonological development involves acquiring the rules of language that govern the sound structure of syllables and words. Infants "break into" the phonology of their language using a range of tactics, including attending to prosodic and phonotactic cues. With ongoing exposure to the phonology of their native language, children acquire a phonemic inventory corresponding to the set of phonemes in the language. They develop a phonemic inventory of both vowels and consonants. The order of consonantal development relates to how frequently the phoneme occurs in the language, the number of words a child uses containing the phoneme, and the articulatory complexity of producing the phoneme. *Phonological awareness* describes a child's explicit sensitivity to or awareness of the phonological segments of spoken language.

Morphological development describes internalization of the rules of language that govern word structure. Key building blocks include acquiring grammatical and derivational morphology. Grammatical morphemes inflect words for grammatical purposes; they include past, future, and present tense markings of verbs and plural and possessive markings of nouns. Derivational morphemes modify root words to change their meaning or class. Children acquire a range of grammatical and derivational morphemes during early and later childhood; such acquisition substantially increases their vocabulary size from a relatively small corpus of root words to a much larger base of derivationally related and grammatically inflected words.

Syntactic development is internalization of the rules of language that govern how words are organized into sentences. There are three key building blocks of syntactic development. The first is an increase in utterance length, typically estimated by calculating the mean length of utterance (MLU) in morphemes. As a child's MLU increases, the internal syntactic sophistication of sentences increases to include the use of articles, conjunctions, and auxiliary verbs. The second building block is the use of different sentence modalities. During early and later childhood, children use a range of sentence types, including the declarative, negative, and interrogative. The third building block is the development of complex syntax, in which children begin to use a variety of phrase types and coordinate clausal structures to produce complex and compound sentences.

Semantic development involves three major tasks. The first is acquiring a mental lexicon of about 60,000 words between infancy and adulthood. *Mental lexicon* refers to the volume of words an individual understands and uses. The mental lexicon includes a variety of word types, which, for young children, includes specific nominals, general nominals, action words, modifiers, and personal–social words. The second task is acquiring words rapidly during word-learning opportunities. After children are exposed to a new word, their representation of the word emerges gradually from an immature state to an adultlike form. Some features of words influence the ease with which children learn them, including the concept represented by the word, the phonological form of the word, and the contextual conditions at initial exposure. The third task is organizing the mental lexicon in an efficient semantic network so entries can be readily retrieved. Children develop links among entries in the semantic network that reflect the strength of associations among words for syntactic, conceptual, and phonological features.

Pragmatic development is acquisition of rules governing how language is used for social purposes. Major building blocks include developing a range of communication functions, acquiring conversational skills, and becoming sensitive to extralinguistic cues in communicative interactions. The development of communication functions involves learning how to communicate "differently in different situations according to the circumstances and communication goals of the participants" (L. Bloom & Tinker, 2001, p. 14). Throughout childhood, children develop a range of functions and become increasingly sophisticated at using language as a social tool. Children's conversational skills emerge in early protoconversations with primary caregivers; through these interactions, children develop a conversational schema specifying the organizational structure of conversations. By late childhood, children are active conversationalists, able to enter conversations skillfully and navigate a topic across many turns. Sensitivity to extralinguistic cues—such as facial expression, posture, intonation, and loudness—also emerges early in childhood. By the end of preschool, children can readily vary their extralinguistic cues for different communicative situations.

 Apply Your Knowledge

Click here to apply your knowledge
to practical scenarios.

BEYOND THE BOOK

1. Diagram this sentence, attributed to the linguist Noam Chomsky: "Colorless green ideas sleep furiously." Analyze it in terms of its syntax and its semantics.

2. Watch a video of a toddler on youtube.com. Describe the child's language in terms of form, content, and use. What do you notice about the toddler's language abilities?

3. Go to the local library or a bookstore. Select two children's picture books from the shelf. Analyze each for the variety of new and interesting words they contain—or, in other words, the number of word-learning opportunities each would provide to a young child. How do the books compare?

4. Play a board game, such as Candy Land, with a 3- or 4-year-old child. Examine the child's pragmatic skills, particularly his or her ability to explain and follow the rules. What do you learn about young children's pragmatic skills?

5. Collect a brief language sample from a child under the age of 5 years using two different techniques. First, ask the child to respond to the question, "Tell me about yourself, such as the things you like to do" and record the child's response. Second, tell the child a brief story about a time when you got hurt, and close the story with "I wonder if anything like this ever happened to you." Record the child's response. Examine both responses for features regarding linguistic form, content, and use. Do you see differences between the two samples? Similarities?

 Check Your Understanding

Gauge your understanding of the
chapter concepts by taking this
self-check quiz.

3

Neuroanatomy and Neurophysiology of Language

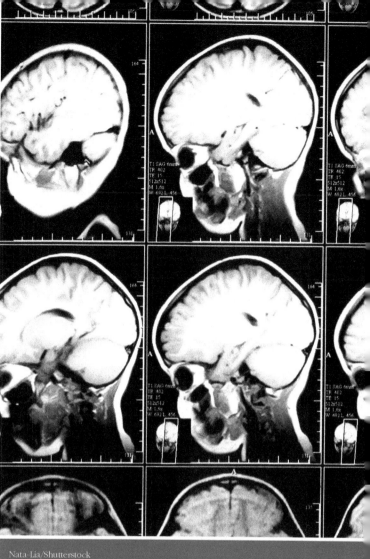

Nata-Lia/Shutterstock

LEARNING OUTCOMES

After completion of this chapter, the reader will be able to:

1. Contrast neuroanatomy and neurophysiology.

2. Identify the major structures and functions of the human brain.

3. Describe how the human brain processes and produces language.

4. Describe major concepts related to neurophysiological and neuroanatomical sensitive periods.

Language is a complex and distinctly human ability that resides in the neuroanatomical and neurophysiological architecture of the human brain. Decades of remarkable technological advances have allowed researchers to study the brain as it performs complex linguistic activities; such studies have increased scientists' understanding of and appreciation for humans' capacity for language. For instance, functional magnetic resonance imaging (fMRI) is a procedure that uses intense magnetic fields to study how the brain functions during various activities, as well as during sleep and rest states. The results of hundreds of studies of the human brain using fMRI have substantially improved what we know about the human brain, to include where and how language is comprehended.

Our knowledge about the neural architecture of the brain—including the neuroanatomy and the neurophysiology of the capacity for language—has grown exponentially during the last few decades. We can credit then-President, George H. W. Bush who proclaimed in 1990, the next 10 years would be the "Decade of the Brain" (Office of the Federal Register, 1990). The advances in knowledge about the brain achieved during the Decade of the Brain and the beginning of the 21st century have provided researchers and students of language development with unprecedented understanding of how the brain processes and produces language, and why, in some cases, language does not develop as expected.

For some students of language development, understanding the neuroanatomical and neurophysiological aspects of language ability may seem difficult; however, such an understanding is critical to fully appreciate and understand the human species' biologically unique capacity for language. In this chapter, we provide a basic introduction to this topic.

WHAT ARE NEUROANATOMY AND NEUROPHYSIOLOGY?

Neuroscience is a branch of science that focuses on the anatomy and physiology of the nervous system, or the neuroanatomy and neurophysiology, respectively. The human nervous system includes the central nervous system (CNS, comprising the brain and the spinal cord) and the peripheral nervous system (PNS, comprising the cranial and spinal nerves, which carry information inward to and outward from the brain and spinal cord). Neuroscientists study the anatomical structures of the nervous system (neuroanatomy), and examine how these structures work together as a complex unit and as separate, distinct biological units (neurophysiology).

Neuroscience is a focused branch of the more general disciplines of anatomy and physiology, which involve the study of body structures and the functions of these structures. More specifically, anatomists study the physical characteristics of body structures and examine how they relate to other structures to form anatomical systems. Physiologists study how body structures function, both individually and in concert with other structures to form physiological systems. The fields of anatomy and physiology date back hundreds of years. Many of the terms in current use were introduced by Hippocrates, the "Father of Medicine" (c. 460 B.C.–c. 380 B.C.). In early modern universities, such as the University of Bologna in Italy and Leiden University in The Netherlands, students learned about anatomy and physiology in the universities' anatomy theaters, where dissections occurred with the corpse placed on a central slab surrounded by tiers of students and other observers.

Matters have changed greatly in the last 500 years, not the least being the emergence of the field of modern neuroscience. Neuroscientists study the structures and functions of the nervous system; their work has benefited tremendously from the rapid and remarkable advances in imaging technologies that allow researchers to study nervous system functions and structures at the level of the neuron.

TABLE 3.1
Areas of study in neuroscience

SUBDISCIPLINE	AREA OF STUDY
Developmental neuroscience	Branch of neuroscience focused on identifying how the structures and functions of the nervous system develop and change with time as a function of aging and experience.
Cognitive neuroscience	Branch of neuroscience focused on identifying how the brain structures and functions support higher-level cognitive functions, such as memory, reasoning, problem solving, and language processing.
Neurology	Branch of medicine focused on the nervous system. Neurologists diagnose and treat diseases that disrupt the normal functioning of the nervous system.
Neurosurgery	Branch of surgery focused on the nervous system. Neurosurgeons conduct surgery to prevent and correct diseases of the nervous system, including diseases of the brain and spinal column.
Neuroanatomy	Branch of neuroscience focused on the structures of the nervous system. Neuroanatomists study the architecture of the central and peripheral nervous systems, including the brain, to determine how their individual components work as single units and together as parts of a complex system.
Neurophysiology	Branch of neuroscience focused on the functions of the nervous system structures. Neurophysiologists study how the various units of the nervous system work both as single units and together as parts of larger systems.
Neuropathology	Branch of neuroscience and of medicine focused on identifying diseases of the nervous system, including their causes. Clinical neuropathologists are trained medical doctors who study tissues of the nervous system to identify whether a disease is present.
Neurolinguistics	Branch of neuroscience focused specifically on human language, with a particular interest in understanding how the brain develops and processes spoken, written, and signed language.

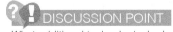

DISCUSSION POINT

What additional technological advances might improve scientists' understanding of the capacity of the brain for language?

Technologies such as magnetic resonance imaging (MRI), positron emission tomography (PET), computerized tomography (CT) scanning, and magnetoencephalography (MEG) provide detailed images of the anatomy and/or physiology of the nervous system. Although commonplace today, researchers only began using MRI to examine the brain's functioning in the early 1990s (Belliveau et al., 1990). Now, there are entire conferences and organizations devoted to sharing research findings that involve neuroimaging of the brain (e.g., the Organization for Human Brain Mapping). See Research Paradigms: *fMRI Studies* for information on a brain-imaging technique that allows researchers to examine brain activity when an individual is engaged in a specific processing task.

Neuroscience has several subdisciplines, including developmental neuroscience, cognitive neuroscience, neurology, neurosurgery, neuroanatomy, neurophysiology, neuropathology, and neurolinguistics. The foci for these various subdisciplines appear in Table 3.1. Of particular interest to the study of language acquisition is the work of neurolinguists, who study the structures and functions of the nervous system that relate to language. Some neurolinguists study the neuroanatomy of language to identify the nervous system structures involved with language processing. Other neurolinguists study the neurophysiology of language to identify the specific ways in which the nervous system functions, such as how the

RESEARCH **PARADIGMS**

fMRI Studies

Functional magnetic resonance imaging (fMRI) is a type of brain imaging that allows researchers and clinicians to identify the brain structures involved in specific mental functions. fMRI is a noninvasive procedure that maps neural activities (i.e., functions) to specific neural regions (i.e., structures) according to changes in blood oxygen levels that correspond to changes in neural activity (Brown, Cheng, Haacke, Thompson, & Venkatesan, 2014). fMRI uses MRI technology, which provides structural scans of the brain (e.g., measurements of anatomical regions of the brain). However, fMRI differs from MRI in that it maps brain functioning by examining brain activity when individuals are engaged in a specific processing task (e.g., listening to yes–no questions) or in a resting state. fMRI has significant benefits over other types of brain-imaging technologies, such as PET scans, because it requires no injections of radioactive materials, images can be collected relatively quickly (often with a single pass), and the resultant images are of extremely high resolution.

An example of an image obtained by using fMRI is presented in the figure accompanying this box.

One example of the potential for fMRI to improve understanding of language functions in the brain is described in a study by a team of scientists in the Netherlands (Groen et al., 2010). In Chapter 2, we noted that children with autism spectrum disorder (ASD) exhibit difficulties with social aspects of communication. One such difficulty involves the ability to integrate information that is important for communicating socially. For instance, when communicating with others, we must integrate our knowledge about the speaker with our knowledge of what words to use to communicate effectively. This is called linguistic-context integration (we must match our language to the context in which we are communicating). When speaking to a 3-year-old, we might choose to use the word "frog" rather than "amphibian" because we understand a young child is more likely to be familiar with the former than the latter. Persons with ASD have difficulty integrating these and

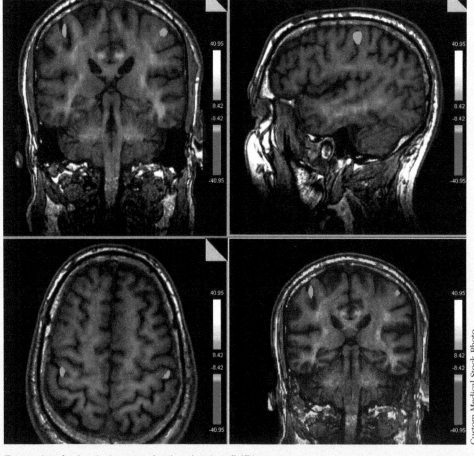

Example of a brain image obtained using fMRI.

Custom Medical Stock Photo

other types of information, which leads to difficulties with social communication.

Few studies have sought to determine whether there is a neural basis for this difficulty. That is, whether differences exist in the brain functions of persons with ASD compared to those without ASD that cause difficulties with social communication. Groen and colleagues sought to determine whether this was the case by using fMRI to study the brain functions of 30 adolescents with ASD and 31 adolescents who were typically developing (TD). The participants listened either to sentences that involved integrating congruent information (the integrated information made sense) or incongruent information (the integrated information didn't make sense). For instance, the participants heard the sentence "If only I looked like Britney Spears in her latest video" as spoken by both a male and a female (Groen et al., 2010, p. 1939). When spoken by a female, the linguistic-context integration is congruent; when spoken by a male, it is not. The researchers identified several regions of interest (ROIs) near Broca's area to examine brain functions while participants heard these congruent and incongruent sentences. They found adolescents with ASD showed less activation in the ROIs when hearing linguistic-context incongruent sentences than the TD participants. Adolescents with ASD do not seem to process incongruent information in the way their typical peers do, suggesting that social-communication difficulties of persons with ADS may have a neural basis.

human brain processes language. Still, other neurolinguists study the neuropathology of language to identify the ways in which diseases and injuries affect the functioning of the human nervous system; for example, some study how various brain structures reorganize and assume new language functions after injury.

Linguistics and psycholinguistics are additional disciplines that have yielded considerable advances in understanding language. *Linguistics* is a broad field concerned specifically with language as a developmental and ecological phenomenon, whereas *psycholinguistics* is a more focused field dealing with the cognitive processes involved in developing, processing, and producing human language. Psycholinguistics is the study of the psychology of language, an integration of the fields of psychology and linguistics. It also involves studying the language and communicative capacities of other species, such as nonhuman primates.

Terminology

Students of language development require knowledge of the specific terminology, or *nomenclature*, to describe anatomy and physiology, as well as the neuroanatomy and neurophysiology of language. Much of this terminology has its roots in ancient Latin and Greek.

Nervous System Axes

The human nervous system is organized along two axes: the horizontal axis and the vertical axis. Together, these axes compose the T-shaped neuraxis. The horizontal axis runs from the anterior (frontal) pole of the brain to the posterior (occipital) pole. The vertical axis extends from the superior portion of the brain downward along the entire spinal cord. Figure 3.1 depicts the horizontal and vertical axes of the neuraxis.

When experts describe specific nervous system structures, they often use the horizontal and vertical axes as reference points. They use four terms to specify locations on a specific axis: rostral, caudal, dorsal, and ventral. On the horizontal axis, *rostral* refers to the front of the brain, whereas *caudal* refers to the back of the brain. *Dorsal* refers to the top of the brain, and *ventral* refers to the bottom of the brain. On the vertical axis, *rostral* refers to the top of the spinal cord (near the brain), and *caudal* refers to the bottom of the spinal cord (near the coccyx, or tailbone). *Dorsal* refers to the back of the spinal cord (the side nearest the back), whereas *ventral* refers to the front of the spinal cord (the side nearest the belly).

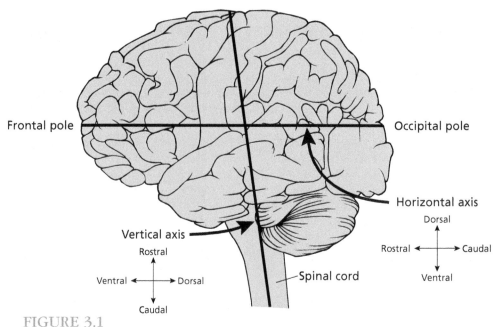

FIGURE 3.1

Vertical and horizontal axes of the neuraxis.

Source: From *Communication Sciences and Disorders: A Contemporary Perspective* (2nd ed., p. 84) by L. M. Justice, 2010, Upper Saddle River, NJ: Pearson Education, Inc. Copyright 2010 by Pearson Education, Inc. Reprinted with permission.

Directional and Positional Terms

Neuroscientists use several additional terms to discuss the directional and positional relationships among various anatomical and physiological structures. *Proximal* refers to structures relatively close to a site of reference, whereas *distal* refers to structures relatively far from a site of reference. Other common terms are *anterior* (toward the front) and *posterior* (toward the back), *superior* (toward the top) and *inferior* (toward the bottom), *external* (toward the outside) and *internal* (toward the inside), and efferent (away from the brain) and afferent (toward the brain). The last two terms often describe the pathways of information as it moves to and from the brain. Efferent pathways (also called *descending pathways*) move away from the brain, carrying motor impulses from the central nervous system to more distal body structures. Afferent pathways (also called *ascending pathways*) move toward the brain, carrying sensory information from the distal body structures to the brain.

Neuroscience Basics

The human nervous system, like that of many other species, is a complex anatomical and physiological structure that includes the brain, the spinal cord, and sets of nerves that carry information to and from the brain and spinal cord. The human nervous system mediates nearly all aspects of human behavior, with few exceptions. In this section, we provide a basic introduction to the major structures of the human nervous system, emphasizing the aspects of the nervous system most relevant to understanding and appreciating language development.

Neurons

The billions of highly specialized cells that compose the nervous system are called neurons. A neuron is functionally divided into four components: cell body, axon, presynaptic terminal, and dendrites. The cell body is the center of the neuron, containing its nucleus; the nucleus contains DNA material (genes, chromosomes) and proteins. The human brain uses an estimated 30,000–40,000 genes, more than

Efferent pathways carry motor impulses away from the brain, whereas afferent pathways carry sensory information toward the brain.

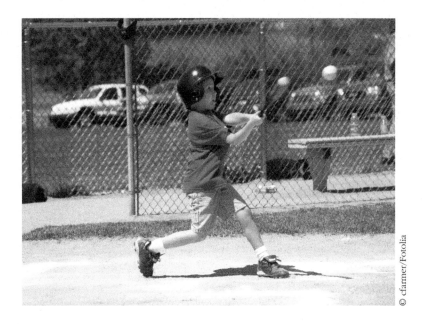

© cfarmer/Fotolia

any other organ of the body (Noback, Strominger, Demarest, & Ruggiero, 2005). The axon and the dendrites are extensions from the cell body, serving as vehicles for the cell body to receive and transmit information from other neurons, as shown in Figure 3.2. The information carried by neurons is in the form of electrochemical nerve impulses; these impulses transmit information to and away from the cell body. Each neuron has a single efferent nerve extension, the axon, which carries nerve impulses away from the cell body. The axon extends from the cell body for a distance of 1 mm to 1 m, at which point it arborizes into a number of terminal branches (Noback et al., 2005). The distal end of each terminal branch is a presynaptic terminal. These terminals are the sites at which the axonal connection of one neuron corresponds with the dendritic extension of another neuron. Dendrites are the afferent extensions of a neuron, meaning they bring nerve impulses into the cell body from the axonal projections of other neurons. A single cell body contains a number of dendritic extensions; many dendrites are studded with small protuberances (called *spines*), which increase the surface area of the afferent connections of the neuron (Noback et al., 2005).

Neurons communicate by means of electrochemical nerve impulses that travel along the dendrite of one neuron and into its cell body, then along the axon to the dendrite of another neuron. The synapse is the site where two neurons meet. For the two neurons to communicate, the nerve impulse must cross the synapse. Neurotransmitters are chemical agents that help transmit information across the synaptic cleft, which is the space between the axon of the transmitting neuron and the dendrite of the receiving neuron. When a synapse is created, that is, when one neuron forges a connection with another neuron, this is referred to as *synaptogenesis*.

The tissue formed by the linkages of thousands of neurons is called *nervous tissue*. The two primary types of nervous tissue are gray matter and white matter. Gray matter consists of the cell bodies of neurons and the dendrites. White matter is the tissue that carries information among gray matter, consisting primarily of axonal fibers that carry information among gray matter tissues. Thus, gray matter is where information is generated and processed, whereas white matter serves as an information conduit.

Neurons are sheathed in a coating called myelin. The myelin sheath contributes to the rapid relay of nerve impulses, particularly within white matter. This sheath also helps protect the neuron. Myelinization refers to the growth of the myelin sheath, a slow process that is not complete until late childhood.

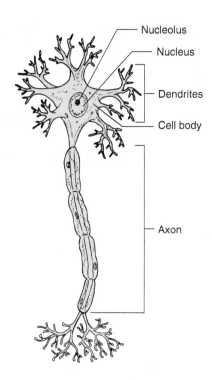

FIGURE 3.2

The neuron.

Source: From *Communication Sciences and Disorders: A Contemporary Perspective* (2nd ed., p. 84) by L. M. Justice, 2010, Upper Saddle River, NJ: Pearson Education, Inc. Copyright 2010 by Pearson Education, Inc. Reprinted with permission.

Learn More About 3.1

As you watch the video titled "The Nervous System, Part 1: Crash Course A&P #8," consider how every level of the nervous system can (and most likely does) impact communication processes. https://www.youtube.com/watch?v=qPix_X-9t7E

Nervous System Divisions

As we mentioned previously, the human body has two major nervous systems: the CNS and the PNS. The CNS consists of the brain and the spinal cord. The PNS comprises the nerves that emerge from the brain and the spinal cord to *innervate* the rest of the body. Innervate is the term in neuroscience that means "to supply nerves" to a particular region or part of the body. The 12 pairs of nerves that emerge from the brain are the cranial nerves. The 31 pairs of nerves that emerge from the spinal cord are called spinal nerves. The cranial and spinal nerves carry information back and forth among the brain, the spine, and the rest of the body. This information includes sensory information carried to the brain by afferent pathways and motor information carried away from the brain by efferent pathways. Figure 3.3 illustrates the major structures of the CNS and PNS.

Central Nervous System. The CNS consists of the brain and the spinal cord. The brain is essentially the chief executive operator of the entire CNS: It initiates and regulates virtually all motor, sensory, and cognitive processes. The spinal cord acts primarily as a conduit of information, carrying not only sensory information from the body to the brain through afferent pathways, but also motor commands from the brain to the rest of the body through efferent pathways.

Given the importance of the CNS to many human functions, its design includes a number of protective shields. The first shield is bone. Both the brain and the spinal cord are protected by bone; the skull covers the brain, and the vertebral column covers the spinal cord.

The second shield is a series of layered membranes: These meninges, which comprise three layers, completely encase the CNS. These are sometimes called the *meningeal envelope.* The inside layer of membrane, called the pia mater, tightly wraps around the brain and spinal cord and carries the blood vessels that serve the

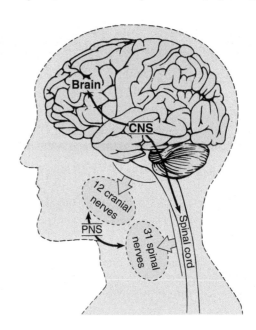

FIGURE 3.3

Major structures of the central nervous system (CNS) and peripheral nervous system (PNS).

Source: From *Communication Sciences and Disorders: A Contemporary Perspective* (2nd ed., p. 83), by L. M. Justice, 2010, Upper Saddle River, NJ: Pearson Education, Inc. Copyright 2010 by Pearson Education, Inc. Reprinted with permission.

brain. It is a thin, transparent shield that gives the brain its bright pink color. The second layer is the arachnoid mater, a delicate membrane separated from the pia mater by the subarachnoid space. The third and outermost layer is the dura mater (literally, "hard mother"). The dura mater consists of thick, fibrous tissue that completely encases the brain and the spinal cord.

The third shield is a layer of fluid called cerebrospinal fluid (CSF). CSF circulates between the two innermost layers of the meninges—the pia mater and the arachnoid mater—within the subarachnoid space. CSF carries chemicals important to metabolic processes, but it is also an important buffer against jolts to the CNS. Perhaps you have heard of a procedure called a spinal tap (not the fictional rock band, which is perhaps a more amusing connotation). Also called a *lumbar puncture*, a spinal tap involves inserting a needle between two of the lower (lumbar) vertebrae and extracting CSF from the subarachnoid space. It is a procedure often used to diagnose meningitis, which is an infection or inflammation of the meninges. [Meningitis is also very serious, so it is important to know the symptoms. Typically, these include headache, neck stiffness, high fever, and altered mental state (Glimåker et al., 2015).]

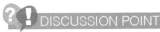

DISCUSSION POINT

The CNS is not totally impervious to injury. What types of accidents or illnesses pose the most risk to the CNS?

Peripheral Nervous System.   The PNS is the system of nerves connected to the brainstem and the spinal cord. These nerves carry sensory information to the CNS and motor commands away from the CNS, thus controlling nearly all voluntary and involuntary activity of the human body.

The PNS consists of two sets of nerves: cranial nerves and spinal nerves. The 12 pairs of cranial nerves run between the brainstem and the facial and neck regions and are particularly important for speech, language, and hearing. The cranial nerves transmit information concerning four of the five senses (vision, hearing, smell, and taste) to the brain. They also carry motor impulses from the brain to the face and neck muscles, including those activating the tongue and the jaw, both of which are

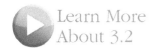

Learn More About 3.2

As you watch the video titled "Central Nervous System: Crash Course A&P #11," think about how the different areas of the brain are associated with language skill, and consider how other areas of the brain may compensate for damage or injury. https://www.youtube.com/watch?v=q8NtmDrb_qo

3.1

Check Your Understanding

Click here to gauge your understanding of the concepts in this section.

involved with speech. The seven cranial nerves most closely involved with speech and language production are the following:

- *Trigeminal* (V): Facial sensation; jaw movements, including chewing
- *Facial* (VII): Taste sensation; facial movements, including smiling
- *Acoustic* (VIII): Hearing and balance
- *Glossopharyngeal* (IX): Tongue sensation; palatal and pharyngeal movement, including gagging
- *Vagus* (X): Taste sensation; palatal, pharyngeal, and laryngeal movement, including voicing
- *Accessory* (XI): Palatal, pharyngeal, laryngeal, head, and shoulder movement
- *Hypoglossal* (XII): Tongue movement

The 31 pairs of spinal nerves run between the spinal cord and all peripheral areas of the human body, including the arms and the legs. These nerves mediate reflexes, sensory activity, and conscious (volitional) motor activity. An important feature of the CNS and PNS is that almost everything is organized to be contralateral. This means the right side of the brain processes information from the left side of the body, and vice versa. In the simplest terms, damage to the left side of the brain will affect the functioning of the right side of the body.

WHAT ARE THE MAJOR STRUCTURES AND FUNCTIONS OF THE HUMAN BRAIN?

The brain is the commander in chief, or mediator, of the entire human body, and it is viewed as the most complex and sophisticated organ of the human body. The relatively small volume and murky gray appearance of the brain belie its significance to the human species' capacity for thought and language. Weighing only about 2 lb (1,100–1,400 g) and comprising about 2% of the total weight of

The relative size of the human brain and its sheer demand for energy—it consumes one-fifth of the metabolic resources of the body—far exceed those of any other mammal.

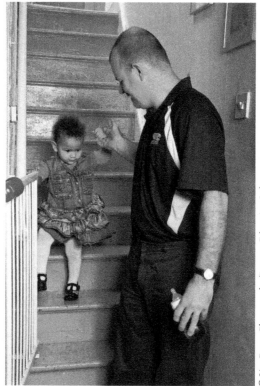

© Lisa Payne Photography/Pearson Education Ltd

the body (Jerison, 2012), the brain is extraordinarily important to the entire functioning of the human body and mind. In fact, the human brain—and its capacity for abstract thought and language—differentiates humans most significantly from other species. The growth of the human brain in both size and weight is one of the most important evolutionary changes in the anatomy of the human species. Proportionally, the relative size of the human brain and its sheer demand for energy (consuming one-fifth of the metabolic resources of the body) far exceed those of any other mammal (Jerison, 2012).

The most important evolutionary change in the human brain, accounting for these increases in weight and mass, is the enlargement of the outer layers of the brain. These enlarged regions are called the neocortex, meaning "new cortex" (or, more literally, "new rind"), which has grown over the original human brain. The neocortex controls most of the functions that exemplify human thought and language, including speech, language, reasoning, planning, and problem solving. Recent research has exposed deficits in regions of the neocortex of children with autism spectrum disorder, which may help us understand why these brain-based functions are so impaired in this population (Stoner et al., 2014).

The brain includes three major sections: the cerebrum, the brainstem, and the cerebellum (see Figure 3.4). Next, we briefly examine these brain sections and identify the major structures and functions of each.

Cerebrum

The cerebrum, or cerebral cortex, is the location of the most unique human qualities: reasoning, problem solving, planning, and hypothesizing, to name only a few. Of the three major divisions of the brain, the cerebrum is the largest, comprising 40% of the weight of the brain and containing more than 100 billion neurons (Noback et al., 2005). The cerebrum includes both the allocortex and the neocortex; the former comprises the original and older human brain (taking up about 10% of brain matter), and the latter consists of the more newly evolved outer structures, corresponding to about 90% of brain matter.

? ! DISCUSSION POINT

You have probably heard of the three major brain divisions: cerebrum, brainstem, and cerebellum. Before reading further, identify what you know about each in terms of where it is located and what functions it serves.

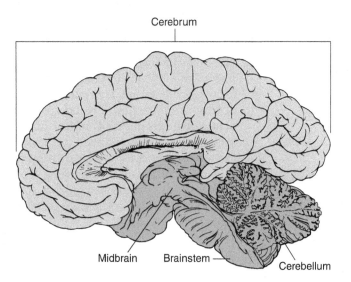

Cerebrum

Midbrain   Brainstem   Cerebellum

FIGURE 3.4

Cerebrum, brainstem, and cerebellum.

Source: From *Communication Sciences and Disorders: A Contemporary Perspective* (2nd ed., p. 86), by L. M. Justice, 2010, Upper Saddle River, NJ: Pearson Education, Inc. Copyright 2010 by Pearson Education, Inc. Reprinted with permission.

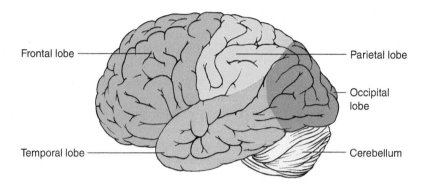

FIGURE 3.5

Lobes of the human brain.

Source: From *Communication Sciences and Disorders: A Contemporary Perspective* (2nd ed., p. 87) by L. M. Justice, 2010, Upper Saddle River, NJ: Pearson Education, Inc. Copyright 2010 by Pearson Education, Inc. Reprinted with permission.

Cerebral Hemispheres

The cerebrum consists of two mirror-image hemispheres, aptly named the right hemisphere and the left hemisphere. The two hemispheres are separated by a long cerebral crevice (or fissure) called the longitudinal fissure. The corpus callosum is a band of fibers that connects the two hemispheres, serving as a conduit for communication between them.

Cerebral Lobes

The cerebrum is organized into six lobes of four types: one frontal lobe, one occipital lobe, two temporal lobes, and two parietal lobes. Each lobe has functional specializations, as discussed in the next sections, although the neural circuitry of the brain features numerous intricate associations among the lobes that result in organized, complex behavior. Figure 3.5 identifies the locations of these lobes.

Frontal Lobe.   The frontal lobe is the largest lobe of the human brain; it resides in the most anterior part of the brain, behind the forehead. Two key functions of the frontal lobe are (a) activating and controlling both fine and complex motor activities, including speech output, and (b) controlling human "executive functions." Executive functions include reasoning, problem solving, planning, hypothesizing, being socially aware, and rationalizing. These unique and important human qualities are *executive* functions because they govern the organized, goal-directed, and controlled execution of critical human behaviors. These are sometimes called *higher-order* cognitive abilities. Executive functions provide humans with the ability to monitor and control their own purposeful behaviors, to override impulses, and to control information processing (Fernandez-Duque, Baird, & Posner, 2000). In short, executive functions are what allow you to stop your arm from reaching for a second piece of chocolate cake or, alternatively, reasoning through why it might be a good choice after all.

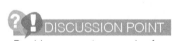

Provide a concrete example of a specific task that requires executive functioning.

The frontal lobe is also important to a critical human attribute called theory of mind (ToM). ToM is one's ability to attribute mental states to others, which is necessary to take the perspective of another (Carlson, Koenig, & Harms, 2013). Basically, ToM is the understanding that other people have thoughts and feelings of their own, and it appears to be a human-specific attribute. Research on baboons, for instance, indicates that even these very intelligent primates do not recognize their own behaviors can have an impact on the mental states of others (Rendall, Cheney, & Seyfarth, 2000). Young children, on the other hand, do show ToM, as when they tell a white lie so as to not upset their parents. For instance, a 4-year-old child might tell a stranger that she looked good in a photo even if she had a smudge on her cheek (Talwar & Lee, 2002), because the child realizes that telling the truth might be upsetting. This involves ToM because the child understands the stranger's mind (and desires) is different than her own. Persons who have brain injuries that affect the frontal lobe typically have difficulties with ToM, such as an inability to take the perspectives of others (Dennis et al., 2013). We discuss children's achievements in ToM as they relate to language development in chapters 5, 6, 7, and 8.

Several sites within the frontal lobe are very important to human language. The prefrontal cortex is the most anterior portion of the frontal lobe. It is the part of the brain that evolved most recently in the human species and is most developed relative to that of other species (Lieberman, 2000). The prefrontal cortex is connected with all other sensory and motor systems of the brain, which allows it to synthesize the vast stores of information necessary for complex, goal-directed human behavior (Stuss & Knight, 2013). This part of the brain is involved with the affective aspects of sensations, including gloom, elation, calmness, and friendliness; it thus serves as a "regulator of the depth of feeling" (Noback et al., 2005, p. 452).

Much knowledge of prefrontal cortex functions has been learned from studies of persons with damage to this area of the brain. Such persons may superficially appear normal (e.g., they can carry on a conversation; they can perform well on perceptual and memory tests), but are likely to have profound difficulties with organization, self-control, and goal-oriented tasks. Their creativity, outlook, disposition, and drive may suffer (Noback et al., 2005).

Also located in the frontal lobe are the primary motor cortex and the premotor cortex, both important for human speech, as well as other motor functions. The primary motor cortex controls the initiation of skilled, delicate voluntary movements, including not only movements of the extremities (e.g., fingers, hands, toes), but also movements used in speech. The premotor cortex is also involved with control of skilled motor functions, including control of musculature and programming patterns and sequences of movements (Noback et al., 2005). These motor areas are organized topographically, in that specific motor functions correspond to specific sites in the cortices. A *homunculus* is a map that illustrates the location of specific human functions; the motor homunculus presented in Figure 3.6 shows the location of various motor functions in the motor cortex. Because the motor functions are organized along a strip, the motor cortex is sometimes called the *motor strip*. Located on both the left and right sides of the frontal lobe, the connections that run from the motor strip in the brain to the motor functions they control throughout the body are contralateral: The right premotor cortex controls the left side of the body, and vice versa.

The motor cortex of the left frontal lobe is also home to Broca's area, an especially important region of the brain for spoken communication. Broca's area, named after the French physician Paul Broca, is responsible for the fine coordination of speech output. In the mid-1800s, Paul Broca was among the first researchers to recognize the functional specializations of the brain: He identified the site of motor control of speech by performing an autopsy on a patient who had lost the ability to speak following brain damage.

Occipital Lobe. The occipital lobe comprises the posterior portion of the brain. This lobe is functionally specialized for visual reception and processing. Located at the posterior pole of the occipital lobe is the *primary visual cortex*. This cortex receives and processes visual information received from the eyes, fusing information on depth, space, shape, movement, and color into a single visual image. Nerve fibers running from the visual cortex and associated areas project to the temporal and parietal lobes for further analysis and interpretation.

Parietal Lobes. The two parietal lobes reside posterior to the frontal lobe on the left and right sides (above the ears). Key functions of the parietal lobes include

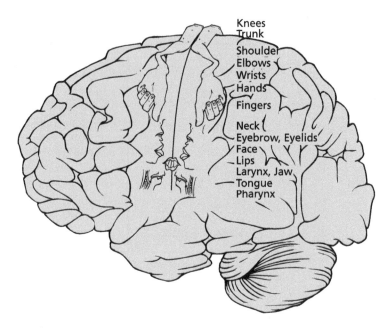

Knees
Trunk
Shoulder
Elbows
Wrists
Hands
Fingers
Neck
Eyebrow, Eyelids
Face
Lips
Larynx, Jaw
Tongue
Pharynx

FIGURE 3.6

Location of various motor functions in the left-hemisphere motor cortex of the human brain.

Source: From *Communication Sciences and Disorders: A Contemporary Perspective* (2nd ed.) by L. M. Justice, Upper Saddle River, NJ: Pearson Education, Inc. Copyright 2010 by Pearson Education, Inc. Reprinted with permission.

perceiving and integrating sensory and perceptual information, comprehending oral and written language, and performing mathematical calculations.

The parietal lobes contain the locations where sensory information received from areas throughout the body is processed. Such processing occurs mainly in the primary somatosensory cortex (or, more simply, the *primary sensory cortex*) and the sensory association cortex, both of which reside just posterior to the primary motor cortex in the frontal lobe. The primary somatosensory cortex is sometimes called the *sensory strip*. It receives and processes sensory experiences of pain, temperature, touch, pressure, and movement from receptors throughout the body. These receptors convert sensory stimuli (e.g., heat) into neural signals and transmit this information to the sensory cortices in the parietal lobes.

The inferior part of the sensory system of the left parietal lobe is tied to language ability, particularly reading and naming abilities, as well as mathematic ability (Buchweitz, Mason, Meschyan, Keller, & Just, 2014; Matejko, Price, Mazzocco, & Ansari, 2013). These functions may occur there because of the important role of the parietal lobes in integrating incoming sensory information with the executive functions of the frontal lobe. In addition, the parietal lobe is especially important to working memory, a complex system that permits individuals to hold in memory certain information while executing a given task, such as a seven-digit phone number while dialing on the phone. Working memory is considered essential for most higher-order executive functions and for acquiring and accessing the lexicon (or store of vocabulary words). See Theory to Practice: *Differential Diagnosis of Language Disorders Using Neurophysiological Models of Language Processing* for a discussion of language disorders and working memory.

Temporal Lobes. The two temporal lobes also sit posterior to the frontal lobe but inferior to the parietal lobes (behind the ears). The temporal lobes are important sites for human language because they contain the functions for processing auditory information and language comprehension. Auditory processing, which

THEORY TO PRACTICE

Differential Diagnosis of Language Disorders Using Neurophysiological Models of Language Processing

Theories of language development propose that many children who exhibit difficulties with language acquisition do so due to a weakness in verbal working memory, specifically its processing capacity. These theories hold that the ability to comprehend and produce language (particularly more complex language) requires active engagement of working memory; working memory is akin to a storage device that maintains the linguistic stimulus while it is being processed (Weismer, Plante, Jones, & Tomblin, 2005). You can engage in a working memory task by seeing if you can hold these ten words in your memory for 5 minutes (without peeking or cheating!).

Bottle-Rain-Erase-Pin-Handle-Ask-Ripe-Street-Elbow-Angry

Such a task can be difficult for many of us, but it is especially difficult for children with language disorders.

Differential diagnosis is an important aspect of psychologists' and speech-language pathologists' clinical decision-making when identifying language impairment. Differential diagnosis, as the name implies, is the act of differentiating a suspected disorder from all other possible disorders. Differential diagnosis is important so that children who have language differences (e.g., who speak a nonstandard dialect) are not mistaken as having a disorder; differential diagnosis is also important for setting treatment goals and developing approaches that effectively remediate the disorder. This noted, differential diagnosis can be tricky. For instance, a child who has had limited exposure to language because of early institutionalization may look similar in his or her grammatical development to a child with a neurologically based neurologically-based language impairment.

Scientific understanding of the neurophysiological correlates of language impairment can be informative in designing tasks that identify neurologically based neurologically-based disorders of language and differentiate them from other conditions or circumstances that affect language development. Consider, for example, the scientific finding that deficits in verbal working memory may serve as a marker of neurologically based, neurologically-based language impairment. In addition to recent fMRI data (Weismer et al., 2005), earlier studies of children with language impairment have shown that verbal working memory capacity predicts their performance on standardized language tests. Thus, measures of working memory (e.g., identifying the number of letters or digits one can hold in working memory) have become a routine part of diagnostic procedures for identifying language impairment (e.g., Weismer & Thordardottir, 2002). By incorporating measures that examine a child's verbal working memory into language assessments, clinicians are better able to differentially diagnose neurologically based language impairment and to develop treatment protocols that address working memory limitations in addition to deficits in language comprehension and expression.

involves analysis of auditory input and recognition of speech sounds, occurs in the primary auditory cortex in the superior portion of the two temporal lobes. Heschl's gyrus, named after Richard L. Heschl (an Austrian anatomist who identified critical functions of the auditory area of the temporal lobe), is a small left temporal lobe region that appears to be specialized for processing speech, particularly its temporal (time) aspects. However, evidence from brain studies shows that at least some aspects of speech processing occur bilaterally in both the right and the left temporal lobes (Frackowiak et al., 2004). Bilateral damage to both the right and the left auditory cortices can result in *word deafness*, in which an individual has intact processing of nonword auditory stimuli, but cannot understand spoken words. However, word deafness does not necessarily occur following unilateral damage (even to the left temporal lobe); thus, speech processing appears to occur in both the right and the left temporal lobes (Frackowiak et al., 2004).

The left temporal lobe also contains Wernicke's area, sometimes called the receptive speech area, which is a critical site for language comprehension. Wernicke's area (named after German neurologist and psychiatrist, Karl Wernicke) is located in the superior portion of the left temporal lobe near the intersection of

The parietal lobe is important for working memory, the complex system that allows humans to keep information in mind while completing a task.

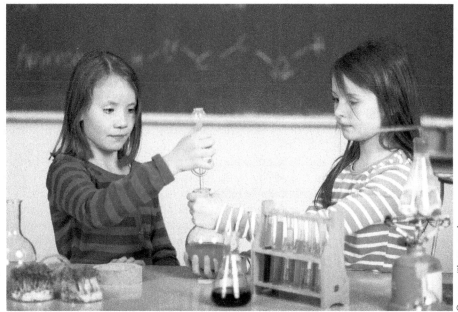

© racorn/Shutterstock

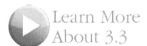

Learn More About 3.3

As you watch the video titled "Meet Your Master: Getting to Know Your Brain – Crash Course Psychology #4," consider the way in which brain function is localized and consider how this anatomical structuring can affect language production and processing. Furthermore, consider how different areas of the brain and different systems can influence each other and how this can impact the multiple aspects of communication. https://www.youtube.com/watch?v=vHrmiy4W9C0

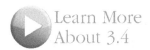

Learn More About 3.4

As you watch the video titled "Introduction to Brain Structure and Function," try to identify the locations in the brain for the major centers of language. https://www.youtube.com/watch?v=Ux_Dr5rvH3Y

the parietal, occipital, and temporal lobes. Consequently, its location is sometimes called the *parieto-occipitotemporal junction*.

Models of language circuitry identify Wernicke's area as a significant point of convergence for receiving and integrating associations from throughout the brain, including the prefrontal cortex, the sensory areas of the parietal lobes, the auditory-processing areas of the temporal lobe, and the visual-processing systems of the occipital lobe. This convergence is also important for language comprehension and production. For instance, language circuitry models detailing how a person sees an object and then names it, propose that visual images are conveyed to Wernicke's area, where the name of the image is generated and then transmitted to Broca's area in the frontal lobe. There, the speech output is organized and then coordinated into motor commands for the articulators (e.g., lips, tongue; Noback et al., 2005). When Wernicke's area is damaged by stroke or other brain injury, individuals typically exhibit significant difficulty with processing and producing coherent language in both spoken and written form. This condition is called *Wernicke's aphasia*. Although persons with Wernicke's aphasia may produce relatively fluent and intelligible speech, their spoken language may not make any sense because it contains a large number of idioms, revisions, errors, and jargon; for this reason, it is often called "jargon aphasia" (Schwartz, 2013). Here is an example of the response made by a person with Wernicke's aphasia when asked to look at a picture and describe what the girl in the picture is doing (Schwartz, 2013, p. 172):

"Anything. I mean she is a beautiful girl. And this is the same with her. And now it's coming there. Now what about here or anything like that."

As this example shows, this individual is speaking fluently but there is little about it that makes sense.

Brainstem

The brainstem sits directly on top of the spinal cord and serves as a conduit between the rest of the brain and the spinal cord. It consists of the midbrain, the pons, and the medulla oblongata, which together perform three primary functions (Noback et al., 2005). First, the brainstem is a key transmitter of sensory information to the brain and of motor information away from the brain. Second, the brainstem is a major relay station for the cranial nerves supplying the head and face, and for controlling the visual and auditory senses. Third, the brainstem structures and functions are associated with metabolism and arousal. Three major reflex centers are located in the brainstem: the cardiac center, which controls the heart; the vasomotor center, which controls the blood vessels; and the respiratory center, which controls breathing.

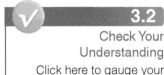

Cerebellum

The cerebellum is an oval-shaped "little brain" that resides posterior to the brainstem. The cerebellum is primarily responsible for regulating motor and muscular activity, and has little to do with the rational part of the brain that involves conscious planning and responses. The motor-monitoring functions of the cerebellum include coordinating motor movements, maintaining muscle tone, monitoring movement range and strength, and maintaining posture and equilibrium.

HOW DOES THE HUMAN BRAIN PROCESS AND PRODUCE LANGUAGE?

Current perspectives on the anatomical and physiological organization of the brain rely on connectionist models. Connectionist models attempt to represent the computational architecture of the brain as it processes various types of information, particularly that which is specific to higher-order human cognition (e.g., reasoning, problem solving). Although historical perspectives on the neuroanatomy and neurophysiology of the brain suggested that specific structures (e.g., Broca's area) were specialized to fulfill specific functions (e.g., motor planning for speech), current scientific knowledge of how the brain works contradicts strict modularity perspectives. Rather, the results of more recent brain research challenge perspectives that isolate highly specific brain functions to specific brain structures, showing that a given brain structure (or cortical area) can vary its functions according to the other cortical areas with which it is interacting (Frackowiak et al., 2004). At the same time, studies also show that specific brain structures can take on other functions in the event of injury (Kolb, 2013). An emergent current perspective of the brain is that is has a "dynamic functional architecture" that emerges over one's lifespan; brain functions are dynamic in that they emerge in response to experiences (both positive and negative, such as injuries) (Blumstein & Amso, 2013, p. 45).

In this regard, the structures of the brain are not necessarily hard-wired for a given role, as was long believed. Thus, most contemporary perspectives of how the brain works is that most higher-level cognitive functions, including that of language, involve numerous brain areas in their execution, several of which are identified in Figure 3.7.

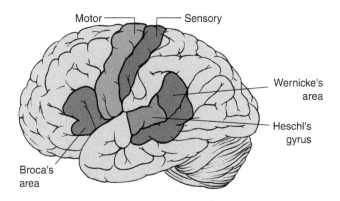

FIGURE 3.7
Areas of the brain involved with language and other functions.

Source: From *Communication Sciences and Disorders: A Contemporary Perspective* (2nd ed., p. 91) by L. M. Justice, 2010, Upper Saddle River, NJ: Pearson Education, Inc. Copyright 2010 by Pearson Education, Inc. Reprinted with permission.

In connectionist models, information processing within the brain (including language processing) is described as involving a network of distributed processors that interact with one another by means of excitatory and inhibitory connections (Kiefer & Pulvermüller, 2012). Connectionist models emphasize that the connectivity among units is critical to understanding how information is processed. Lieberman (1991) used the analogy of electrical power networks to discuss connectivity: "Through a complex interconnected network of generators and 'switching centers', the system adjusts and redirects power from other generators, and apportions output to different units" (p. 33). As Lieberman described, in electrical power networks (and other models based on connectionist principles), power is not located in a single, discrete location, but is distributed throughout an entire network.

In contrast to the current emphasis on connectionism as a means for understanding language processes in the brain, much of the historical literature on the neuroanatomy and neurophysiology of language emphasized the correspondences between specific language functions and specific brain structures. This emphasis was the result, at least in part, of scientists' inability to closely examine the brain while it is engaged in various language tasks. In the past, knowledge of brain structures and functions was based primarily on studies of what went wrong when a person's brain was damaged. Currently, because of technological advances, researchers have the tools to study exactly what happens in the brain when individuals engage in highly specific tasks, such as retrieving words corresponding to concrete or abstract labels. Although research results suggest that particular regions of the brain correspond to certain aspects of language processing or speech production, many basic language processes (e.g., word retrieval) are distributed throughout the sensory and motor cortices of the brain and are not confined to a single structure (Frackowiak et al., 2004). In the next sections, we briefly summarize the neuroanatomical and neurophysiological correlates of language processing for semantics, syntax and morphology, phonology, and pragmatics. The relevance of connectionist models to current representations of how language in each domain occurs in the human brain should be apparent.

Semantics

Semantics involves an individual's knowledge of words, or internal lexicon. A person's internal lexicon comprises thousands of words, varying in semantic features, or feature categories. For example, some words reference animate objects (e.g., *girl*), whereas others reference inanimate objects (e.g., *canoe*). Likewise, some words reference abstract concepts (e.g., *faith*), whereas others represent tangible concepts, such as size, color, and shape. Given the abundance of conceptual categories represented in a person's lexical store of words, you should not be surprised to learn that lexical knowledge is distributed across the brain. This fact has been substantiated by brain-mapping studies that identify the parts of the brain that activate when individuals engage in such tasks as retrieving newly learned words, or accessing words during a decision-making task (e.g., producing a verb in response to a noun stimulus). The aggregated results from numerous studies reveal the following three findings:

1. *Semantic knowledge is a distributed modality.* Word storage involves distributed neural networks transcending the frontal and temporal lobes, with some activation in the parietal lobes. The neural networks in the various lobes seem to serve different functions in semantic processing. The frontal lobe is involved with the executive elements of word knowledge (e.g., evaluation of semantic information), and the temporal lobe is involved with the storage and organization of semantic memories and categories (Bookheimer, 2002; Frackowiak et al., 2004).

2. *Semantic knowledge is left-lateralized* Semantic processing consistently activates left-hemisphere regions, particularly left inferior portions of the frontal lobe and regions across the entire left temporal lobe. At least one region of the left

temporal lobe, mapping to storage locations for semantic information, is larger than its companion site in the right hemisphere (Frackowiak et al., 2004).

   3.   *Some aspects of semantic knowledge involve right-hemisphere processing.* Although many aspects of semantic knowledge are left-lateralized functions, the right hemisphere also contributes to semantic processing, particularly the processing of figurative and abstract language. For instance, when processing an idiom (e.g., "He'll *bend over backward* to help you"), an individual must consider the connotative meaning of the phrase rather than the strict, literal meaning (Bookheimer, 2002). Processing idioms and other types of figurative language (e.g., metaphors, proverbs) activates right-hemisphere regions, including those that correspond anatomically to the left-hemisphere Broca's and Wernicke's areas (Bookheimer, 2002). Thus, although semantic knowledge is mostly a function of the left hemisphere, when processing involves a more holistic interpretation of meaning (rather than one-to-one mappings of words to meanings), the right hemisphere becomes involved.

Although brain-imaging studies add more precision to understanding of lexical organization and retrieval, current models of semantic processing are consistent with 19th-century neurological models (Frackowiak et al., 2004). Nineteenth-century models identified Wernicke's area in the left temporal lobe as a critical site for word recognition and lexical retrieval; these models further proposed that the left hemisphere was specialized for language processing. The left hemisphere and, more particularly, Wernicke's area remain an important locus for word storage, although advances also show semantic knowledge is more widely distributed across the left hemisphere than was previously understood.

Syntax and Morphology

An individual's ability to rapidly and automatically process the rules of syntax and morphology (morphosyntax) has long been viewed as something that is hard-wired in the brain, referred to as a *language instinct* (Pinker, 1994), or, alternatively, the *language acquisition device* (Chomsky, 1978). By many accounts, this uniquely human faculty is possible because of the genetically-based adaptation of the human brain for processing the universal grammar of language. As some experts contend, evolutionary history has equipped humans with an innate, species-specific ability to represent the discrete rule-governed syntactic rules of a universal grammar. This remarkable neurophysiological capacity explains young children's uncanny ability to rapidly and effortlessly acquire the small, finite set of morphosyntactic rules that ultimately allow them to produce and understand an infinite variety of sentences, regardless of the specific language they develop.

The possibility of a distinct morphosyntactic brain module is supported by at least three lines of research. First, studies of language learning in nonhuman primates revealed that other species can develop a reasonably sized lexicon, but that grammatical learning eludes them, a finding that supports the likelihood of a specialized neurophysiological module for morphosyntactic acquisition in the human brain (Aboitiz & Ricardo, 1997). Second, the likelihood of a specialized morphosyntactic processor is supported by study results showing specific impairments in morphosyntax as a function of focal brain damage, particularly in Broca's area (see Bookheimer, 2002). Individuals with damage to Broca's area can retain the ability to produce syntactically correct speech "automatisms" (or clichés; e.g., "Oh, my goodness!" "Good morning"), which suggests that well-rehearsed sentences and phrases are represented as whole units in the right hemisphere (Glezerman & Balkoski, 1999), whereas processing discrete morphosyntactic elements of language involves a specialized brain function in Broca's area.

   Third, the results of a number of studies of morphosyntactic processing showed increased activation of the language areas of the left hemisphere, notably Wernicke's area (for grammatical processing) and Broca's area (for formulating grammatically

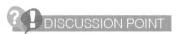

DISCUSSION POINT

Provide several additional examples of sentences with legal syntactic structures that are devoid of meaning.

ordered speech output), as well as the parietal lobes. Likewise, the results of studies involving attempts to isolate semantic processing from syntactic processing showed distinct neuroanatomical correlates for processing complex syntax; these correlates correspond to the inferior left frontal lobe in Broca's area (Bookheimer, 2002). This region appears to be specialized for not only processing the morphosyntactic elements of language, but also selectively attending to syntax, such as examining whether a sentence uses a "legal" syntactic structure even when the sentence is devoid of meaning (e.g., "Twas brillig, and the slithy toves . . ."; Friederici, Opitz, & von Cramon, 2000).

Nonetheless, researchers heartily disagree as to whether morphosyntactic processing should be represented as the function of a single domain-specific module, or by connectionist models that emphasize interactivity of various regions of the brain. Grammatical production and comprehension requires a person to combine fixed semantic representations into novel and complex representations of sentences; it also involves nonlinguistic symbolic and conceptual thought, as well as planning and reasoning (Glezerman & Balkoski, 1999). When individuals engage in complex linguistic tasks, left-hemisphere frontal, temporal, and parietal regions are activated, which shows an interaction of executive, semantic, and morphosyntactic processing (Bookheimer, 2002). In light of such evidence, morphosyntactic processing might best be conceived as a complex cognitive ability served by a variety of separate and specialized cortical areas transcending the right and left hemispheres. In evolutionary terms, a primitive human grammar may have once resided in a distinct language area of the brain (e.g., Broca's area). However, the higher-level complex grammar in modern-day language requires integration of the traditional language areas of the brain with other cognitive systems via complex interconnections of the parietal, temporal, and frontal lobes (Brennan & Pylkkänen, 2012).

Phonology

Processing speech sounds is qualitatively and quantitatively different from processing nonspeech sounds because speech comprises a series of overlapping, rapidly changing, and rapidly produced phonetic segments (Golumbic, Poeppel, & Schroeder, 2012). Whereas, the capacity of the human brain to process sequences of nonspeech sounds is fairly limited (about 7–9 units/second), speech processing occurs at much higher rates (50–60 units/second; Lieberman, 1991). Some experts contend that the human brain has evolved a specialized processor, sometimes called the phonetic module, designed specifically for processing the phonetic segments of speech (Liberman & Mattingly, 2014). Experts view this specialized processor as a "biologically coherent system, specialized from top to bottom" to process the phonetic segments of speech (Liberman, 2000, p. 115). The phonetic segments of spoken language are channeled through the human ears along the auditory pathway that culminates in the primary and secondary auditory cortices of the temporal lobe. Rapid analysis of the temporal characteristics of the speech sounds occurs in the auditory centers of the left temporal lobe, whereas the spectral characteristics of speech sounds are processed in the right temporal lobe. Therefore, both hemispheres seem to be involved in speech–sound processing, although the auditory regions of the left temporal lobe appear to be critical locations for phonetic analyses of speech sounds (Frackowiak et al., 2004).

Once speech sounds are phonetically analyzed, they must be processed as linguistic units, or phonemes. This level of processing, which occurs in Broca's area, is termed *phonological processing*; it involves analyzing phonological segments and working memory. Neuroimaging data confirm historical neuroanatomical models in which phonological processing and speech production are located at the site of Broca's area in the motor cortex of the left hemisphere. Nevertheless, Broca's area does not work alone to process and produce speech. Heschl's gyrus,

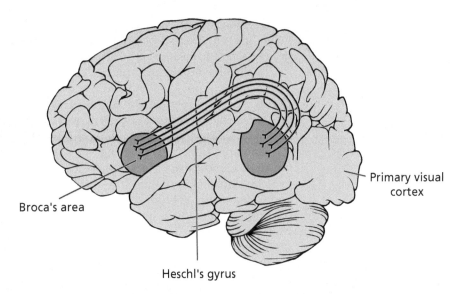

FIGURE 3.8

Anatomical connections among language areas of the brain.

Source: From *The Human Nervous System: Structure and Function* (6th ed., p. 450), by C. R. Noback, N. L. Strominger, R. J. Demarest, and D. A. Ruggiero, 2005, Totowa, NJ: Humana Press. Copyright 2005 by Humana Press, Inc. Reprinted with permission.

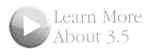

Learn More About 3.5

As you watch the video titled "Language and the Brain," be aware of how different areas of the brain (specifically Broca's and Wernicke's areas) contribute to forming, producing, and understanding language. Additionally, notice how functions differ depending on whether someone is receiving or producing a signal. https://www.youtube.com/watch?v=Yq7ozVixqDs

Wernicke's area, and Broca's area of the left hemisphere are connected by a series of anatomical pathways, even though they are anatomically remote, as shown in Figure 3.8 (Frackowiak et al., 2004). These interconnections support the interactions of processing mechanisms involved with auditory processing (Heschl's gyrus), language comprehension (Wernicke's area), and phonological processing (Broca's area). Recall from previous sections that Broca's area is also the site of sensorimotor encoding of phonological (speech) output, with efferent pathways to organize the controlled, voluntary production of speech sounds. The shared neurophysiology for both phonological processing and phonological production suggests that the motoric production of speech may play a role in phonological development (Bookheimer, 2002).

Although theoretical models of speech perception continue to emphasize the likelihood of a specialized phonetic module (likely corresponding to Broca's area), researchers have failed to identify a single structure or location in the brain specialized solely for speech processing. For instance, Broca's area activates for some nonlinguistic tasks, which suggests its functions are not dedicated solely to phonological processing or speech production. Thus, although the human brain has a specially designed phonological processor, this processor is not exclusive to this task, which casts "doubt on the concept of the language-specific [phonetic] processing module" (Bookheimer, 2002, p. 167).

Pragmatics

The pragmatics of language involves using language as a social tool. It concerns understanding the rules of communication, which include following conventions related to the quantity, quality, manner, and relevance of language during communication. Although the aspects of language discussed thus far involve a significant investment of the traditional language areas of the brain (e.g., Heschl's gyrus, Wernicke's area, Broca's area), pragmatic ability draws primarily on frontal lobe functions. In other words, an individual who sustains damage to the language areas of the brain that results in significant impairment of semantic, phonological, and morphosyntactic abilities may have fully intact pragmatic skills. Conversely, an individual with frontal lobe damage may have intact semantic, phonological, and morphosyntactic abilities, yet use language in odd and idiosyncratic ways.

As discussed previously, one major function of the frontal lobe is to control human executive functions, including reasoning, problem solving, planning, hypothesizing, social awareness, and rationalizing. These functions involve the organized, goal-directed, and controlled execution of critical human behaviors. Pragmatic abilities involve the organized, goal-directed, and controlled use of language as a means for communication with other people. Thus, when these more general executive functions are impaired, the social use of language is often undermined.

The results of brain-imaging studies indicate that many human executive functions involve not only the frontal lobe, but also other neurophysiological functions of the brain. For example, consider the case of willful attention. *Willful attention* is what people use to maintain attention to a given task when competing stimuli are present (Frackowiak et al., 2004). Your attention to reading this chapter likely involves some degree of willful attention if competing thoughts (e.g., thinking about an upcoming exam) or events in the environment (e.g., friends talking, music playing) exist. Both parietal and frontal lobe regions are involved in willful attention. Together, they impose a hierarchy of control over the competing forces for attention in that the parietal lobe is involved with processing incoming stimuli, whereas the frontal lobe forces attention to the particular stimulus selected for attention (e.g., the words you are reading; Frackowiak et al., 2004). Consider an individual whose frontal lobe functions are compromised, perhaps as a result of frontal lobe injury. During communication with another person (one competing force for attention), he or she may be distracted by other competing forces for attention (e.g., noises in the environment), which thus degrades his or her ability to sustain the communication topic. Therefore, the pragmatic aspects of language are compromised.

WHAT ARE NEUROPHYSIOLOGICAL AND NEUROANATOMICAL SENSITIVE PERIODS?

Thus far in this chapter, we have presented the brain as if it were a static neuroanatomical structure. This representation is far from the truth. As a human develops prenatally and postnatally, the brain undergoes significant changes as a result of experience. In short, our experiences change our brain over time. In this section, we consider the brain as a dynamic organ that changes during growth, dealing specifically with the concept of neurophysiological and neuroanatomical sensitive periods, with a particular focus on how these periods affect the capacity for language.

Sensitive Periods Defined

As applied to the development of the human brain, a sensitive period is a time frame of development during which a particular aspect of neuroanatomy or neurophysiology underlying a given sensory or motoric capacity undergoes growth or change. For instance, the results of a classic study showed that depriving kittens of visual input during the first 6 weeks of life resulted in permanent blindness, indicating this developmental time frame is a critical window of opportunity for visual development in kittens (Hubel & Wiesel, 1970). In a human analog, studies of birth defects in children born to pregnant women exposed to radiation in Nagasaki and Hiroshima during World War II showed brain damage (i.e., mental retardation, microcephaly) to be most serious when radiation exposure occurred between 56 and 105 days postovulation (Huttenlocher, 2002). This time frame corresponds to a period of significant prenatal growth in neuron numbers in the forebrain (Schull, 1998). Thus, at least for in utero humans, the period between 56 and 105 days

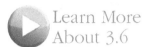

Learn More About 3.6

As you watch the video titled "Neurolinguistic Processing," pay special attention to the order in which language signals are processed in the brain. https://www.youtube.com/watch?v=wi5mQs7c56c

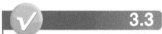

3.3
Check Your Understanding
Click here to gauge your understanding of the concepts in this section.

postovulation corresponds to a window of opportunity for supporting the child's neural development prenatally; it is also a time of significant risk.

As these examples show, sensitive periods have the following three features:

1.   Sensitive periods correspond to a time of active neuroanatomical and neurophysiological change. Other terms used to describe this time include critical period, window of opportunity, critical moment, and sensitive phase (Bruer, 2001). Although the term critical period is prevalent in the literature, it carries the connotation that changes occurring in a critical period are irreversible and permanent, which is often not the case. For instance, monkeys that experience visual deprivation during a visual critical period can regain nearly normal visual function with intense remediation (e.g., suturing closed the normal eye; Bruer, 2001). Therefore, many scientists prefer the term sensitive period, which carries the "window of opportunity" connotation, but allows that change is possible beyond the sensitive period (Bruer, 2001).

2.   *Sensitive periods are a phase not only of opportunity but also of risk.* Some experts identify critical periods as a phase in which "normal development is most sensitive to abnormal environmental conditions" (Bruer, 2001, p. 9). Studies of sensitive periods are important not only for improving researchers' fundamental understanding of human brain development, but also for identifying periods during which the brain is most vulnerable to risks. This knowledge is useful for prevention—for instance, ensuring that women prior to and in the several months following conception ingest adequate levels of folic acid to support the embryo's neural tube development. Sensitive periods therefore correspond to times in which an individual's developmental trajectory can be changed for better or for worse.

3.   Sensitive periods have a beginning and an end point, and the length of a period varies for different aspects of neuroanatomy and neurophysiology. In the previous example, the sensitive period for neural tube development in prenatal human embryos is about 32 days; thus, this period is one of significant risk to the developing embryo if neural tube development is compromised in some way, which occurs with inadequate folic acid consumption by the mother (Huttenlocher, 2002). In contrast, the sensitive period for language acquisition is much longer, perhaps as long as 12 years for the development of grammar.

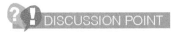

DISCUSSION POINT

Consider additional risks to prenatal development, such as maternal alcohol and tobacco use. For each risk you identify, consider what it might tell you about corresponding sensitive periods in prenatal development.

Neuroanatomical and Neurophysiological Concepts Related to Sensitive Periods

Synapses provide the means for neurons within the CNS to communicate, and the synaptic connections forged among neurons during development result in the complex neural circuitry that allows information processing in the human brain (Huttenlocher, 2002). Most synaptic connections do not arise randomly, nor are humans born with them already in place in the brain. Rather, synaptogenesis (the formation of synaptic connections) is driven by sensory and motoric experiences after birth and occurs most rapidly in the first year of life (Huttenlocher, 2002). At about the end of the first year, the infant's brain contains approximately twice as many synaptic connections as an adult's; from this time to adolescence, excess synapses are pruned, a process called synaptic pruning.

Neural plasticity is a term pertaining to the malleability of the CNS, and it relates primarily to the capacity of the sensory and motor systems to organize and reorganize themselves by generating new synaptic connections or by using existing synapses for alternative means. Consider that infants with significant left-hemisphere brain damage that destroys the language areas can achieve typical or near-typical language abilities by recruiting other neural functions to serve the purposes of language; neural plasticity accounts for this possibility (Huttenlocher, 2002). Older children and adults who sustain a similar type of brain damage often cannot achieve normal language in their lifetime, which suggests that brain plasticity varies with time. Hence, plasticity relates to sensitive periods because the plasticity of the brain for reorganizing itself and for resolving injury or damage to its neurophysiology and neuroanatomy varies during development.

Plasticity is often categorized into two types: experience-expectant plasticity and experience-dependent plasticity. These two types of plasticity differentiate the effects of the environment on changes in the brain (Lent & Tovar-Moll, 2015). Experience-expectant plasticity refers to the ongoing sculpting of brain structures that occur as a result of normal experiences. As the infant develops, multitudes of synapses are present in the brain, expectantly waiting for certain normal experiences to occur for them to organize themselves into functioning circuits. This type of plasticity uses the basic hardware that is provided to sculpt the brain as experiences amass. This type of plasticity develops "obligatory cortical functions" (Huttenlocher, 2002, p. 176) that organize basic sensorimotor neural systems, such as vision, hearing, and language. Most infants develop these experience-expectant functions because the basic stimuli needed to foster their development are present in the typical environment. Once the sensitive period for a given experience-expectant brain function has passed, though, environmental experiences no longer readily modify cortical circuits, possibly because few (if any) unspecified synapses remain. Acquisition of language grammar occurs as a function of experience-expectant plasticity.

In contrast with experience-expectant plasticity, experience-dependent plasticity is unique to a given individual; this type of functional brain modification requires highly specific types of experiences for change. This type of plasticity is what permits humans to "learn from our personal experience, and store information derived from that experience to use in later problem solving" (Bruer & Greenough, 2001, p. 212). Learning new information (whether it is novel information or information that must be relearned after brain injury) requires three mechanisms: the formation of new synaptic connections among neurons (dendritic sprouting), the generation of new neurons, and an increase in synaptic strength (Huttenlocher, 2002). Unlike experience-expectant plasticity, experience-dependent plasticity is a brain capacity available independent of age because, through time, the human brain retains most of its capacity to learn through experience and to adapt to change.

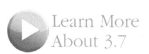

Learn More About 3.7

As you watch the video titled "The Growth of Knowledge: Crash Course Psychology #18," consider how language and communication concepts change as a child's cognitive abilities grow and mature. https://www.youtube.com/watch?v=8nz2dtv--ok

Sensitive Periods and Language Acquisition

You probably have some knowledge of how sensitive periods relate to language acquisition. For instance, if you attempted to learn a new language in high school and found it exceedingly difficult, you may have attributed the difficulty to your being past the "window of opportunity" for learning a new language. Moreover, you are likely aware of (or have even attended) an *immersion* preschool program, in which children are exposed to two or more languages (e.g., English and Spanish) simultaneously in an effort to take advantage of sensitive periods for language acquisition.

In this section, we consider the evidence on whether sensitive periods for language acquisition are a scientific reality, that is, whether humans have a relatively brief window of time in which to acquire language, beyond which language cannot be learned. In some respects, identifying sensitive periods for language acquisition is a scientific challenge because of the ethical impossibility of actively manipulating children's language-learning environments to study the effects of language deprivation at different points to identify such periods. Nonetheless, some "natural" experiments have occurred that help scientists identify sensitive periods for language acquisition by the brain.

Linguistic Isolation

Linguistic isolation occurs when a child develops with little or no exposure to a spoken or sign language. A few cases of "feral children" (children deprived of language exposure as a result of abuse and neglect) provide support for a sensitive period for language acquisition. The most notable case is that of Genie, an adolescent in California who was discovered by social workers after having been locked in a bedroom for her entire life and presumably beaten for her attempts to vocalize or communicate. Despite substantial language therapy in subsequent years, Genie never developed age-appropriate grammatical skills. However, the extent to which concomitant cognitive disabilities combined with years of neglect may have affected Genie's capacity for language cannot be determined; thus, her case provides inconclusive support for sensitive periods for language.

Evidence on sensitive periods for language acquisition is more conclusive in studies of children who are deaf who are not exposed to a language, whether spoken or sign (e.g., American Sign Language [ASL]), until sometime beyond infancy and toddlerhood. Newport and her colleagues examined ASL fluency for three groups of individuals who were deaf: those who learned ASL from birth, those who learned it between ages 4 and 6 years, and those who learned it after age 12 years. They found that age of ASL learning was associated with ASL fluency: Individuals who acquired ASL at birth exhibited nativelike language fluency, whereas those who acquired it later in life exhibited significant deficits in language ability, particularly in the area of grammar (see Newport, Bavelier, & Neville, 2001). Such evidence points to the period of birth through early adolescence as a sensitive period for language acquisition. Although language skills can be acquired after this period, many individuals are unlikely to acquire nativelike fluency.

There are, regrettably, also situations today in which children are reared in institutionalized environments in which they receive very little linguistic stimulation (van Ijzendoorn, Luijk, & Juffer, 2008). Children most typically left to institutionalized care are those who are born with a developmental disability that makes care for them difficult (e.g., blindness, cerebral palsy, Down syndrome), or creates a social stigma, when the parents do not have the financial or emotional resources to care for the child, or when the parents are deceased (as in cases of orphans with AIDS/HIV). Countries with high rates of poverty, and that experience traumatic events are particularly affected. In Haiti, for instance, it is estimated that there are more than 750,000 orphans since the major earthquake of 2010. Although the provision of institutionalized care for young children, whether in orphanages or foster homes, has long been a reality, the linguistic environments of some of these children may well constitute a type of linguistic isolation. This stems from cultural patterns of care within institutionalized settings (in which adult–child conversation seldom occurs), but is also due to discontinuity in care, in which a child may receive care from up to 50 different caregivers in a 24-hour period and have little opportunity to form stable attachments (Vorria et al., 2003).

Second Language Learners

One interesting approach to estimating sensitive periods for language acquisition is to compare the language abilities of groups of individuals who learned a second language at different times of life. Flege and colleagues conducted such an investigation (Flege, Yeni-Komshian, & Liu, 1999) by examining two aspects of language skill among Koreans who varied in their age of arrival (AOA) to the United States: phonology (specifically, the extent to which they exhibited a foreign accent) and grammar (that is, skills in applying syntactic rules). Interestingly, accents seemed to be governed by a sensitive period, in that later AOAs were associated with stronger foreign accents. On the other hand, this was not the case for syntax. AOA was less strongly associated with English syntactic skill than other variables, such as one's use of English and one's amount of education in the United States. The authors suggest that experience using one's second language, as well as educational experience are more important to second language acquisition than constraints imposed by a sensitive period.

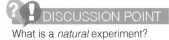

DISCUSSION POINT

What is a *natural* experiment? How are natural experiments different from "true" experiments?

THEORY TO PRACTICE

Sensitive Periods and Early Intervention

Children exhibit tremendous growth in their language abilities in the first several years of development. This period largely coincides with the explosion of synaptogenesis within the cerebral cortex, which begins in the weeks just prior to birth (during the third prenatal trimester) and then declines around the third birthday. In this so-called sensitive period of development, children exhibit the greatest ease in acquiring language. As discussed in Chapter 2, children examine the child-directed speech (CDS) that occurs around them to develop their lexicon, grammar, and phonology and to learn how language is used pragmatically as a social tool within their cultural community. However, after the third birthday, synapses that were not formed begin to be eliminated through the process of synaptic pruning. Consequently, children's ability to acquire language also declines as their brains become less plastic.

What does the notion of sensitive period mean to the practice of early intervention? Early intervention is the implementation of practices and programs to enhance the early development of children experiencing risk. This risk may be *environmental*, such as being reared in extreme poverty, or it may be *developmental*, such as having a profound hearing loss. Regardless, the sensitive period implies that intervention should be implemented as early as possible so it coincides with the explosion of synaptogenesis within the developing brain. Theoretically, early intervention implemented intensively in the first few years of life will

capitalize upon the natural advantages that synaptogenesis affords and therefore will be more effective.

Scientists have tested whether this is indeed the case when applied to early intervention practices. In the Bucharest Early Intervention Project (Nelson et al., 2007), which we discussed in Chapter 1, scientists tested the hypothesis that early intervention implemented earlier in children's lives has greater impacts on children's language and cognitive abilities as compared to intervention offered later. In this study, 136 abandoned children residing in Romanian orphanages were randomly assigned to either stay in institutionalized care (68 children) or be moved into foster homes. For the latter group, the age of placement occurred at different times: from birth to 18 months (14 children), between 18 and 24 months (14 children), between 24 and 30 months (22 children), or after 30 months (9 children). When the children were 42 and 54 months of age, the scientists assessed their language and cognitive abilities and found that children placed in foster homes earliest received significantly higher scores than those placed in foster homes later. In general, placement prior to 2 years of age seemed to provide the greatest developmental advantage (a difference of about 10 IQ points), a finding consistent with what we might expect based on development of the cerebral cortex. This study provides exceedingly strong evidence of the importance of early intervention as a means for mitigating early risks to development of language and cognition.

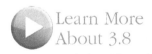

Learn More About 3.8

As you watch the video titled "Transfer in Child L2 Acquisition," recognize the differences in language production that are dependent on when an L2 is acquired and how production of a language can differ between children and adults.
https://www.youtube.com/watch?v=MgTEpTJiREA

Other studies, including those on the language development of children who must acquire a new language (and lose their first) following a foreign-birth adoption, have also failed to identify a sensitive period for language acquisition, relative to learning a second language. In fact, these studies have shown that "even by 7 or 8 years of age, plasticity in language areas is still sufficiently high to promote an essentially complete recovery of normal language" (Pallier et al., 2003, p. 159). Thus, although young children unequivocally exhibit a unique propensity for learning language, and although the capacity of the brain for rapid language acquisition slows with time, a growing number of scientists argue that "the view of a biologically constrained and specialized language acquisition device that is turned off at puberty is not correct" (Hakuta, 2001, p. 204). See Language Diversity and Differences: *International Adoption and Language Acquisition* for a discussion of foreign-birth adoption and sensitive periods.

Plasticity and Language

Evidence on sensitive periods for language acquisition suggests that researchers must consider both experience-expectant and experience-dependent plasticity

LANGUAGE DIVERSITY AND DIFFERENCES

Foreign-birth adoptions in the United States—an estimated 7,000 such cases occurred in 2013 (U.S. Department of State, 2014)—provides an important avenue for scientists to explore the possibility of identifying sensitive periods for language acquisition. In a foreign-birth adoption, a child is adopted from overseas, often from an institution. In the United States, most foreign-birth adoptions are from China, Ethiopia, Russia, South Korea, and Ukraine (U.S. Department of State, 2014). In addition to the developmental challenges children experience during institutionalized care, in which they may have relatively little contact with adults and thus few experiences with healthy attachment and language–cognitive stimulation, these children often come from countries plagued by limited prenatal care and maternal exposure to infectious diseases (Glennen, 2015). Although the risks these children encounter early in life are substantial, the results of studies of outcomes for foreign adoptees suggest that many will achieve healthy developmental outcomes in cognitive and physical achievements (Glennen, 2015).

In this chapter, we discuss the concept of experience-expectant brain plasticity. In contrast with experience-dependent plasticity, experience-expectant plasticity is the developmental mechanism of the brain for achieving basic processes, including language, in relatively short time periods. Experts have failed to identify a specific end point for the sensitive period for language acquisition, which would presumably correspond to a loss of experience-expectant plasticity. Nevertheless, this sensitive period extends from at least birth to age 5 years, if not beyond, and during this period the brain exhibits an amazing capacity to make amends for early delays in language, as shown by studies of foreign-birth adoptees.

Studies of children adopted from Eastern European orphanages into homes within the United States reveal that most of these children exhibit early and significant lags in language development, corresponding to their apparently limited exposure to language stimulation during their period of institutionalized care (Glennen & Masters, 2002). However, when these children are followed over time, studies tend to show that their skills in their second language eventually become in line with typical non-adopted children. Glennen (2015) has followed 44 children who were adopted from Russia, Kazakhstan, Hungary, and Romania into American homes. All had lived in institutionalized care for at least one year prior to being adopted. At ages 5 to 7 years, the children were given a battery of language assessments; as a group, the children had language skills in the average range across multiple measures of vocabulary, syntax, and morphology. What's particularly remarkable about these children's performance on language assessments in the early primary grades is that a larger percentage of children than would be expected scored in the *above average* range on these measures. For instance, on a grammar test, nearly 25% of children scored in the above average range; normative references would suggest that 16% of children would score in this range. Among this group of international adoptees, a large proportion of children had superior language skills than would be expected! To understand this phenomenon, it is important to point out that children who are adopted internationally tend to be adopted into homes that are quite advantaged. Parents who adopt children internationally tend to be financially well off and highly motivated towards parenting. Consequently, the language advantages for international adoptees may, in part, reflect their arrival to highly stimulating language-learning environments. Nonetheless, data such as these reveal the experience-expectant plasticity of the brain for acquiring language during the sensitive period, even when it has a late start.

✓ 3.4

Check Your Understanding

Click here to gauge your understanding of the concepts in this section.

to understand the capabilities of the brain for language during the life span. Whereas experience-expectant plasticity provides the immature brain with capacities well beyond those evident as people age, experience-dependent plasticity provides the human brain—even at advanced ages—with the capacity to grow and adapt not only to new experiences, but also to illness, disease, and injury to the brain. Although some development periods correspond to time frames in which language learning is easiest (particularly infancy through early adolescence), researchers' inability to identify a putative end point to the sensitive period for language acquisition likely reflects the experience-dependent abilities of the human brain to adapt and modify itself in response to the environment.

SUMMARY

Language, a complex and distinctly human behavior, resides in the neuroanatomical and neurophysiological architecture of the human brain. *Neuroscience* is a branch of science that focuses on the anatomy and physiology of the nervous system, described respectively as *neuroanatomy* and *neurophysiology*. The human nervous system includes the *central nervous system* (comprising the brain and the spinal cord) and the *peripheral nervous system* (comprising the cranial and spinal nerves, which carry information inward to and outward from the brain and the spinal cord). The billions of highly specialized cells that compose the nervous system are *neurons*. A neuron is functionally divided into four components: *cell body, axon, presynaptic terminal*, and *dendrites*. The cell body is the center of the neuron, containing its nucleus. The axon and the dendrites are extensions from the cell body. The axon transmits information away from the cell body; *the presynaptic terminals* of the axon are the sites at which the axonal connection of one neuron corresponds with another neuron. Dendrites are the afferent extensions of a neuron, bringing nerve impulses into the cell body from the axonal projections of other neurons. The *synapse* is the site where two neurons meet. For two neurons to communicate, the nerve impulse must cross the synapse.

The brain, which contains more neurons than any other organ in the human body, consists of two mirror-image hemispheres. Aptly named, the *right hemisphere* and the *left hemisphere* are separated by a long cerebral crevice (or fissure) called the *longitudinal fissure*. The *corpus callosum* is a band of fibers that connects the two hemispheres, serving as a conduit for communication between the hemispheres. The brain is further divided into six lobes: one frontal lobe, one occipital lobe, two temporal lobes, and two parietal lobes. Each lobe has functional specializations. The frontal lobe is the site of complex executive behaviors (e.g., reasoning, planning, problem solving), and contains in its left hemisphere an important site for speech production and phonological processing: Broca's area. The occipital lobe is the site of visual perception and processing. The two parietal lobes are the site for not only perceiving and integrating sensory and perceptual information, but also comprehending oral and written language and performing mathematical calculations. The two temporal lobes contain sites critical to auditory processing, as well as language comprehension; language is lateralized to the left hemisphere in Wernicke's area.

Many theorists have argued that the brain exhibits a sensitive period for language acquisition because the *experience-expectant brain plasticity* used in language development is available for a relatively short duration. In contrast, *experience-dependent plasticity* is the ability of the brain to adapt itself to new information with time. Some evidence—including that attained from studies of feral children, children who are deaf, and second language learners—suggests that birth to early adolescence is a sensitive period for language acquisition. Nevertheless, researchers have not yet been able to identify a putative end point for this sensitive period, probably because the experience-dependent plasticity of the brain endures (more or less) throughout life. Thus, although infants, toddlers, and young children acquire language remarkably easily, the capacity to learn language (or relearn language following brain damage) is present for the entire human life span.

 Apply Your Knowledge

Click here to apply your knowledge to practical scenarios.

BEYOND THE BOOK

1. There are a number of commercial programs on the Internet that claim to boost brain functioning, including computer games and even vitamins. Search the Internet to find a few such examples. How convincing are the claims for each of the commercial programs that the brain will actually improve?

2. International adoption rates have decreased in the last few years in the United States. Explore patterns of international adoption to see why rates increase and decrease with time.

3. A classic study by Hubel and Wiesel in 1970 involving kittens was instrumental in improving our understanding of neural plasticity. What can you find out about this study? How was the research conducted, and what did it tell us about the brain's plasticity? In your opinion, is this work worthy of the Nobel Prize the authors received?

4. The frontal lobe is responsible for executive functions. In small groups, discuss the notion of *executive functions* and identify specific activities in which one draws upon these functions in daily life.

5. The Bucharest Early Intervention Project involved the random assignment of children to remain in institutionalized care or to be placed in foster care. Discuss the ethical issues of research of this type and why, in your opinion, random assignment of children to such conditions is appropriate or not.

 Check Your Understanding

Gauge your understanding of the chapter concepts by taking this self-check quiz.

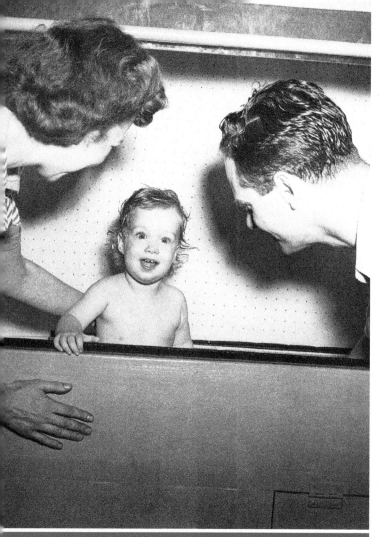

Psychologist and Behaviorist, B.F. Skinner (pictured with his wife and his daughter, Deborah), invented a baby tender – a temperature- and humidity-controlled box with a door and glass window front that was designed to keep babies warm and comfortable, without the use of excess clothing or blankets. Skinner's invention aimed to reduce a mother's laundry load, and to keep babies clean, comfortable, and free from excess household noise during the first few years of life.

4

The Science and Theory of Language Development

LEARNING OUTCOMES

After completion of this chapter, the reader will be able to:

1. Explain who studies language development and why.

2. Describe some major approaches to studying language development.

3. Compare and contrast some major language-development theories.

4. Explain how language-development theories influence practice.

In this chapter, we introduce the theory and science of language development. Theory refers to descriptive statements or principles devised to explain a group of facts or phenomena. In essence, a theory is a claim or hypothesis that may be tested repeatedly with an array of scientific methods; when the accumulated evidence consistently supports a given theory throughout time, it becomes an accepted part of the knowledge base in a particular discipline, and we can then use the theory to make predictions about natural phenomena. In the area of language development, theories provide explanations for how and why children develop their capacity for language across the different domains. For example, one language-development theory we discuss later in this chapter suggests that children's environments (rather than genetics or innate abilities) influence their language achievements.

Theory and science complement each other in intricate ways. Science is the process of generating and testing theories and can be considered the "final court of appeal for the viability of a scientific hypothesis or conjecture" (Shavelson & Towne, 2002, p. 3). Researchers who study language development use the scientific method to examine the adequacy of theories about how and why language develops and to generate new theories. Ultimately, the goal of science is to generate "cumulative knowledge by building on, refining, and occasionally replacing, theoretical understanding" (Shavelson & Towne, 2002, p. 3). Therefore, theories provide the foundation for scientific studies, and the outcomes of scientific studies help experts refine and even replace their theories with time. All the concepts and understandings we present in this textbook are based on the accumulated theoretical and scientific knowledge of language-development scholars.

After reading the preceding paragraphs, you might be wondering why it is important to learn about the science and theory of language development or even, more generally, why one should study language development at all. For starters, because language use is an ability unique to humans, knowing more about language development helps to satisfy the curiosity about what it means to be human. Practically speaking, studying language development is helpful to students pursuing a variety of specializations and career paths. For example, those considering a career in education will benefit from an understanding about such issues as how phonological awareness (awareness of the sound structure of language) contributes to children's later reading skills. Students considering a career in speech–language pathology will benefit from understanding about typical language milestones and the range of normal individual variation in achieving those milestones. (Future parents will likely benefit from an understanding of these areas as well.) Those considering a profession in neuroscience will benefit from understanding about brain processes that contribute to the production and comprehension of language.

No matter which career field you ultimately pursue, it will be important to learn about the specific practices the field endorses and uses. Currently, many fields, including those mentioned in the previous paragraph, emphasize the use of evidence-based practice (EBP). EBP involves integrating theoretical knowledge with scientific inquiry (which may include reviewing existing scientific literature) to inform decision-making. It is thus important that practitioners in a variety of areas understand why their particular field engages in certain practices (and avoids others); science and theory are important foundations for EBPs, and for this reason, this chapter presents an overview of the theories that provide a foundation for the scientific studies that inform practice in the area of language development.

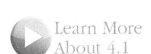

Learn More About 4.1

As you watch the video titled "What is a Scientific Theory?" consider how theory and science complement one another and think about why they are so important to studying language development. https://www.youtube.com/watch?v=3vKJMFta6v1

WHO STUDIES LANGUAGE DEVELOPMENT AND WHY?

Language has fascinated people for thousands of years. The ancient philosophers Plato and Aristotle questioned the relationships among language, thought, and reality, whereas early linguists such as Dionysius Thrax studied the form

TABLE 4.1

Scientific disciplines, major foci, and research questions about language development

DISCIPLINE	MAJOR FOCUS	SAMPLE RESEARCH QUESTIONS
(Developmental) psychology	Human mind and behavior and the changes that occur in humans as they age	To what extent do individuals experience word naming challenges as they age? (Verhaegen & Poncelet, 2013)
Linguistics	Aspects of human language, including phonetics, phonology, morphology, syntax, and semantics	How do the phonological features of one's native language affect the perception of phonemes in nonnative languages? (Pajak & Levy, 2014)
Psycholinguistics	Psychological and neurobiological factors that enable humans to acquire, use, and understand language	To what extent can electrophysiological studies reveal how infant phonetic representations develop into adult representations? (C. Phillips, 2001)
(Linguistic) anthropology	Relationship between language and culture; social use of language; language variation across time and space	How does the way in which a person expresses information verbally relate to how they encode information in gesture? (Kita & Özyürek, 2003)
Speech–language pathology	Prevention, diagnosis, and treatment of speech and language disorders	To what extent does evidence support the use of commercially available tests of child language for identifying language impairment in children? (Spaulding, Plante, & Farinella, 2006)
Education	Aspects of teaching and learning	To what extent does comprehensive language and literacy intervention promote language and literacy development in preschool children? (Wasik, Bond, & Hindman, 2006)
Sociology	Aspects of society such as cultural norms, expectations, and contexts	In what ways does the presence of an interpreter contribute to communication patterns between a physician and a patient? (Aranguri, Davisdon, & Ramirez, 2006)

and structure of language. In the 21st century, experts continue to ponder and investigate many of these same issues as they work to expand and refine the theoretical understanding of language development, and to seek answers to practical questions about how to support children's early and later language achievements.

Scientists who conduct language-development research are from many disciplines, including psychology, linguistics, psycholinguistics, anthropology, speech–language pathology, education, and sociology. Each discipline has a different major focus and different research questions with respect to language development (see Table 4.1 for some examples). However, because many disciplines include specializations in language, identifying a one-to-one correspondence between specific areas of study and a given discipline is difficult. For example, researchers in each of the previously listed disciplines might have an interest in investigating the relationship between parental language use and children's language growth. Scientists in all of these disciplines, as well as others, are making important improvements to existing language-development theories.

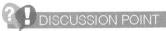 DISCUSSION POINT

Why are you studying language development? How might knowing about language development help you in your career?

People study language development for many reasons. Some do so to further basic understanding about language as a human phenomenon. This type of research is called *theoretical research*, or basic research: It focuses primarily on generating and refining the existing knowledge base. Other people do so to address specific problems in society and to inform practices relevant to language development. This type of research is called applied research: People typically conduct applied research to test different approaches and practices that pertain to real-world settings. Basic and applied research provide important complementary contributions to the study of language development, and many language scientists conduct both types of research.

Basic Research

Many language-development scholars conduct basic research, the outcomes of which advance fundamental understanding of human learning and development. In this type of research, experts develop, test, and refine theories about language development. When the outcomes of basic research consistently confirm a theory, the theory becomes an accepted explanatory principle—akin to knowledge.

Scientists who conduct basic research on language development do so primarily to improve understanding of this particular phenomenon. Basic research topics in language development include the ways children learn the meanings of words, the order in which children acquire the grammatical structures of their native language, and the ages by which children typically produce speech sounds. One example of basic research is a study by Saylor and Sabbagh (2004), which investigated how children learn new words. These researchers studied how children coordinate different types of information present in the environment to facilitate learning new words. Basic research in language development, such as Saylor and Sabbagh's work, not only helps build a knowledge base concerning how children develop their language abilities, but also provides an important foundation for applied research, which we discuss in the next section of this chapter. See Language Diversity and Differences: *Dialect Discrimination* for an example of basic research that uncovers how individuals may face discrimination on the basis of the English dialect they speak.

LANGUAGE DIVERSITY AND DIFFERENCES

Dialect Discrimination

One important avenue for basic research in the area of sociolinguistics concerns the investigation of differential treatment of persons because of their language or dialect. In a series of four experiments, Purnell, Idsardi, and Baugh (1999) identified relations between speech characteristics and housing discrimination. In this study, a tridialectal experimenter—using Standard American English (SAE), African American Vernacular English (AAVE), and Chicano English (ChE)—placed telephone calls to make appointments to discuss apartments for rent in five geographic areas. Results showed that the experimenter secured appointments between 60% and 70% of the time in all regions when he used the SAE dialect. However, when he used the AAVE and ChE dialects, his success rates were significantly lower. Furthermore, the experimenter's success rate when he used the AAVE and ChE dialects was related to the local population composition. For example, in a geographic area with a 95% White population, the experimenter confirmed 70% of his appointments by using SAE and only 29% and 22% of his appointments by using AAVE and ChE, respectively. Results of other experiments in this study verified that average listeners can discriminate among dialects with as little information as a single word. The results of this study provide compelling evidence that discrimination against individuals on the basis of speech characteristics and in the absence of visual cues is a valid concern in the housing market, and it may occur in other social arenas as well.

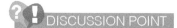
DISCUSSION POINT

What other legal or civil rights
issues may benefit from sociolinguistic research? How might researchers systematically test the
questions you raise?

Although much basic research focuses specifically on developing, testing, and refining theories, one type concentrates on building connections between theory and practice. This kind of research, called use-inspired basic research, addresses useful applications of research findings (Stokes, 1997). For example, use-inspired basic research in language development might explore how and when children acquire particular language abilities to inform interventions for children lagging in language growth. As a specific example of use-inspired basic research, Charity, Scarborough, and Griffin (2004) studied the language skills of African American children ages 5–8 and considered how children's familiarity with the English dialect used in their school (School English) contributed to their success in reading. Researchers found that children who were more familiar with School English performed better on measures of reading achievement than children who were less familiar with School English. Theoretically, the findings of this study are informative to understanding the relationship between spoken dialects and reading development. Moreover, these findings have some useful applications to practice by suggesting the need to design and study programs that promote children's familiarity with the school dialect to determine whether such familiarity improves their reading achievement.

Applied Research

More than 200 years ago, philosopher Jean-Jacques Rousseau (1712–1778) offered the following advice to parents about speaking to their children: "Always speak correctly before them, arrange that they enjoy themselves with no one as much as with you, and be sure that imperceptibly their language will be purified on the model of yours without your ever having chided them" (A. Bloom, 1979, p. 71).

Assuredly, Rousseau's practical advice was based on then-current language-development theories, particularly the influence of language models on children's language acquisition. Just as theories must be tested and refined to build a knowledge

Jean-Jacques Rousseau's theory of language development emphasized the role of the environment, especially the language input parents provide to children.

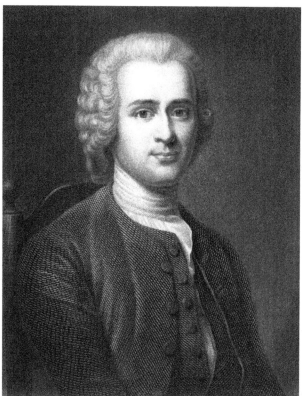

© Georgios Kollidas/Alamy

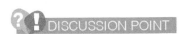

DISCUSSION POINT

Applied research focuses on responding to specific societal needs. What are some additional societal needs that might involve the study of language development?

base, specific practices require direct testing by science. Applied research contributes to specific societal needs by testing the viability of certain practices and approaches (Stokes, 1997). It typically involves using experimental research designs to examine the causal relationship between a specific approach, program, or practice and a specific language outcome.

The results of applied research are important for various reasons. As we discussed in Chapter 1, language is a critical tool that members of all world societies use to establish relationships with other people and to negotiate needs and wants. In many societies, language is an essential tool for learning in academic contexts at all levels, from early childhood through adulthood. Persons with poor language skills risk not achieving their full academic potential. In most societies, language is also a tool used in many employment contexts, and persons with poor language skills may face challenges to obtaining and maintaining gainful employment. Scientists who study language development for applied purposes respond to such societal needs by determining why some individuals progress relatively slowly in language development. They do so in two ways: by learning how to identify persons at risk for or exhibiting disordered language development, and by developing ways to remediate delays and disorders in language when they do occur. The consumers of such research include, among others, teachers, psychologists, pediatricians, special educators, child care providers, social workers, physicians, speech–language pathologists, and teachers of English as a second, or foreign, language.

Scientists who conduct applied research on language development are from the same disciplines as scientists who conduct basic language research. Applied researchers usually test language-development practices relevant to three main contexts: homes, clinical settings, and schools. In studies of the home environment, researchers examine the effectiveness of specific practices or approaches parents can use to help their children develop language during home activities. For instance, applied researchers may study whether a specific style of parent–child book reading improves children's vocabulary more or less than a different style does (e.g., Whitehurst et al., 1988), or whether parents who view a training video subsequently engage in significantly different reading interactions with their children compared to parents who do not view the training video (Blom-Hoffman, O'Neil-Pirozzi, Volpe, Cutting, & Bissinger, 2007). In studies of the clinical environment, applied researchers examine the effectiveness of different approaches that clinical professionals, such as speech–language pathologists and clinical psychologists, may use with specific populations of patients. For instance, Thompson, Shapiro, Kiran, and Sobecks (2003) studied the effectiveness of different approaches for improving the sentence comprehension of adults with language disorders due to stroke. In studies of the school environment, applied researchers examine the effectiveness of different approaches that educators may use in the classroom to build children's language skills. For example, Throneburg, Calvert, Sturm, Paramboukas, and Paul (2000) revealed elementary-grade students with language impairment learned more vocabulary words during lessons team-taught by a speech–language pathologist and a classroom teacher than during lessons delivered in a "speech room" by only the speech–language pathologist. As all these examples show applied research provides particularly valuable information for parents and professionals with a vested interest in ensuring the language achievements of children, adolescents, and adults.

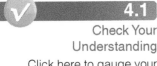

4.1

Check Your Understanding

Click here to gauge your understanding of the concepts in this section.

WHAT ARE SOME MAJOR APPROACHES TO STUDYING LANGUAGE DEVELOPMENT?

In the previous sections, we discussed why persons in a range of disciplines study language development. We also emphasized the integrative relationship between theory and science, as well as how people generate language-development theories and refine them through both basic and applied research. In this section, we discuss a sample of approaches scientists use to study three aspects of language development: speech perception, language production, and language comprehension. In Chapters 5–8, which address major achievements in language development during the infant, toddler, preschool, and school-age years and beyond, respectively, we describe these approaches in more detail.

Approaches to Studying Speech Perception

Goal of Speech Perception Studies

When infants enter the world, they bring with them a keen capacity to attend to speech and other auditory stimuli in the world around them. In Chapter 5, we discuss some theories on how infants begin to parse the speech stream to begin to learn the sounds and words of their native language. *Speech perception* studies help researchers learn about how children use their speech perception to draw information from and ultimately learn language.

Methods for Studying Speech Perception

The study of speech perception has improved dramatically during the past few decades as a result of a range of technological advances, one of which is digitization. Researchers who study speech perception typically present auditory stimuli to participants and measure their response to the stimuli. With digital technologies, researchers have an important tool for preserving media, for ensuring high-quality presentations of auditory stimuli, and for allowing fine manipulation of the stimuli. Using specially developed computer software, speech perception researchers can record a specific speech sound and carefully manipulate it into a series of fine-grained variants to determine how much auditory information an individual needs to hear to recognize the sound. Researchers examining speech perception in infants frequently use digital media to manipulate the speech stream. For instance, Saffran, Aslin, and Newport (1996) developed digitized sequences of made-up three-syllable words to reveal 8-month-old infants are able to detect statistical patterns in running speech and thereby, segment words from the speech stream.

In addition to benefiting from digital technologies, researchers who study speech perception in very young children have profited from another cutting-edge technology. While infants are still in the womb, scientists can measure their heart rates and kicking rates as a response to different auditory stimuli and examine, for example, the extent to which infants differentiate speech sounds from non-speech sounds (Karmiloff & Karmiloff-Smith, 2001). Although studies of prenatal speech perception are relatively new, a long, rich history of infant speech perception research has substantially improved our general understanding of speech perception development (see Galle & McMurray, 2014 and see Gerken & Aslin, 2005 for a review of 40 years and 30 years of research on infant speech perception studies, respectively). Research Paradigms: *Psycholinguistics and the Head-Turn Preference Procedure* provides a description of one type of speech perception study, the *head-turn preference procedure*, and in Chapter 5, we describe another type of speech perception study, the *high-amplitude nonnutritive sucking (HAS) procedure*. Researchers using these procedures take advantage of natural human reflexes (orientation to sound in the case of the *head-turn preference procedure* and sucking in the case of the HAS procedure) to learn about how people perceive speech.

Speech perception researchers have also long relied on behavioral testing, in which children or adults respond by speaking, pointing, or pressing buttons in response to different speech stimuli. An important complement to behavioral testing is brain-imaging technologies, such as magnetic resonance imaging (MRI), functional magnetic resonance imaging (fMRI), electroencephalography (EEG), magnetoencephalography (MEG), the event-related potential (ERP) technique, and optical topography (OT). These technologies allow researchers to conduct direct, real-time investigations of speech perception by presenting individuals with specific speech sounds and identifying the exact areas of the brain where speech perception occurs. Researchers can then develop *tonotopic maps* that link the brain areas to the types of auditory stimuli they process (Fitch, Miller, & Tallal, 1997).

Approaches to Studying Language Production
Goal of Language Production Studies

Language production studies help inform practitioners of children's ability to use language expressively. In these studies, researchers examine children's emergent form, content, and use capabilities. Such studies may involve normative research, in which experts compile data from multiple individuals on a certain aspect of language development and from these data determine and chart the ages (or grades) by which children typically meet certain milestones. For example, Justice et al. (2006) published descriptive data on the narrative productions of kindergartners through sixth graders, providing the average number of words and the average length of utterances for children's fictional stories at each grade level. Normative data such as these are useful for many professionals who need to know children's typical language production skills at a given age or grade.

One of the most well-known normative studies of early language production was used to develop a communication development checklist: the MacArthur–Bates Communicative Development Inventories (CDI; formerly the MacArthur Communicative Development Inventories). Dale and Fenson (1996) gathered language production information from more than 1,800 infants and toddlers, and from it developed the CDI. Parents, educators, and clinicians consult the CDI norms to determine how many words typically developing children understand and produce at various ages. Subsequent research has examined the validity of the CDI

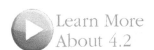

Learn More About 4.2

Watch the video titled "Head-Turn Preference Procedure" (see 5:21–9:09 of the video) to learn how researchers conduct the Head-Turn Preference Procedure to study speech perception. This video also demonstrates the High Amplitude Sucking Procedure (0:00–5:21) and the Preferential Looking Procedure (9:09–12:19), which we discuss in subsequent chapters. https://www.youtube.com/watch?v=EFlxiflDk_o

---

🔍 RESEARCH **PARADIGMS**

Psycholinguistics and the Head-Turn Preference Procedure

Psycholinguistics is a field that lies at the intersection of psychology and linguistics. Psychologists who study language aim to uncover how humans learn and use language, whereas linguists aim to learn more about language form (syntax, phonology, morphology) and content (semantics).

One research paradigm psycholinguists use to investigate speech perception is the *head-turn preference procedure,* which takes place in a three-sided booth. On the front wall of the booth are a green light and a hole through which the researcher can view the inside of the booth. The left and right sides of the booth each contain a single red light with an audio speaker behind each light. An infant sits on a caregiver's lap in the center of the booth.

The experiment begins when the researcher flashes one or the other red light in the booth to attract the infant's attention. Once the infant is attending, a sound stimulus begins to play through the speaker and continues to play until the infant looks away for a specified amount of time (e.g., 2 seconds). This sequence of events continues as the infant listens to different stimuli on the right side and left side of the booth. Because the infant controls the length of time he or she listens to the audio stimuli, researchers conclude that a preference for one of the two sounds indicates the infant can distinguish between the two sounds. The head-turn preference procedure has revealed that infants learning English prefer the stress patterns of the English language to other stress patterns (Jusczyk, Cutler, & Redanz, 1993), can segment familiar words from passages of speech (Jusczyk & Aslin, 1995), and are sensitive to the phonotactics (acceptable combinations of sounds) of their native language (Mattys, Jusczyk, Luce, & Morgan, 1999). See Kemler Nelson et al. (1995) for a thorough description of this research method.

? ! DISCUSSION POINT

Scholars generally use the head-turn preference procedure to answer basic research questions. Can you think of any use-inspired basic research questions about language development this procedure might help answer?

for identifying the language abilities of late-talking toddlers (Heilmann, Weismer, Evans, & Hollar, 2005), young children with profound hearing loss who use cochlear implants (Thal, DesJardin, & Eisenberg, 2007), and young children with autism spectrum disorder (Luyster, Qiu, Lopez, & Lord, 2007), among other groups.

Sander conducted a similarly well-known normative study in 1972 and identified when children typically acquire specific speech sounds, or *phonemes*. Sander's norms (see Figure 4.1) describe the ages by which children can produce particular phonemes, as well as the order in which children master them. Other normative studies have, for the most part, provided similar results, as shown in Table 4.2.

Methods for Studying Language Production

Language production studies are generally either observational or experimental. In *observational studies*, researchers examine children's language use in naturalistic or semistructured contexts, usually by using a tape recorder or another audio recording device to capture children's language for a certain period. In naturalistic settings, the researcher does not manipulate the context. For instance, a researcher may observe the language occurring between parents and children while the family is eating dinner together. One of the most well-known naturalistic observational studies is that of Hart and Risley (1995), who collected monthly audio

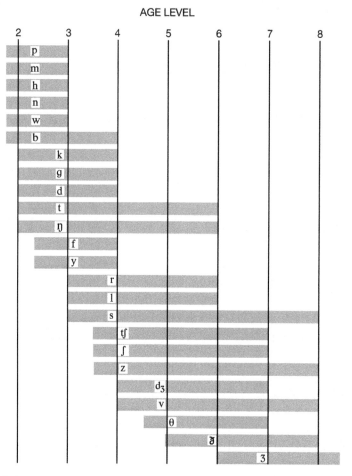

FIGURE 4.1

Sander's (1972) customary ages of production of English consonants.

Source: Reprinted with permission from "When are speech sounds learned?" by E. K. Sander, 1972. *Journal of Speech and Hearing Disorders, 37,* p. 62. Copyright 1972 by American Speech-Language-Hearing Association. All rights reserved.

TABLE 4.2
Normative references for English speech sound acquisition from six sources

CONSONANT	ARLT AND GOODBAN[a]	PRATHER ET AL.[b]	POOLE[c]	SANDER[d]	TEMPLIN[e]	WELLMAN ET AL.[f]
/m/	3–0	2	3–6	<2	3	3
/n/	3–0	2	4–6	<2	3	3
/h/	3–0	2	3–6	<2	3	3
/p/	3–0	2	3–6	<2	3	4
/ŋ/	3–0	2	4–6	2	3	*
/f/	3–0	2–4	5–6	2–6	3	3
/j/	—	2–4	4–6	2–6	3–6	4
/k/	3–0	2–4	4–6	2	4	4
/d/	3–0	2–4	4–6	2	4	5
/w/	3–0	2–8	3–6	<2	3	3
/b/	3–0	2–8	3–6	<2	4	3
/t/	3–0	2–8	4–6	2	6	5
/g/	3–0	3	4–6	2	4	4
/s/	4–0	3	7–6	3	4–6	5
/r/	5–0	3–4	7–6	3	4	5
/l/	4–0	3–4	6–6	3	6	4
/ʃ/	6–0	3–8	6–6	3–6	4–6	—
/tʃ/	4–0	3–8	—	3–6	4–6	5
/ð/	5–0	4	6–6	5	7	—
/ʒ/	4–0	4	6–6	6	7	6
/dʒ/	4–0	>4*	—	4	7	6
/θ/	5–0	>4*	7–6	4–6	6	—
/v/	3–6	>4*	6–6	4	6	5
/z/	4–0	>4*	7–6	3–6	7	5
/ʍ/	3–0	>4*	7–6	*	*	—

* = Sound not produced correctly by 75% of subjects at the oldest age tested; — = sound not tested or not reported.

[a] Arlt, P. B., & Goodban, M. T. (1976). A comparative study of articulation acquisition as based on a study of 240 normals, aged three to six. *Language, Speech, and Hearing Services in Schools, 7,* 173–180. (Criterion: 75% of children tested for initial, medial, and final word positions)

[b] Prather, E. M., Hedrick, E. L., & Kerin, C. A. (1975). Articulation development in children aged two to four years. *Journal of Speech and Hearing Disorders, 40,* 179–191. (Criterion: 75% of children tested; average for initial and final word positions)

[c] Poole, I. (1934). Genetic development of consonant sounds in speech. *Elementary English Review, 11,* 159–161. (Criterion: 100% of children tested for initial, medial, and final word positions)

[d] Sander, E. K. (1972). When are speech sounds learned? *Journal of Speech and Hearing Disorders, 37,* 55–63. (Criterion: 51%, based on average from Templin [1957] and Wellman, Case, Mengert, and Bradbury [1931])

[e] Templin, M. C. (1957). *Certain language skills in children* (Institute of Child Welfare Monograph Series 26). Minneapolis: University of Minnesota Press. (Criterion: 75% of children tested for initial, medial, and final word positions)

[f] Wellman, B., Case, I., Mengert, I., & Bradbury, D. (1931). Speech sounds of young children. *State University of Iowa Studies in Child Welfare, 5,* 2. (Criterion: 75% of children tested for initial, medial, and final word positions)

Source: From *Reference Manual for Communicative Sciences and Disorders: Speech and Language* (pp. 285–286), by R. D. Kent, 1994, Austin, TX: PRO–ED. Copyright 1994 by PRO–ED, Inc.. Reprinted with permission.

Researchers can observe children interacting with other people in naturalistic settings, make an audio recording of the interaction, transcribe the recording, and then analyze the transcript to learn how children's language develops.

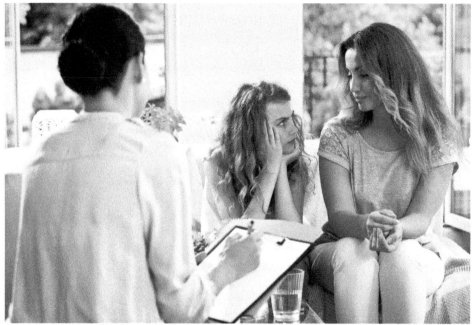

© Izabela Habur/E+/Getty Images

samples of parents' and children's language in the home environment for more than 2 years. In addition to illuminating the relationship between features of parental language and children's language growth, the results of this study provided useful references for the number and types of words children use as they develop their vocabulary skills.

Alternatively, in semistructured settings, researchers manipulate the environment in which they are observing children's language form, content, and use. Typically, researchers manipulate contexts to elicit the aspects of language they are interested in studying. We previously noted the Justice and colleagues (2006) study, which examined the fictional narratives of kindergartners through sixth graders. In this study, researchers were interested in examining characteristics of children's fictional narratives in each of seven grades. Therefore, they created a condition for eliciting narratives from children using different types of stimuli (e.g., a sequence of pictures).

In observational studies, researchers typically record children's language for a certain period, after which they transcribe the language and analyze it for specific properties or qualities. Hart and Risley's (1995) study involved transcribing hundreds of hours of parent–child conversation, then analyzing the transcripts for the number and types of words used. Although the observational aspect of this research may require only a few minutes or hours, the subsequent transcription and analysis of language can take hundreds to thousands of hours. Some computer software is available to support the analyses, but typically transcription requires listening and relistening to audiotapes and videotapes and typing the transcription by hand into the computer programs.

Experimental studies differ from observational studies in that the researcher actively manipulates variables of interest. One classic experimental design for language production studies involves manipulating the context in which, or the conditions under which children experience new words and examining how children's production of these words varies by context. For instance, Saylor and Sabbagh (2004) exposed 3- and 4-year-old children to a series of new words and systematically varied the way in which the children were exposed to them. After the children heard the new words, researchers used a puppet to ask them questions about each new word and recorded their responses to examine how the conditions of exposure influenced the children's learning of the new words. Many experimental studies of language production occur in a research laboratory and follow strict protocols so researchers can accurately determine the extent to which children can produce specific language structures.

Experimental studies of language production vary widely and may examine many aspects of production, including vocabulary, morphology, syntax, phonology, and pragmatics. Researchers are inventive in designing experiments to assess children's production abilities in these various areas. In some studies, researchers may use *pseudowords* (nonsense words) to assess children's morphological skills or vocabulary skills. Pseudowords allow control over children's previous experience with words; because these words are invented, researchers can assume children have no experience with them. A classic pseudoword task used to examine children's morphological skills was designed by Jean Berko (1958; now Jean Berko Gleason), who presented pseudowords to children and asked them to produce plural forms of these words. For example, children might demonstrate their understanding of the English plural morpheme by producing the plural form of *glorp* as *glorps* and the plural form of *dax* as *daxes*. We provide a complete description of this pseudoword task in Chapter 6.

Language production studies may also require children to repeat sentences so researchers can determine whether they have a grasp of certain grammatical structures. For example, an examiner may ask a child to repeat the sentence, *She is going to the party*. A child who has not yet mastered the auxiliary verb *is* will likely omit it ("She going to the party") and not produce an exact repetition of the sentence. Researchers may also ask children to correct erroneous sentences as another way to gauge their ability to produce more complex grammatical structures.

Approaches to Studying Language Comprehension

Goal of Language Comprehension Studies

Many times, researchers would like to understand what children know about language, even if they cannot express what they know. Language comprehension studies specifically tap into what children understand about language, and with the assistance of some creative research paradigms, experts can measure children's language comprehension even before children speak their first word.

Methods for Studying Language Comprehension

Language comprehension research requires a different set of tools and techniques than language production studies. In studying comprehension, researchers try to estimate what children or adults understand rather than produce. For prelinguistic infants, researchers generally use visual fixation (looking time) on a stimulus as a measure of language comprehension. For example, a researcher can determine whether an infant knows the words *mommy* and *daddy* by placing pictures of the infant's mother and father side by side and asking the infant to look at either "mommy" or "daddy." The researcher must take into account other considerations as well to ensure the validity of the experiment. In Chapter 5, we provide additional details on research paradigms that use visual fixation as a measure of language comprehension.

For older children, researchers can use pointing as a measure of language comprehension instead. For instance, the researcher may present a word or sentence and ask the child to select from an array of pictures the one that matches the word or sentence. This technique is common in standardized language assessments and researchers can use it to study children's comprehension of morphology, such as the plural form ("Point to the picture of two cats"); syntax, such as passive sentences ("Point to the picture showing *The boy was kicked by the girl*"); and vocabulary ("Point to the picture of the compass").

Alternatively, researchers may ask children to act out a series of sentences with toy props. For instance, to assess children's comprehension of the semantic roles

4.2

Check Your Understanding

Click here to gauge your understanding of the concepts in this section.

agent and *recipient*, the researcher could provide the child with a toy dog and a toy cat; say "The dog is pulling the cat's tail"; and instruct the child to act out the scenario with the dog and cat props. Likewise, to test a child's comprehension of passive sentences, a researcher could give the child a set of farm animals and ask the child to show the sentence, *The horse is being kicked by the cow.*

WHAT ARE SOME MAJOR LANGUAGE-DEVELOPMENT THEORIES?

Questions Language Theories Should Answer

Recall from the beginning of this chapter that theories provide testable explanations concerning children's language development. In large part, language-development theories attempt to explain *how* children learn their native language, a question of great interest for both theoretical and practical reasons. Researchers are interested in theories to build on knowledge about language development as a uniquely human phenomenon that is remarkable for various reasons (see Chapter 1). Likewise, practitioners are interested in language development to better help children and adults who may have difficulties with language. Professionals who work with children and adults with language difficulties draw on theory to make informed decisions about the practices and programs they use with these individuals.

Theories about language development are both abundant and varied in focus. Some theories address specific language accomplishments, such as word learning or question formation (e.g., Hirsh-Pasek, Golinkoff, & Hollich, 2000; Hollich, Hirsh-Pasek, & Golinkoff, 2000). Other theories focus on language development at particular ages (c.f. Nippold, 2007) or in the context of specific disabilities. The extent to which a theory helps *in general* to provide an explanation of language development is an important consideration. Some theories are too limited in scope to provide a useful explanation of language development in general, whereas others are so broad they fail to account for variability in language development when considering different language domains or achievements across the life span. Next, we present three questions you may use to consider each theory appearing subsequently in this chapter (Hirsh-Pasek & Golinkoff, 1996). We consider an adequate theory to provide some type of explanation for each question:

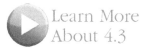

Learn More About 4.3

As you watch the video titled "Nativist, Learning, and Interactionist Theories of Language Development Explained," think about how nature-inspired (nativist), nurture-inspired (learning), and interactionist theories of language development differ.

https://www.youtube.com /watch?v=RRGwdfQV8kU

1. What do infants bring to the task of language learning?
2. What mechanisms drive language acquisition?
3. What types of input support the language-learning system?

What Do Infants Bring to the Task of Language Learning?

Some theorists propose infants arrive in the world essentially preprogrammed to acquire language. Other theorists contend infants learn language through their experiences and are not born with innate language capabilities. These divergent views fuel what is called the *nature versus nurture* debate or the *nativist-empiricist* debate (see Landau, 2009). Most language-development theories lie somewhere between the *nature* and *nurture* ends of the continuum and assert that language development results from the interaction of a number of factors, including biological, social, cognitive, and linguistic factors.

What Mechanisms Drive Language Acquisition?

The question of what mechanisms drive language acquisition addresses the processes by which language develops from infancy forward. For example, some theorists propose the processes people use to learn language are *domain specific*, or dedicated solely to the tasks of comprehending and producing language. Other theorists contend that people use processes for learning language that are domain

?! DISCUSSION POINT

What are some other fundamental questions you would use to guide a comparison of language-development theories?

general, or the same as processes they use in other situations, such as solving problems and perceiving objects and events in the environment. Recall from Chapters 1 and 3 our brief discussion on the concept of modularity. *Modularity* is a theoretical account of how the brain is organized for various cognitive processes. A strict modularity perspective includes a domain-specific account of language acquisition, whereas a nonmodularity perspective provides a domain-general account.

What Types of Input Support the Language-Learning System?

The final question concerns the kinds of input that drive language development after birth as children grow and develop. Some theorists suggest that increasing knowledge of social conventions and a child's desire to interact with others are the most important supports for language development. Other theorists propose that when children simply hear more and more language, they use "positive evidence" that other people provide to make assumptions about the structure of their native language.

Major Language-Development Theories

We can generally group language-development theories into those that are relatively nurture inspired, those that are relatively nature inspired, and those that acknowledge the interaction of multiple contributions. *Nurture-inspired theories* are often called *empiricist theories*, and they rest on the notion that humans gain all knowledge through experience. The extreme empiricist position is that an infant arrives in the world as a "blank slate," with no innate language abilities. In contrast, *nature-inspired theories*, also called *nativist theories*, generally hold that much knowledge is innate and genetically transmitted rather than learned by experience. The extreme nativist position is that an individual's underlying language system is in place at birth and children use this system to extract rules about their native language apart from other cognitive abilities. Between the nature and nurture ends of the continuum are *interactionist* theories. Interactionist theories acknowledge that language develops through the interaction between nature-related and nurture-related factors.

See Table 4.3 for an overview of some prominent language-development theories (some historical and others more contemporary). Table 4.4 presents answers

TABLE 4.3
Overview of language development theories

THEORY (PROPONENT)	NATURE–NURTURE CONTINUUM	MAJOR TENETS	KEY CONCEPTS
Behaviorist theory (Skinner)	Nurture inspired	Language is like any other human behavior and does not reflect any special innate endowment.	Operant conditioning; Reinforcement.
		Children learn language through operant conditioning and shaping; some verbal behaviors are reinforced and others are suppressed.	
		Complex behaviors (e.g., speaking in complete sentences) are learned as a series of steps in a chain, in which each step stimulates each successive step.	
Universal grammar (Chomsky)	Nature inspired	Children are born with general grammatical rules and categories common to all languages.	Language acquisition device; Parameters

THEORY (PROPONENT)	NATURE–NURTURE CONTINUUM	MAJOR TENETS	KEY CONCEPTS
		Children use input to discover the parameters their language uses to satisfy the general grammatical rules and categories they are born with.	
Modularity theory (Fodor)	Nature inspired	Language is organized in highly specific modules in the brain.	Localization; Encapsulization
		Language modules perform dedicated functions but can interact with one another to produce combinations of functions.	
Bootstrapping theories (Syntactic - Gleitman; Semantic - Pinker; Prosodic - Wanner & Gleitman)	Nature inspired	Children use their knowledge of syntactic categories, word meanings, or the prosodic structure of language to make inferences about other aspects of language.	Bootstrapping; Syntax; Semantics; Prosody; acoustics
Social-interactionist theory *(Vygotsky)*	Interactionist	Language emerges through social interaction with peers and adults. Language skills move from a social plane to a psychological plane. Initially, language and cognition are intertwined processes, but they become separate capabilities by about age 2 years.	Social plane–psychological plane; Zone of proximal development
Cognitive theory (Piaget)	Interactionist	Children's cognitive development and interactions with the physical environment drive language development. Children's speech begins as egocentric because children can view the world only from their own perspective.	Cognition hypothesis; Egocentric speech
Intentionality model (Bloom)	Interactionist	The tension between the desire to communicate intentions to other people and the effort required to communicate these intentions drives language development.	Intentionality
Competition model (MacWhinney)	Interactionist	Repeated exposure to reliable language input strengthens children's "correct" representations of the morphology, phonology, and syntax of their language.	Reliable input; Strengthened representation
Connectionist theories (Rumelhart & McClelland)	Interactionist	Language is organized in a network containing nodes and connections.	Nodes; Connections
		The network of nodes and connections undergoes constant transformation in response to language input.	
Usage-based theory (Tomasello)	Interactionist	Children attend to and understand other people's intentions and then imitate other persons' intentional communicative actions to learn language.	Joint attention; Intention reading

TABLE 4.4

Answers to three questions about the nature of language development theories

THEORY	QUESTIONS		
	WHAT DO INFANTS BRING TO THE TASK OF LANGUAGE LEARNING?	WHAT MECHANISMS DRIVE LANGUAGE ACQUISITION?	WHAT TYPES OF INPUT SUPPORT THE LANGUAGE-LEARNING SYSTEM?
Behaviorist theory	No mention	Operant conditioning by parents and adults—a domain-general process	Reinforcement of desirable verbal behavior and punishment of undesirable verbal behavior
Universal grammar	Explicit, domain-specific linguistic knowledge	Discovery of the parameters a person's language encompasses—domain-specific processes	General linguistic input (even of an impoverished quality)
Modularity theory	Specialized modules in the brain	Functions performed by dedicated language modules—domain-specific processes	Input that promotes parameter setting of modules and interactions among language modules
Bootstrapping theories	Syntactic categories, semantic categories, or sensitivity to prosodic or acoustic structure of language	Domain-general processes to understand how language works, domain-specific processes to notice correlations between syntax and meaning (syntactic bootstrapping), to make hypotheses about new words (semantic bootstrapping), or to notice correlations between acoustic properties of speech and syntactic categories (prosodic bootstrapping)	Syntactic input, semantic input, or acoustic input
Social interactionist theory	General social structure	Social interactions with others—a domain-general process	Linguistic input that is within the child's zone of proximal development
Cognitive theory	General cognitive structure	General cognitive processing abilities—a domain-general process	Understanding events, relations, and phenomena in a nonlinguistic sense
Intentionality model	General social structure	Engaging with other people and objects—a domain-general process	The tension between the desire to engage with other people and the effort required to express elaborate intentional states
Competition model	Ability to attend to and organize linguistic data	Induction and hypothesis testing—domain-general processes	Reliable and frequent input patterns
Connectionist theories	Ability to attend to and organize linguistic data	Pattern detection—a domain-general process	Reliable and frequent input patterns
Usage-based theory	Intention reading, which emerges during infancy	The child's interpretation of the social environment—a domain-general process	Reproducing intentional communicative actions through cultural or imitative learning

THEORY TO PRACTICE

Applied Behavior Analysis

Applied behavior analysis (ABA) is an umbrella term encompassing several methods stemming from Skinner's behaviorist theory. It is often used as an intervention approach for children with autism. The principles of operant conditioning—stimulus, response, and reinforcement—are common to ABA interventions for autism. In such interventions, an adult or a therapist first makes a request of the child. The request may consist of asking the child to repeat a word or phrase or to fill in the blank of a *cloze* statement (e.g., "I want to eat _____"). The request serves as the stimulus for the behavior that follows. When the child responds by performing the requested behavior, the adult or therapist immediately reinforces the child to promote such linguistic behavior in the future.

ABA interventions can be intensive and time-consuming, sometimes requiring training in ABA and several to many hours per week of one-on-one therapy. Some ABA interventions use *discrete trial training* (DTT), which consists of a series of distinct trials the adult or therapist repeats until the child masters the target skill. Subsequent trials build on these skills to shape more complex skills. To build language skills, DTT moves from eliciting simple behaviors, such as direct imitation, to more advanced behaviors, such as forming *wh-* questions (e.g., "What?" "When?" "Where?"). The results of some research suggest children with autism who undergo ABA-inspired therapy make significant gains in their academic, intellectual, and language functioning in both the short term and the long term (Lovaas, 1987; Peters-Sheffer, Didden, Korzilius, & Sturmey, 2011). However, this approach to language intervention is not without controversy (Heflin & Simpson, 1998).

to the questions concerning what infants bring to the task of language learning, the mechanisms that drive language acquisition, and the types of input that support the language-learning system, for each theory.

Nurture-Inspired Theory

Behaviorist Theory. B. F. Skinner (1904–1990), who appears in the chapter-opening photo with his wife and his daughter Deborah, popularized the notion of *behaviorism*, according to which all learning is the result of operant conditioning (Skinner, 1957). In operant conditioning, behaviors that are reinforced become strengthened, and behaviors that are punished become suppressed. To Skinner, language is not a special behavior; rather, it is a behavior like any other behavior humans can learn. Thus, Skinner's theory of language learning is essentially identical to his general learning theory in that it focuses on observable and measurable aspects of language (the behavior) children produce as they interact with the environment. See Theory to Practice: *Applied Behavior Analysis* for a practical application of behaviorist theory.

According to this language-development theory, children arrive at the task of language learning without innate knowledge; rather, environmental stimuli elicit verbal responses, or language, from children. Children then "learn" language as adults reinforce their verbalizations, as in the following example:

Eight-month-old Dresden would shriek loudly when he was hungry and wanted to be fed. Dresden's mother would grab his bottle and say; "You want your bottle? Baaaaah-ttle." On one occasion, Dresden imitated his mother by saying "ba." Dresden's mother was so excited at his attempt that she laughed and smiled as she fed Dresden his bottle, reinforcing Dresden's use of this "word." Dresden then began to say "ba" when he wanted his bottle, and Dresden's mother would retrieve it more quickly than when Dresden simply shrieked. Because Dresden's mother rewarded him quickly with a bottle each time he uttered "ba," Dresden eventually stopped shrieking and continued to say "ba" when he was

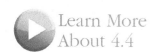

Learn More About 4.4

As you watch the video titled "ABA Therapy to Elicit and Reinforce Verbal Behavior," notice how the therapist uses applied behavior analysis techniques to elicit and reinforce a child's verbal behavior.

https://www.youtube.com/watch?v=5H6E4BEBZ1U

❓❗ DISCUSSION POINT

Describe the link among theory, science, and practice in ABA interventions. How might subscribing to a different language-development theory influence language therapy techniques for children with autism?

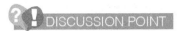

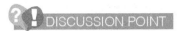

DISCUSSION POINT

Skinner equates language to other human behaviors such as learning to walk. How are learning to talk and learning to walk similar? How do they differ?

hungry. Dresden's mother eventually began to accept only close approximations of the word *bottle*, including "ba-ba" and later "ba-bble" before she hurried to get a bottle.

You may wonder how children ever learn to speak in complete sentences if reinforcement is the key to learning, but Skinner's theory of verbal behavior accounts for complex linguistic behavior as well. Complex behavior consists of a series, or chain, of behaviors, in which each step in the process stimulates each successive behavior. In the case of even complex verbal behavior, operant conditioning is the mechanism that drives language learning.

Nature-Inspired Theories

Universal Grammar.   Noam Chomsky (1965) popularized the term universal grammar (UG), which describes the system of grammatical rules and constraints consistent in all world languages. Chomsky postulated that language acquisition depends on an innate, species-specific module dedicated to language and not to other forms of learning. Unlike Fodor (see modularity theory), who postulated language to involve a series of modules, Chomsky theorized the existence of one language module, called the language acquisition device.

According to UG theory, children are born with a basic set of grammatical rules and categories that exist in all languages, and the input they receive sets parameters (options) to match those of their native language. In UG, the implicit knowledge children have about language is called *linguistic competence*, whereas the actual comprehension and production of language in specific situations is called *linguistic performance*. UG posits that children are born with linguistic competence and that mistakes and omissions in their speech indicate performance difficulties and not a lack of competence. The disconnect between children's performance and their grammatical competence may result from limitations in their processing capacities and other contextual factors that may mask competence (Brooks, 2004).

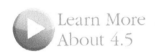

Learn More About 4.5

As you watch the video titled "Chomsky's View of Language Development Explained," consider ways in which Chomsky's view is nature-inspired.

https://www.youtube.com/watch?v=3gU-B0-DCKI

Modularity Theory.   Fodor's (1983) modularity theory is a popular cognitive approach emphasizing the organization of the cognitive infrastructure of the brain as comprising a series of highly specified modules, including modules for various aspects of language processing. A modularity perspective of language views it as an innate capacity localized to domain-specific processors that are encapsulated in their functions from other processors. To say that language is *localized* means the modules composing the language system each operate by using a dedicated neural system. The concept of *encapsulization* means the processors operate independently of one another. Thus, language modules operate independently to perform dedicated functions, yet can interact with one another at higher levels to produce combinations of functions. Because language modules operate independently, different types of input drive language development forward in different areas (e.g., the lexicon, syntax, morphology). For example, the number and kinds of words a young child hears form an environmental influence that helps shape the lexicon, whereas innately given syntactic rules help shape the child's sentence formation abilities.

Because modularity theory stipulates separate areas of language can develop independently of one another, it has implications for understanding language development. This phenomenon is most obvious in children who have an impairment in one or more language areas (e.g., receptive language, expressive language). In Chapter 3, we presented neurological evidence concerning the modularity perspective.

Bootstrapping Theories.   You may have heard some people refer to *bootstrapping* their way to a particular accomplishment. This term means the individual

The bootstrap idiom for language development is derived from the process of pulling your boots on with only the assistance of the small loop sewn onto the top, back portion of the boot.

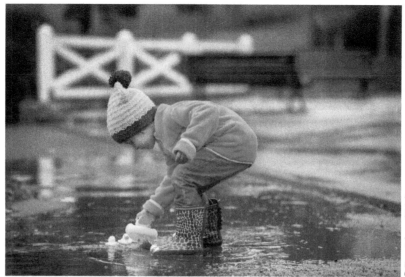

© Tomsickova/Fotolia

accomplished a goal by personal effort or with minimal outside assistance. The bootstrap idiom is derived from the process of pulling a boot on with only the assistance of the small loop sewn to the top, back portion of the boot. Syntactic bootstrapping describes the process by which children use the syntactic frames surrounding unknown verbs to successfully constrain or limit the possible meanings of the verbs. This theory is a nature-inspired account of language development focused specifically on syntactic development. Nurture-inspired theorists suggest children learn the meaning of an unfamiliar verb by examining extralinguistic cues, such as observing their own actions or the actions of other people nearby, to narrow the meaning of the verb. However, as Gleitman and Landau argued, the extralinguistic context will most likely not reveal a single, clear meaning (Gleitman, 1990; Landau & Gleitman, 1985). For example, the extralinguistic context surrounding the request, "Are you *bringing* me the remote control?" might prompt a child to interpret the verb in the sentence to mean "hold," "carry," "walk," or "bring." Therefore, children probably use additional linguistic information—particularly the syntax of the sentence—as they learn the meanings of new verbs.

In the preceding example, information about the meaning of *bring* is available in the syntax in which *bring* appears. In this example, an indirect object (*me*) and then a direct object (*remote control*) follow the word *bring*, which suggests *bring* is a verb of transfer (because transfer involves both the thing transferred and the person to whom it is transferred). Therefore, the meanings of *hold*, *carry*, and *walk* would not be good candidates. Syntactic bootstrapping is a nature-inspired language-development theory because it proposes children arrive at the task of language learning with knowledge of syntactic categories and use this knowledge to understand the meanings of words that fill various positions in sentences.

Semantic bootstrapping is another type of bootstrapping theory. Like syntactic bootstrapping, semantic bootstrapping uses the bootstrap metaphor to illustrate how children acquire particular linguistic concepts with minimal outside assistance. However, the difference lies in what children bootstrap. With semantic bootstrapping, children deduce grammatical structures by using word meanings they acquire from observing events around them (Pinker, 1984). After children acquire a large, diverse lexicon from their observations of objects and events in the world, they use correspondences between semantics and syntax to determine the syntactic category to which each word belongs. For example, once a child learns *bird* describes a solid object, he or she may infer *bird* is a count noun. Later, when the child understands the determiner *a*, he or she may infer other words that include the determiner a (*a watch, a clock*) are also count nouns.

Prosodic bootstrapping is a third type of bootstrapping theory; it suggests infants use their sensitivity to the acoustic properties of speech (e.g., pitch, rhythm, pauses, stress) to make inferences about units of language, including clauses, phrases, and words. When infants are sensitive to the acoustic patterns of their native language, they may be better able to isolate important language units from running speech, and eventually they begin to assign meaning to those units. As one example of how researchers tested the prosodic bootstrapping theory, Jusczyk et al. (1993) demonstrated that 9-month-old infants showed a significant preference for bisyllabic (two-syllable) words with a strong-weak stress pattern (e.g., ba-by, mo-ther) compared to words with a weak-strong stress pattern (e.g., be-lieve, cre-ate). The researchers supposed that because the strong-weak stress pattern is the dominant pattern for English bisyllabic words, this likely contributed to infants' preference. English-learning infants who are sensitive to the dominant stress patterns of their native language may use this information to their advantage as they attempt to isolate single words from the speech they hear around them.

Interactionist Theories

Social-Interactionist Theory.   In the early 20th century, Soviet psychologist, Lev Vygotsky (1896–1934) stressed the importance of social interaction for children's language development. Vygotsky contended that all concepts are introduced first in the context of social interaction (the *social plane*); then, with time, these concepts are internalized to the *psychological plane*. Social interaction between an infant and other, more capable persons (parents, siblings, teachers, etc.) is a critical mechanism for children's language acquisition. Vygotsky viewed language as a uniquely human ability that exists independent of general cognition starting at about age 2 years: He believed prior to this time, general cognition and language are intertwined, but at about age 2 years, these two processes begin to develop as separate (albeit interrelated) capabilities.

One critical concept in Vygotskian theory is the zone of proximal development (ZPD), which is the difference between a child's *actual developmental level*, as determined by independent problem solving, and his or her *level of potential development*, as determined through problem solving in collaboration with a more competent adult or peer (Vygotsky, 1978). The ZPD concept characterizes development dynamically by describing abilities in children that are in the process of maturing rather than by focusing solely on abilities that have already matured. Consider this example:

Lori and her 4-year-old son, Alexander, are having a conversation about rhyming words in a storybook. Without assistance from Lori, Alexander cannot produce rhymes. For instance, she asks him, "What is a word that rhymes with *cat?*" and receives no response. However, when Lori provides Alexander with support, by telling him three words that rhyme with *cat* (*bat, fat, mat*), he can produce a rhyming word (*rat*).

You might ask whether Alexander can actually recognize rhymes. On the one hand, he cannot do so independently; on the other hand, with some help from his mother, he can complete the task. From a Vygotskian perspective, examining what children can do with mediated assistance from others is necessary for identifying maturing capabilities, which provides an important window into development. Vygotsky's position is that as children learn language through social interactions, their general cognitive abilities are subsequently propelled forward.

Cognitive Theory.   Jean Piaget (1896–1980), a Swiss psychologist, is best known for his observational studies of his three children's development and his theories

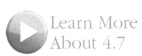

Learn More About 4.6

As you watch the video titled "Steven Pinker on How Children Learn Language," consider how the examples reflect a nature-inspired view of language development. https://www.youtube.com/watch?v=ir7arILiqxg

Learn More About 4.7

As you watch the video titled "Vygotsky's Theory of Development," consider how the examples reflect an interactionist view of language development. https://www.youtube.com/watch?v=lnzmZtHuZPY

on genetic epistemology, or the study of the development of knowledge. One important element of Piaget's work is his emphasis on stages of learning and development. Piaget hypothesized a series of cognitive stages children experience and emphasized that achievements in one stage must occur before a child can move on to the next stage.

Piaget (1923) did not believe language to be a domain-specific ability, but rather a domain-general ability that closely follows children's general cognitive development. His perspective on the subservience of language to cognition has been referred to as the *cognition hypothesis* because certain cognitive achievements must be in place for language achievements to emerge (see Sinclair-de-Zwart, 1973). In essence, Piaget did not view language as a special faculty but as an ability that reflects developments in other areas of growth, such as perceptive, cognitive, and social processes. He viewed language as following the same stages he proposed for general cognitive development.

Piaget viewed children as active agents in constructing their understanding of language. According to Piaget, children are egocentric and developmentally predisposed to view the world from only their perspective. For this reason, conversations between young children are essentially collective monologues, in which each child produces a monologue but cannot respond contingently or take turns with each other. The following dialogue between two preschoolers is an example of how egocentric speech plays out in conversations with young children:

KEVIN: Watch me score a goal!

PETE: The ground is squishy and muddy.

KEVIN: Ok, here goes. Are you watching?

PETE: My socks are getting wet!

According to Piagetian theory, children do not replace egocentric speech with true dialogue until they develop the ability to see others' perspectives. This contention supports the idea that cognitive development gives way to language achievements.

Intentionality Model.   According to the intentionality model, children's abilities in language, emotional expression, cognition, social interaction, and play develop in tandem (L. Bloom, 2000; L. Bloom & Tinker, 2001). The child is responsible for driving language learning forward. This model differs from other interactionist theories that propose the child's environment or peers have the most influence in driving language development. In fact, in this model, children learn language when what they have in mind differs from what other individuals around them have in mind because they must express themselves to share this information. For example, a young girl cannot assume her mother will always know when she is thirsty and offer her a drink. Therefore, the girl must learn to express this intention with language. To acquire language, then, children must be intentional, they must take strides to engage in social interaction, and they must put forth effort to construct linguistic representations for the ideas they want to express and then act to express these ideas.

Competition Model.   The competition model describes specific mechanisms through which children acquire the acceptable morphological, phonological, syntactic, and lexical forms that compose their native language (MacWhinney, 1987; MacWhinney, 2004). Children acquire language forms that they hear frequently and reliably early in life, and later in life they acquire forms that they hear rarely or inconsistently. In the competition model, multiple language forms compete with one another until the input strengthens the correct representation and the child no longer produces an incorrect form.

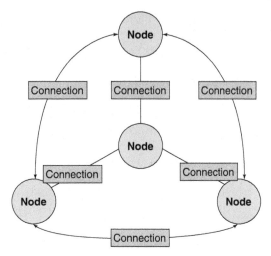

FIGURE 4.2

A connectionist network.

A common child language phenomenon that illustrates how the competition model works is overgeneralization. You have probably heard children say "I goed" instead of "I went", or "I runned" instead of "I ran." When children who are learning language make an irregular past tense verb regular by adding a /d/, /t/, or /ld/ sound, they are overgeneralizing the past tense rule that applies to most verbs in the English language. Eventually, though, with ongoing reliable exposures to an irregular form such as *went*, the correct past tense representation of the word is strengthened, and the incorrect form (*goed*) dies out.

Connectionist Theories. Connectionist models of language development attempt to visually approximate the inner workings of the brain, and they model and simulate the mechanisms responsible for language growth in relationship to input. Connectionist theories are relevant to modeling an array of cognitive processes, but, in the area of language, they focus on modeling how language is organized across the brain and on describing how connections are forged among words within the lexicon, or store of words in the brain (see Chapter 2 for a discussion of the mental lexicon).

Connectionist researchers use models to represent nonlinear, dynamic, and complex development in language and other areas. One important aspect of language development that connectionist researchers have modeled is the process by which children learn both the regular (e.g., *walk–walked, cook–cooked*) and the irregular (e.g., *eat–ate, fly–flew*) forms of past tense verbs (Rumelhart & McClelland, 1986). Connectionist models are simulations of how nodes and connections are organized in larger networks (Figure 4.2). *Nodes* are simple processing units that can be likened to brain neurons. Nodes receive input from external sources through *connections*. The connections between nodes vary in strength, depending on the connection weight. The network of nodes and connections adapts and transforms itself continually in response to the input it receives. For example, connections between some nodes may weaken with time from reduced input or counterevidence, and connections between other nodes may become stronger with time and contribute to a reorganization of the entire network. Elman, Bates, Johnson, Parisi, and Plunkett (1996) provide a more detailed introduction to connectionist models.

Usage-Based Theory. Engaging in social interactions is undoubtedly a strong impetus for attending to and learning language. Prelinguistic infants provide substantial evidence for this claim. You have probably experienced a situation similar to this scenario:

While two women were talking, the 8-month-old daughter of one of them began to interject some babbling sounds into the conversation as if to indicate that she, too, wanted to take part in the social exchange.

Usage-based theories of language acquisition, a term Tomasello (2003) coined, emphasize the social nature of language as an impetus for furthering children's language abilities, contending that children learn language because they have reason to talk (e.g., Budwig, 1995).

Tomasello's (2003) usage-based theory of language development is based on evidence concerning the emergence of intentionality during the first year of life. For example, in their first year, infants engage in periods of sustained joint attention with other individuals, actively direct the attention of other people to objects and events, and begin to use communicative intentions to achieve various ends. Usage-based theories suggest children's knowledge of language form and meaning emerges from their use of language, during which they induce patterns of form and meaning. A critical premise of this theory is the child's skills in intention reading. *Intention reading*, which emerges during infancy, refers to the child's ability to recognize the intentions and mental states of other people, corresponding to the increasing capacity of the infant to engage communicatively with other persons. As a child becomes aware of others' intentions, he or she begins to actively manipulate them—for example, by drawing his or her mother's attention to an object of interest. As children repeatedly and increasingly use their awareness of social conventions to engage with other people, their more general language abilities emerge.

4.3

Check Your Understanding

Click here to gauge your understanding of the concepts in this section.

HOW DO LANGUAGE-DEVELOPMENT THEORIES INFLUENCE PRACTICE?

Linkage of Theory to Practice

To this point, we have discussed some of the people who study language development and why they do so. We have described some general approaches for studying language development. We have also examined several language-development theories and their premises about the predetermined abilities of infants, the mechanisms that drive language development, and the kinds of input that support language development. Next, we bridge the gaps between language-development theory, science, and practice. Linking theories to practices is not a novel idea. People routinely let their ideas about particular phenomena guide their practices. You can witness this occurrence in diet trends, the medicine people take, and child-rearing practices, to name a few areas. In some cases, the connection between theory and practice is clear. For instance, Newton's first law states an object in motion will remain in motion until acted on by an outside force. Many people, not wanting their bodies to remain in motion long enough to pass through the windshield upon impact in a car crash, faithfully wear seat belts when they travel.

However, in the case of language development, the connection between theory and practice is not always so transparent. For this reason, practitioners must make every effort to understand the theories that guide particular practices. Also important is determining whether a theory offers ample support to guide the practices in question. In the following section, we provide examples of the connection between language-development theories and practice in the context of two historical second language–learning methods. Then, in the next section, we discuss three types of practices language-development theories inform. Finally, we discuss the concept of evidence-based practice, focusing on the links between theory, science, and practice in education and clinical decision-making.

The audiolingual method, created during World War II, was derived from behaviorist theory and emphasizes drilling of language skills.

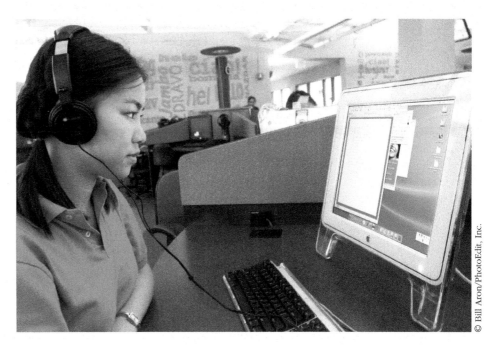

© Bill Aron/PhotoEdit, Inc.

Instruction in English as a Second Language: Theory and Practice

Theories of language learning influence language-teaching practices in a number of ways, although, as we mentioned previously, the link between theory and practice is not always direct. Rather, the connection between theory and practice is mediated by principles of instruction, including cognitive, affective, and linguistic principles. *Cognitive principles* include ideas governing language processing and automaticity and the role of tangible and intangible rewards the speaker gains through language use. *Affective principles* are related to the individual's confidence with language learning and his or her propensity to take risks with respect to language. *Linguistic principles* describe the role of a person's native language in simultaneously facilitating and interfering with second language acquisition. (See H. D. Brown, 2001, for a thorough discussion of language instruction principles.) When teachers of English as a second language select particular instructional practices, they consider not only language-learning theories but also relevant principles concerning all the preceding factors.

Two historical methods for teaching English as a second language that stem from distinct language theories are the audiolingual method and the Silent Way. Although these methods are no longer widely used, we describe them because they provide clear examples of the link between language-development theories and practice. The *audiolingual method* was developed in response to an increasing need for translators during World War II. It emphasizes imitation, repetition, and memorization of language forms to create automatic and habitual language responses. Teachers using the audiolingual method engage students in language drills that include positive reinforcement for target verbal behavior. For example, the teacher might present lines of dialogue for students to repeat and then praise them for pronouncing the lines correctly. Teachers target more complex linguistic behavior only after students have mastered smaller, simpler chunks of language. This method has roots in behavioral psychology—more specifically in Skinner's nurture-inspired behaviorist theory—in that it emphasizes eliciting a learner's rote, habitual responses to language forms.

The *Silent Way* is a language-teaching method that was popular during the cognitive revolution of the early 1970s. It emphasizes the importance of allowing

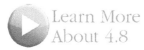

Learn More About 4.8

As you watch the video titled "Audiolingual Method Demonstration," consider how nurture-inspired theories of language development have contributed to this historical (and no longer widely used) practice for second language instruction. https://www.youtube.com/watch?v=isalagL8LAQ

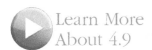

Learn More About 4.9

As you watch the video titled "Silent Way Demonstration," consider the ways in which interactionist theories of language development have contributed to this historical (and no longer widely used) practice for second language instruction. https://www.youtube.com/watch?v=E2UbkYo7ufY

students to generate hypotheses about language rules and then to apply the rules and discover errors. Using the Silent Way, teachers facilitate students' discovery of language rules, remaining mostly silent and using color-coded rods rather than words to represent vocabulary words, grammatical forms, and pronunciation rules. The Silent Way values the learner's ability to process and detect patterns in linguistic input, to generate and test hypotheses, and to correct errors by personal effort, as well as the learner's native language abilities and knowledge—all characteristics of interactionist theories of language development.

Despite relatively limited use in the 21st century, both the audiolingual method and the Silent Way illustrate how language-development theories can be translated into educational practice. These examples also show how extremely different practices can be used in the field on the basis of a particular theory that is in vogue at the time. Sometimes, however, the connection between theory and practice is not so transparent. In Chapter 9, we discuss theories of second language development and describe additional (and more contemporary) second language–teaching practices.

Practices Language Theories May Inform

Many professionals are interested in applying language-development theories to practice, including clinical psychologists, speech–language pathologists, audiologists, social workers, and teachers. Parents are also interested in how they may connect theories to practice so they may promote their children's language achievements. In this section, we consider three direct applications of language theory (and research) to practice: prevention, intervention and remediation, and enrichment.

The goal of *prevention* is to inhibit language difficulties from emerging and thus reduce the need to resolve such difficulties later in life. Preventing language difficulties is particularly important for children who are at risk for language problems because of their biological predispositions, the family's socioeconomic status, or the quality of language interactions between adults and children in the home. One popular type of prevention activity many preschool programs across the United States use focuses on fostering phonological awareness in young children. Phonological awareness is the ability to focus on the sounds that make up syllables and words; well-developed phonological awareness can help children succeed in later reading instruction. Various programs are available to promote phonological awareness in young children, which may, in turn, prevent children from experiencing later problems in reading achievement. We discuss phonological awareness in greater detail in Chapter 7.

Intervention and *remediation* are programs or strategies to help children, adolescents, and adults who exhibit difficulties with some aspect of language development. Language intervention may be appropriate for toddlers who show delays in acquiring their first words, or who are slow to start combining words to make two-word utterances. For preschoolers, intervention may focus on helping children with language problems communicate more effectively with other people and improving their morphological, phonological, syntactic, and semantic development. Numerous programs and strategies are available for targeting these aspects of language development. For school-age children with language problems, intervention often focuses on helping children improve their academic language skills, such as their understanding of curricular vocabulary or their use of comprehension strategies to better understand what they read. Various interventions are also available for adults who lose their language skills because of disease or illness.

Enrichment is the process through which teachers, clinicians, and other adults provide children, adolescents, and adults with an enhanced language-learning environment that both builds on existing skills and promotes the development of new and more advanced language abilities. One example of a language enrichment program is *Learning Language and Loving It* (http://www.hanen.org). This program teaches preschool educators ways to promote children's language learning in the early education environment. The *Learning Language and Loving It* program, and its accompanying book by Weitzman and Greenberg (2002), takes a child-centered approach to enhancing children's early language, social, and literacy development by training educators to use specific strategies for interacting with children in responsive ways. As other examples, an enrichment program for adolescents might teach appropriate ways to interact with peers. An enrichment program for adults who speak English with an accent (e.g., businesspersons who speak Chinese as a first language but use English for business purposes) may address improved pronunciation.

Evidence-Based Practice: Linking Theory, Science, and Practice

As we mentioned near the beginning of this chapter, evidence-based practice (EBP) involves integrating theoretical knowledge with scientific inquiry to inform decision making. Practitioners incorporate the principles of EBP to inform their everyday decision making in a variety of fields; this chapter focuses on the fields of education and speech–language pathology and audiology, as they are most relevant to the field of language development.

Within school settings, professionals must regularly make decisions about how best to teach children. For example, administrators and curriculum specialists must decide which curricula to adopt (e.g., a first-grade reading curriculum that relies heavily on computer games and technology versus a first-grade reading curriculum that does not incorporate technology), and teachers must decide what kinds of instructional practices to implement within their classrooms (e.g., whether or not to place students in small groups based on their ability level). Because the field of education has increasingly emphasized the importance of identifying and adopting scientifically-based or evidence-based curricula, programs, and practices, many commercial products have responded by claiming to be "evidence-based," "theoretically-driven," "field-tested," "scientifically-proven," or "research-based." Education professionals thus face the challenge of distinguishing between those curricula, programs, and practices that are truly evidence-based and those whose claims are largely or completely unfounded.

The U.S. Department of Education's Institute of Education Sciences (IES) is one organization that provides guidance to education professionals on how to evaluate curricula, programs, and practices to determine the extent to which they are evidence-based (see U.S. Department of Education, 2003). For example, IES describes how professionals can evaluate whether an intervention they are considering for adoption is backed by "strong" evidence of effectiveness. IES considers evidence to be strong when it is from two or more well-designed and well-implemented randomized controlled trials (studies that randomly assign participants to an intervention or control group to measure the intervention's effects) conducted in typical school settings.

There are a number of resources on the Web that education professionals can consult to help guide their decision-making. One example is the IES What Works Clearinghouse (WWC) Web site (http://ies.ed.gov/ncee/wwc/). The WWC Web site evaluates the quality of research evidence for education curricula, programs, and practices in a number of areas (e.g., beginning reading, English learners). As another example, the Campbell Collaboration (C2) Web site (http://www.campbellcollaboration.org) prepares, maintains, and disseminates reviews of research evidence in the areas of education, crime and justice, and social welfare.

With regard to speech–language pathology and audiology, professionals routinely make clinical decisions about the kinds of interventions and practices they will implement to improve the speech, language, and hearing abilities of the children they work with. The American Speech-Language-Hearing Association (ASHA) provides a position statement that describes how professionals should incorporate the principles of EBP in their clinical decision-making by integrating high-quality research evidence with client preferences and values and with their own experience as practitioners (ASHA, 2005). As with the IES guidelines for EBP, ASHA recommends that professionals evaluate the quality of evidence before incorporating such evidence in their decision-making. ASHA further emphasizes five additional areas to consider in making clinical decisions: (a) integrating the needs, values, abilities, preferences, and interests of individuals and their families with research evidence; (b) acquiring and maintaining the knowledge and skills necessary to provide high-quality services; (c) identifying informative and cost-effective screening and diagnostic tools in accordance with the EBP literature; (d) identifying effective clinical protocols for prevention, treatment, and enhancement in accordance with the EBP literature; and (e) continually monitoring and incorporating new high-quality research evidence that has implications for practice. Another resource for clinical professionals is the Cochrane Collaboration (http://www.cochrane.org), which provides systematic reviews of research evidence in the area of health care interventions. Another example is ASHA's National Center for Evidence-Based Practice in Communication Disorders (N-CEP) Compendium of EBP Guidelines and Systematic Reviews (http://www.asha.org/members/ebp/compendium/). This compendium includes guidelines and systematic reviews in more than 100 topic areas, such as pragmatics and written language, to help guide clinical decision-making.

4.4

Check Your Understanding

Click here to gauge your understanding of the concepts in this section.

SUMMARY

In this chapter, we distinguish among theory, science, and practice and demonstrate how the three complement one another in the field of language development. A *theory* of language development is a claim or hypothesis that provides explanations for how and why children develop their capacity for language. In the field of language development, *science* describes the process of generating and testing language theories, and *practice* includes the areas of people's lives that language-development theories and science influence, including second language–teaching methods and methods for the *prevention* of language difficulties, for *language intervention and remediation,* and for language *enrichment.*

Scientists from many disciplines (including psychology, linguistics, psycholinguistics, anthropology, speech–language pathology, education, and sociology, among others) study language development. Some scientists conduct *basic research* in language development, with the goal of generating and refining the existing knowledge base. Other scientists conduct applied research, with the goal of testing approaches and practices that pertain to real-world settings.

Scientists use various approaches to study language development. For example, to study infants' *speech perception* abilities, scientists can measure infants' heart rate, kicking rate, and visual responses to auditory stimuli. To measure young children's *language production* abilities, scientists might use observational studies to examine children's language in naturalistic or semistructured contexts—or experimental studies, in which the researcher manipulates variables of interest. To study children's *language comprehension* abilities, scientists might measure looking time or pointing toward a stimulus.

Language-development theories can be examined in the context of three questions: (a) What do infants bring to the task of language learning? (b) What mechanisms drive language acquisition? (c) What types of input support the language-learning system?

Nurture-inspired, or *empiricist*, theories of language development contend that humans gain all knowledge through experience. The extreme empiricist position is that an infant arrives in the world as a "blank slate," with no innate language abilities. *Nurture-inspired* theories include behaviorist theory. *Nature-inspired*, or *nativist* theories, contend that much knowledge is innate and genetically transmitted rather than learned by experience. The extreme nativist position is that an individual's underlying language system is in place at birth and that children use this system to extract rules about their native language apart from other cognitive abilities. *Nature-inspired* theories include universal grammar, modularity theory, and bootstrapping theories. *Interactionist theories* acknowledge that language develops through the interaction between nature-related and nurture-related factors, including biological, social, cognitive, and linguistic factors. Interactionist theories include social interactionist theory, cognitive theory, intentionality model, competition model, connectionist theories, and usage-based theory.

Language-development theories contribute to practices in several areas. These areas include instruction in English as a second language, prevention of language difficulties, intervention and remediation, and enrichment. Language-development theories and science are crucial to the concept of EBP in both education and clinical decision making.

 Apply Your Knowledge

Click here to apply your knowledge to practical scenarios.

BEYOND THE BOOK

1. In small groups, discuss some of your own interactions or encounters with infants, toddlers, or young children that seem to support either a nature-inspired, nurture-inspired, or interactionist view of language development.

2. With another classmate, discuss some ways in which professionals incorporate the tenets of nature- and nurture-inspired theories and interactionist theories of language development in their practices.

3. Using ASHA's N-CEP Compendium of EBP Guidelines and Systematic Reviews (http://www.asha.org/members/ebp/compendium), navigate to the systematic reviews in the area of "speech and language," choose a review of interest to you, and summarize the findings of the review for a classmate.

4. Using the Internet, search for a commercially available language-related curriculum, approach, or practice that claims to be research-based. Describe the extent to which the Web site substantiates the claim that the product is research-based.

5. In small groups, discuss some potential challenges a clinical professional might encounter when integrating the needs, values, abilities, preferences, and interests of a child's family with research evidence.

 Check Your Understanding

Gauge your understanding of the chapter concepts by taking this self-check quiz.

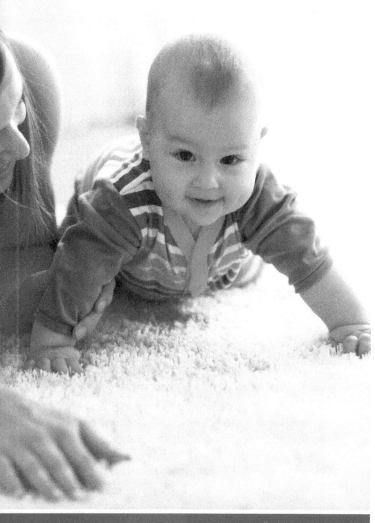

© Alena Ozerova/Fotolia

5

Infancy

Let the Language Achievements Begin

LEARNING OUTCOMES

After completion of this chapter, the reader will be able to:

1. Identify major language-development milestones that occur in infancy.

2. Explain some early foundations for language development.

3. Describe major achievements in language form, content, and use that characterize infancy.

4. Explain factors that contribute to infants' individual language achievements.

5. Describe how researchers and clinicians measure language development in infancy.

The first year of life is packed with spectacular prelinguistic and linguistic developments. Although infants are not yet using their language system productively, their receptive language abilities begin growing by leaps and bounds from the moment they are born. Infants need not waste any of their time maneuvering through traffic jams, preparing dinner, paying bills, walking the dog, or cutting the grass, as their parents do. As a result, they can devote all their waking hours to exploring their environment, engaging in social interactions with other people, and taking in all the sights and sounds surrounding them. In this chapter, we first provide an overview of the major language-development milestones infants achieve during their first year. Such milestones include not only using the prosodic and phonetic regularities of speech to isolate meaningful units from continuous speech, but also gaining the ability to perceive speech sounds in terms of meaningful categories. We also examine infants' awareness of actions and the intentions underlying these actions, their ability to categorize items and events according to perceptual and conceptual features, and their early vocalizations. Second, we discuss some of the early foundations for language development, including infant-directed speech, joint reference and attention, daily routines of infancy, and caregiver responsiveness. In the third section, we describe infants' major achievements in language form, content, and use. In the fourth section, we elucidate some reasons for the intraindividual and interindividual differences among children who are developing language. Finally, fifth, we briefly examine some of the methods researchers and clinicians use to measure language development in infancy.

WHAT MAJOR LANGUAGE-DEVELOPMENT MILESTONES OCCUR IN INFANCY?

Infant Speech Perception

Before infants are ready to speak their first word, they listen attentively to the sounds around them. As you probably know from hearing foreign languages, the speech stream is not divided neatly into words with spaces in the same way many written languages are. For this reason, infants learning language must be able to segment the speech they hear into meaningful phrases and words. Infants are amazingly adept at detecting speech patterns and using these patterns to their advantage as they learn to break continuous speech into smaller units. Infants' *speech perception ability*—their ability to devote attention to the prosodic and phonetic regularities of speech—develops tremendously in the first year as infants move from detecting larger patterns, such as rhythm, to detecting smaller patterns, such as combinations of specific sounds.

Attention to Prosodic Regularities

The prosodic characteristics of speech include the *frequency*, or pitch, of sounds (e.g., a low-pitched hum vs. a high-pitched squeal); the duration, or length, of sounds; and the *intensity*, or loudness, of sounds. Combinations of these prosodic characteristics produce distinguishable stress and intonation patterns that infants can detect. Stress is the prominence placed on certain syllables of multisyllabic words. For example, the first syllable of the word _over_ is stressed, whereas the second syllable of the word *above* is stressed. Intonation, like stress, is the prominence placed on certain syllables, but it also applies to entire phrases and sentences. For instance, compare the patterns you hear in the following two sentences:

"You like sardines."

"Do you like sardines?"

Notice the first sentence, a declarative sentence, ends in a falling intonation, whereas the second sentence, an interrogative, ends in a rising intonation.

How do infants use prosodic regularities to segment the speech stream? One way is by becoming familiar with the dominant stress patterns of their native language. Infants learning English hear many more strong–weak (*over*) stress patterns in bisyllabic words than they hear weak–strong (*above*) stress patterns. By age 9 months, infants learning English prefer to listen to words containing strong–weak stress patterns (Jusczyk, Cutler, & Redanz, 1993). A preference for the dominant stress pattern of their native language can help infants begin to isolate words in continuous speech. For example, infants learning English who hear phrases such as "barking doggie," "smiling baby," or "yellow flower" would be more likely to parse the bisyllabic words within those phrases correctly as barking/doggie, smiling/baby, and yellow/flower and would be less likely to parse the words incorrectly as kingdo, lingba, or llowflo. Coupled with their ability to engage in statistical learning, infants who notice the common stress patterns in their native language learn over time where likely word boundaries occur in running speech.

Attention to Phonetic Regularities

The phonetic details of speech include *phonemes*, or speech sounds, and combinations of phonemes. According to Stager and Werker (1997), infants who are not yet learning words devote much attention to the phonetic details of speech, whereas older children concentrate their efforts on word learning at the expense of fine phonetic detail (but see Yoshida, Fennell, Swingley, & Werker, 2009). Stager and Werker arrived at this conclusion after conducting a series of four creative experiments. In the second experiment of the series, researchers repeatedly presented an object on a television screen, accompanied by the sound "bih," to 8- and 14-month-old infants. Once the infants were accustomed to the object–sound pairing, the researchers tested them using a *switch design*; they presented the original object–sound pairing in half of the test trials and presented the original object paired with a new sound in the other half of the trials using the phonetically similar word "dih." The 14-month-olds did not seem to notice the switch in sound, but the 8-month-olds did: They watched the new pairing for a significantly longer time than they watched the original pairing. Why could the younger infants detect a change the older infants missed? Stager and Werker hypothesized that the 14-month-olds devoted their attention to learning the object name and did not notice the fine sound difference, whereas the 8-month-olds engaged in a simple sound discrimination task and were able to notice the phonetic distinction (Figure 5.1). It is interesting to note that in

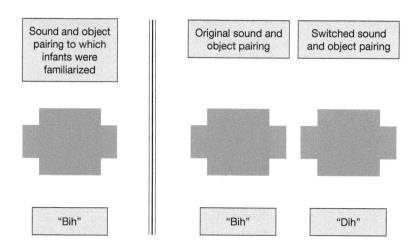

FIGURE 5.1

Illustration of a switch design, similar to the design used in the second experiment of Stager and Werker's (1997) speech perception task.

the third experiment in the series, researchers found when they replaced the phonetically similar words "bih" and "dih" with the phonetically dissimilar words "lif" and "neem," the 14-month-olds noticed the switch in sound. It is also noteworthy that in the fourth experiment in the series, the researchers found if they paired a checkerboard pattern (which infants are unlikely to consider an object that should have a name) with the sound "bih," the 14-month-olds noticed the switch in sound between "bih" and "dih" during the test trials, which indicates they treated this task as a simple sound discrimination task rather than a word learning task. In sum, the researchers concluded that infants listen for more phonetic detail in speech perception tasks than in word learning tasks.

Unlike adults, who are able to group incoming speech sounds into categories that are meaningful in their language, young infants do not yet know which fine-grained sound differences change the meaning of a word. Thus, it is important that they be able to detect even the finest acoustic differences in speech sounds. As infants receive more and more exposure to the phonemes of their native language, they develop categorical perception abilities (which we discuss later in this chapter) that are crucial for speech perception throughout one's life. Categorical perception allows listeners to distinguish between phonemes so they can quickly and efficiently process incoming speech by ignoring those variations that are nonessential or nonmeaningful in their language.

Detection of Nonnative Phonetic Differences.   Infants' ability to notice fine phonetic detail is not limited to their native language. In the first year, they can distinguish among the sounds of all world languages, an ability older children and adults lack. As infants develop and become attuned to the sounds they hear regularly, their ability to distinguish nonnative phonemic contrasts diminishes. For example, up to about 6 months of age, infants learning English can distinguish between two different sounds in the Hindi language that would both sound like "da" to older English-speaking children and adults. Being able to perceive fine phonetic contrasts is crucial, because infants must be prepared to distinguish between sounds that are meaningful in whichever language or languages they encounter regularly in their community.

The process by which infants start to focus more on perceptual differences that are relevant to them (such as the difference between two native phonemes) and focus less on perceptual differences that are not relevant to them, or that they encounter less often (such as the difference between two nonnative phonemes), is called perceptual narrowing. Perceptual narrowing is not limited to speech sounds. In fact, infants experience perceptual narrowing with regard to abilities such as face perception (the ability to discriminate between faces the infant does not encounter regularly) and the perception of musical rhythm (the ability to discriminate between musical rhythms not present in one's culture). Some researchers suggest that because perceptual narrowing occurs over the second half of the first year of life in areas other than the perception of speech sounds, the ability to distinguish nonnative contrasts is likely a domain-general process and not a domain-specific process or one that applies only to language learning (Scott, Pascalis, & Nelson, 2007).

Detection of Phonotactic Regularities.   As infants hear their native language more and more, they also develop the ability to recognize permissible combinations of phonemes in their language, or *phonotactic regularities*. For example, infants acquiring English learn that the combination of sounds /ps/ (as in *maps*) must occur in a syllable-final position and never in a syllable-initial position. They also learn that the /h/ sound (as in *happy*) must begin syllables and never occur in a syllable-final position. Infants' ability to detect phonotactic regularities in their native language helps them segment words from continuous speech (Mattys & Jusczyk, 2001). For instance, in the preceding example, when infants determine that the sequence /ps/ occurs at the end of syllables and words, they can infer the sounds

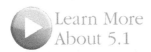

Learn More
About 5.1

As you watch the video titled "Detection of Nonnative Sounds," consider how infants' ability to detect nonnative speech sounds changes across the first year of life. https://www.youtube.com/ watch?v=Ew5-xbc1HMk

From infancy, humans can categorize speech sounds into meaningful categories. Persons who are deaf likewise categorize hand shapes into meaningful categories.

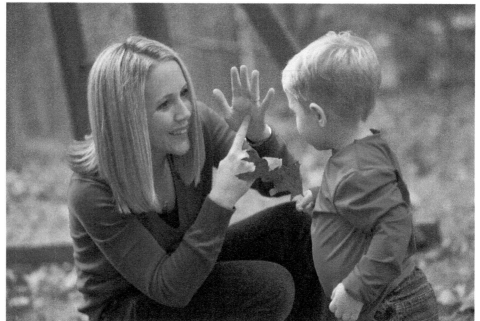

© Huntstock/Getty Images

that precede /**ps**/ are part of the same word and that the sounds following /**ps**/ start a new syllable or word. Infants' ability to differentiate between permissible and impermissible sound sequences in their native language is present by about age 9 months (Jusczyk, Luce, & Charles-Luce, 1994). Some research suggests phonotactic regularities may play a role in later-developing skills, such as word learning, as children seem to learn words with common phonotactic sequences more rapidly than words with rare phonotactic sequences (Storkel, 2001, 2003).

Categorical Perception of Speech

As language users, our perception of speech is *categorical*, which means we categorize input in ways that highlight differences in meaning. Categorical perception is an ability infants develop over the first year of life as they are exposed to language. At a very general level, infants categorize incoming sounds into speech and nonspeech sounds. Then infants learn to categorize speech sounds according to the particular features of the sounds, such as whether the sound is voiced (*doe*) or voiceless (*toe*). Categorical perception of speech sounds allows people to distinguish between sounds in different categories (/p/ vs. /b/), but without special training, people cannot distinguish between variations of sounds within the same category (the first and last /p/ sounds in *pup*). Variations of sounds in the same category, as in the previous example, are called *allophones* of the same phoneme. Allophones of a phoneme are measurably different from one another (such as in the amount of aspiration they contain), but they do not signal a difference in meaning between two words, as phonemes do.

One mechanism humans use to distinguish between sounds in different categories is voice onset time. Voice onset time is the interval between the release of a stop consonant (e.g., *p*, *b*, *t*, *d*) and the onset of vocal cord vibrations. The voice onset time for the sound /b/ is much shorter than that for the sound /p/. This temporal difference helps people distinguish between these two seemingly similar sounds. See Figure 5.2 for an illustration of voice onset time for the phonemes /p/ and /b/. The arrows to the left on the diagrams indicate the point at which the consonant is released, whereas the arrows to the right indicate the point at which the vocal cords begin to vibrate. Notice the wider space between the arrows for the consonant *p*, which reflects the longer voice onset time.

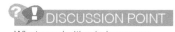

DISCUSSION POINT

What regularities in language might you rely on when studying a foreign language (as an adult) to isolate meaningful units from continuous speech?

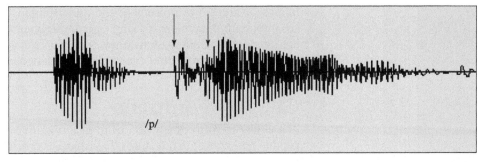

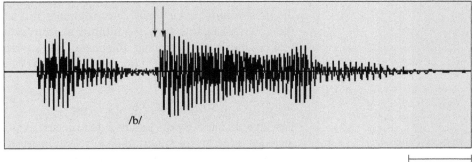

100 ms

FIGURE 5.2
Voice onset time for the consonant sounds /p/ and /b/.

As mentioned previously, infants are equipped with the ability to categorize speech sounds that are and are not a part of the repertoire of their native language. This ability also holds for hand shapes in American Sign Language (S. A. Baker, Idsardi, Golinkoff, & Petitto, 2005). Subsequently in this chapter, we discuss the impact of category formation abilities on language development in more detail.

Awareness of Actions and Intentions

? ! DISCUSSION POINT

Consider the verbs *to chase* and *to flee*. How might an understanding of the goals underlying the actions help an infant distinguish between the two?

Although infants are far less mobile than their toddler counterparts, they are sensitive to actions and movement surrounding them. By age 4 months, infants can distinguish between purposeful and accidental actions, and they appear to focus on the intentions underlying actions rather than the physical details of the actions (Woodward & Hoyne, 1999).

Over the first year, infants learn to view human actions as goal-directed, meaning they pay attention to the outcomes and objects to which humans direct their actions rather than to other superficial perceptual properties of the event. For example, Woodward (1998) familiarized 9-month-old infants with a human hand reaching and grasping one of two toys sitting side by side on a curtained stage (e.g., the actor might repeatedly reach for and grasp a dog on the left side of the stage and not reach for or grab a ball on the right side of the stage). After the infants were familiar with the reaching and grasping event, researchers switched the position of the toys (e.g., the dog was moved to the right side of the stage and the ball was moved to the left side). The infants then watched a series of test events. In the new goal/old path event, infants saw the actor grasp the other toy by taking the same path as before across the stage (e.g., the actor reached for and grasped the ball [new goal] on the left side of the stage [old path]). In the old goal/new path, infants saw the actor grasp the same toy as before by taking a new path (e.g., the actor reached for and grasped the dog [old goal] on the right side of the stage [new path]). During the test trials, infants looked longer at the switch in goal than the switch in path, indicating they were sensitive to the goal directedness of another human's actions.

Infants' awareness of movement and understanding of the goals underlying actions are important precursors for language development because once they understand the intentions behind actions, they, too, can engage in intentional communication by pointing, gesturing, and eventually using language.

Category Formation

The ability to form categories, or to group items and events according to the perceptual and conceptual features they share, is crucial for language development. In fact, this prelinguistic ability is one of the earliest to develop and perhaps one of the most robust predictors of later cognitive and linguistic outcomes. For example, the ability of infants ages 3–9 months to form categories predicts both their general cognitive and language abilities at age 2 years (Colombo, Shaddy, Richman, Maikranz, & Blaga, 2004) and their cognitive outcomes at age 2.5 years (Laucht, Esser, & Schmidt, 1995).

Hierarchical Structure of Categories

Research results support the idea that object category formation is hierarchical and includes three levels: superordinate, subordinate, and basic (Figure 5.3). The *superordinate level* is the uppermost level in a category hierarchy. Superordinate terms describe the most general concept in a particular category and include words such as *food*, *furniture*, and *clothing*. Superordinate terms are among the later words children acquire. Children cannot successfully categorize words at the superordinate level until preschool age unless they have multiple exemplars on which to base their judgment about the appropriate superordinate category (Liu, Golinkoff, & Sak, 2001). For example, to understand grapes are part of the category *fruit*, the child would need to see that other fruits (e.g., oranges, bananas) are part of the same category.

The *subordinate level* is the lowest level in a category hierarchy. Subordinate terms describe specific concepts in a category. For example, *garbanzo*, *pinto*, and *kidney* are subordinate terms for different types of beans.

The *basic level* lies in the center of a category hierarchy. Basic-level terms describe general concepts in a category, including words such as *apple*, *chair*, and *shirt*. Infants' first categories are basic-level categories, just as their first words are basic-level words (Mervis & Crisafi, 1982).

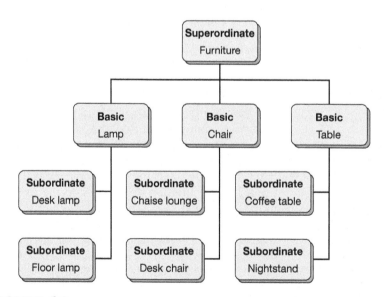

FIGURE 5.3

Hierarchical structure of categories.

Basic Categories at Each Hierarchical Level

In addition to using the hierarchical structure of categories to learn new concepts and words, infants use two types of categories at each level of the hierarchy: perceptual categories and conceptual categories (Mandler, 2000).

Perceptual Categories.   Infants form perceptual categories on the basis of similar-appearing features, including color, shape, texture, size, and so forth. They use perceptual categories to recognize and identify objects around them. Infants begin to form perceptual categories at a very young age: By age 3 months they can distinguish between cats and dogs (Quinn, Eimas, & Rosenkrantz, 1993), and by age 4 months they can distinguish between animals and furniture (Behl-Chadha, 1996).

Conceptual Categories.   Whereas perceptual categorization involves knowing what an object looks like, conceptual categorization requires infants to know what an object does (Mandler, 2000). Infants learn that balls roll, dogs bark, and airplanes fly. When infants have conceptual categories, they can use these categories to make inductive generalizations about new objects without relying on perceptual similarity. For example, suppose you show an infant who has never seen a penguin, both a real penguin and a toy penguin. Although the toy penguin may look much like the real penguin, infants having conceptual category formation abilities would make inferences about the real penguin on the basis of their knowledge about other live animals. Likewise, they would understand the toy penguin in terms of other toys they already know about. They would probably not be surprised to see the real penguin move around, eat, and interact with other penguins, but they would not expect the toy penguin to do such things simply because it looks like the real penguin.

As mentioned previously, children begin to categorize language aspects at a very young age. However, because the many global languages categorize language concepts differently, children learning different languages may perceive the world in different ways (see Language Diversity and Differences: *Concept Categorization Among Languages*).

Early Vocalizations

To this point, we have discussed several milestones of infancy that might go unrecognized without close inspection. No one sees infants processing speech sounds or directly witnesses their category formation abilities at work. Next, however, we discuss some of the more obvious prelinguistic milestones infants achieve during the first year—namely, their early vocalizations. By 5 months of age, infants learn that their noncry vocalizations elicit reactions from social partners, and such responsiveness on the part of caregivers facilitates infants' development of phonology and speech and further promotes their social interactional abilities (Goldstein, Schwade, & Bornstein, 2009).

Infants follow a fairly predictable pattern in their early use of *vocalizations*. Researchers who study early vocalizations often classify these sounds according to a *stage model*, which means they describe infants' vocalizations as following an observable and sequential pattern. One such stage model is the Stark Assessment of Early Vocal Development—Revised (SAEVD-R; Nathani, Ertmer, & Stark, 2006), which parents, researchers, and clinicians can use to classify vocalizations and assess an infant's oral communication abilities. The SAEVD-R includes 23 types of vocalizations grouped into five distinct developmental levels:

1.   *Reflexive (0–2 months).* The first sounds infants produce are called *reflexive sounds*, which include sounds of discomfort and distress (crying, fussing) and vegetative sounds such as burping, coughing, and sneezing. Although infants have no control over the reflexive sounds they produce, adults often respond as if reflexes

LANGUAGE DIVERSITY AND DIFFERENCES

Concept Categorization Among Languages

Cultures do not necessarily represent concepts in the same way. As a result, languages may differ in how they label concepts with words. From a very early age, infants become aware of how their native language represents concepts. Consider the following example of how different languages label concepts differently.

The English language distinguishes between actions that characterize *containment*, or "put in," relationships and those that characterize *support*, or "put on," relationships. In contrast, the Korean language distinguishes between *tight-fit* (*kkita*) relationships and *loose-fit or contact* relationships; English does not represent this distinction (Choi, McDonough, Bowerman, & Mandler, 1999). Children become sensitive to these language-specific spatial categories by age

18–23 months. For instance, when Korean-learning infants see an event in which a book is placed *in* a tightly fitting box, and an event in which rings are placed tightly *on* a pole, they classify these events similarly (as they are both tight-fit relationships). Korean speakers would use the word *kkita* to describe both of these situations. However, English-learning infants classify these events differently because they perceive one event to represent a containment relationship and the other a support relationship. English speakers would use the phrase "put in" to describe the first situation and the phrase "put on" to describe the second situation.

As another example, when English-learning infants see an event in which an apple is placed in a

The English term "put in" describes containment relationships, such as the following:

apple in bowl*   finger in ring**
cigarette in mouth*   pen into its top**
toys in box*   hand in glove**
books in bag*   cassette in case**
bottle in refrigerator*   piece in puzzle**
                            thread into beads**

*Korean speakers would not classify such relationships in a similar way and they would use various verbs to label the situations rather than a single phrase, such as "put in".

**Korean speakers would classify such relationships as tight-fit and they would use the word *kkita* to label the situations.

English = put in

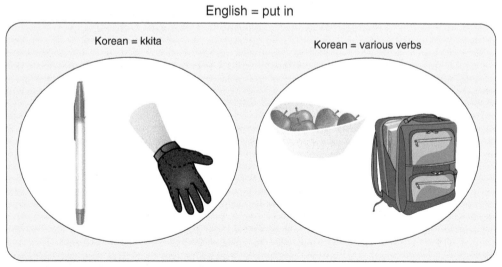

bowl, and an event in which a hand is placed in a glove, they classify these events similarly (as both represent containment) and would use the phrase "put in" to describe both situations. However, Korean-learning infants classify these events differently because they perceive the first event as a loose-fit relationship and the second event as a tight-fit relationship (Korean speakers would use the word *kkita* to describe the second event, but not the first).

Therefore, this example suggests that language guides children from a young age as they perceive the spatial relationships around them. Bowerman and Choi (2003) call this the *language as category maker hypothesis*, as the language one learns (and the way it refers to and differentiates categories) influences the categories one forms. Interestingly, 18-month-old infants learning English can form abstract categories (such as tight-fit) after they view multiple examples of the category in conjunction with a verbal label (Casasola, Bhagwat, & Burke, 2009), which lends further support to the language as category maker hypothesis.

The English term "put on" describes support relationships, such as the following:

ring on finger*	cup on table**
top on pen*	loose-fitting ring on pole**
tight-fitting ring on pole*	hat on**
Lego piece onto Lego stack*	coat on**
glove on*	magnet on refrigerator**
bracelet on*	shoes on**

* Korean speakers would classify such relationships as tight-fit and they would use the word *kkita* to label the situations.

**Korean speakers would not classify such relationships in a similar way and they would use various verbs to label the situations rather than a single phrase, such as "put on".

English = put on

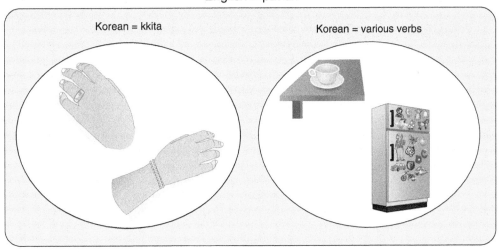

Korean = kkita   Korean = various verbs

Source: Cognitive Development, Vol. 14, S. Choi, L. McDonough, M. Bowerman, and J. M. Mandler, "Early Sensitivity to Language-Specific Spatial Categories in English and Korean," p. 248, Copyright 1999.

DISCUSSION POINT

What is another example of a task researchers might use to determine how infants who are learning different languages (e.g., English vs. Arabic) perceive spatial categories?

are true communication attempts. Parents ascribe communicative functions to even the earliest of infants' vocalizations (C. L. Miller, 1988). They ask infants questions such as "Why so much fussing?" to engage them in dialogue. Parents may even interpret infants' reflexive sounds out loud for them: "Oh, you're saying you want Mommy to hold you, aren't you?" Compared with nonparents, parents are usually more sensitive to infants' reflexive sounds and distress calls and report that they

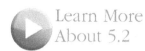

Learn More About 5.2

As you watch the video titled "Stage 1 – Reflexive Sounds," listen for the number of different sounds the newborn makes while stretching and moving around.

http://www.youtube.com/watch?v=VBooggBCKbI

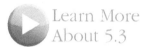

Learn More About 5.3

As you watch the video titled "Stage 2 – Control of Phonation," listen for the vowel-like sounds this 3-month-old makes (such as "ayeah" and "eeey") and the combinations of a consonant-like sound with a vowel-like sound (such as "geee" and "goo").

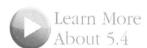

Learn More About 5.4

As you watch the video titled "Stage 3 – Expansion," listen for the vowel-like sounds and squeals the infant makes while interacting with his parents.

http://www.youtube.com/watch?v=VeV2Cq9BrsA

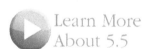

Learn More About 5.5

As you watch the video titled "Stage 4 – Basic Canonical Syllables," listen for reduplicated babbling (such as "ba-ba-ba") and variegated babbling (such as "ga-da-ba") as he interacts with his father.

http://www.youtube.com/watch?v=S8I200dIIIg

base their judgments about an infant's distress level on information they gain from the crying infant's face and voice (Irwin, 2003).

2. *Control of phonation (1–4 months)*. In the control of phonation stage, infants begin to produce *cooing* and *gooing* sounds. Such sounds consist mainly of vowel-like sounds (sounds that approximate vowels but would not be transcribed as adult vowels). Infants in this stage might also combine vowel-like segments with a consonant-like segment (e.g., "aaam"). Other sounds in the control of phonation stage include isolated consonant sounds such as *nasalized* sounds (i.e., airflow is directed through the nose), as well as "raspberries," trills, and clicks. When infants produce consonant-like sounds, they typically do so far back in the oral cavity (e.g., "goooo"). These early consonant sounds are easier for infants to produce than are sounds that require more precise manipulation of the tongue, lips, or teeth (e.g., /t/ and /f/).

3. *Expansion (3–8 months)*. In the expansion stage, infants gain more control over the articulators and begin to produce isolated vowel sounds (those that would be transcribed as adult vowels), as well as *vowel glides* (e.g., "eeeey"). Infants also experiment with the loudness and pitch of their voices at this time, and they may squeal or produce a series of squeals. During this stage, infants may also use marginal babbling, an early type of babbling containing consonant-like and vowel-like sounds with prolonged transitions between the consonant and vowel sounds.

4. *Basic canonical syllables (5–10 months)*. In this stage, infants begin to produce single consonant-vowel (C-V) syllables (e.g., "ba," "goo"). Canonical babbling also emerges in this stage, and it differs from earlier vocalizations in that the infant produces more than two C-V syllables in sequence. Babbling may be reduplicated or nonreduplicated. Reduplicated babbling consists of repeating C-V pairs, as in "ma ma ma," whereas nonreduplicated babbling (or variegated babbling) consists of nonrepeating C-V combinations, such as "da ma goo ga." In many cultures, infants prefer nasal sounds (/m/, /n/, and the final sound in *sing*) and stop sounds (/p/, /b/, /t/, /d/) in their variegated babbling (Locke, 1983), combining such sounds variously with vowels to produce long vocalized sequences. Infants in this stage also produce *whispered vocalizations*, C-V combinations followed by an isolated consonant ("ba—g") and disyllables, which consist of two C-V syllables separated by an audible gap (ba—ba). Often, parents view their children as beginning to talk when the children begin to babble because such syllable combinations resemble adult speech.

Hearing infants are not the only babies to babble. Infants who are deaf, as well as infants who hear but have parents who are profoundly deaf, babble manually—using their hands. Just as the vocalizations of infants who hear speech mimic the specific rhythmic patterns that bind syllables, so do the hand movements of babies born to parents who are deaf. These infants' hand movements have a slower rhythm than that of ordinary gestures, and the infants produce these movements within a tightly restricted space in front of the body (Petitto, Holowka, Sergio, & Ostry, 2001).

5. *Advanced forms (9–18 months)*. In the more advanced stage of early vocalizations, infants begin to produce *diphthongs*, which are combinations of two vowel sounds within the same syllable, as in the combination of sounds in *boy* and the combination of sounds in *fine*. Infants also begin to produce more complex syllable forms, including single-syllable types such as V–C ("am") and C–C–V ("stee"), complex disyllables such as V–C–V ("abu"), and multisyllabic strings with and without varied stress intonation patterns ("odago"). Probably the most noticeable achievement in the advanced forms stage is jargon. Jargon is a special type of babbling containing at least two syllables and at least two different consonants and vowels, as well as varied stress or intonation patterns. Because infants using jargon incorporate stress and intonation patterns, you may think you are hearing questions, exclamations, and commands, even in the absence of recognizable words.

DEVELOPMENTAL TIMELINE

PHONOLOGY

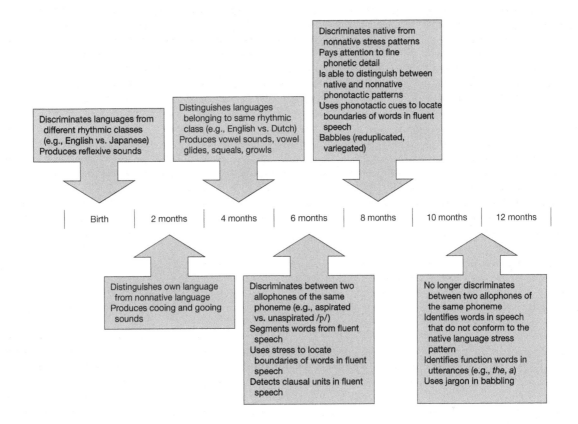

Discriminates languages from different rhythmic classes (e.g., English vs. Japanese)
Produces reflexive sounds

Distinguishes languages belonging to same rhythmic class (e.g., English vs. Dutch)
Produces vowel sounds, vowel glides, squeals, growls

Discriminates native from nonnative stress patterns
Pays attention to fine phonetic detail
Is able to distinguish between native and nonnative phonotactic patterns
Uses phonotactic cues to locate boundaries of words in fluent speech
Babbles (reduplicated, variegated)

Birth | 2 months | 4 months | 6 months | 8 months | 10 months | 12 months

Distinguishes own language from nonnative language
Produces cooing and gooing sounds

Discriminates between two allophones of the same phoneme (e.g., aspirated vs. unaspirated /p/)
Segments words from fluent speech
Uses stress to locate boundaries of words in fluent speech
Detects clausal units in fluent speech

No longer discriminates between two allophones of the same phoneme
Identifies words in speech that do not conform to the native language stress pattern
Identifies function words in utterances (e.g., *the, a*)
Uses jargon in babbling

SEMANTICS

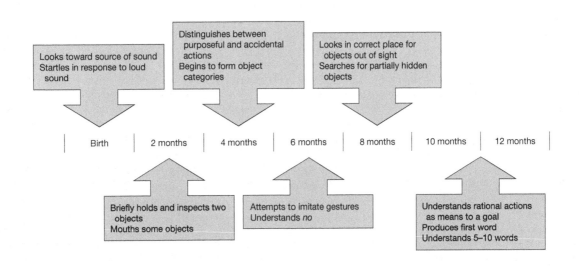

Looks toward source of sound
Startles in response to loud sound

Distinguishes between purposeful and accidental actions
Begins to form object categories

Looks in correct place for objects out of sight
Searches for partially hidden objects

Birth | 2 months | 4 months | 6 months | 8 months | 10 months | 12 months

Briefly holds and inspects two objects
Mouths some objects

Attempts to imitate gestures
Understands *no*

Understands rational actions as means to a goal
Produces first word
Understands 5–10 words

PRAGMATICS

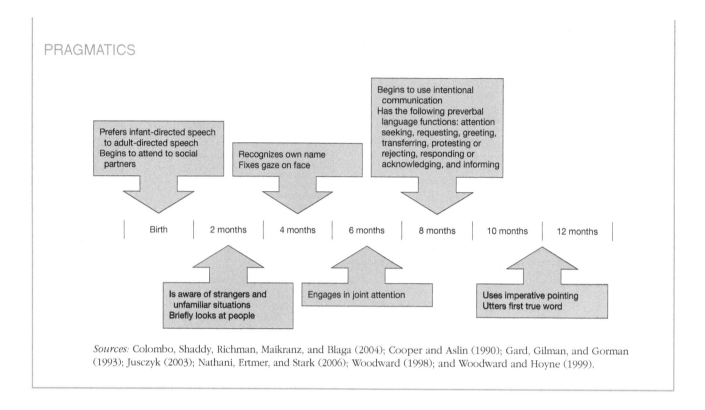

Sources: Colombo, Shaddy, Richman, Maikranz, and Blaga (2004); Cooper and Aslin (1990); Gard, Gilman, and Gorman (1993); Jusczyk (2003); Nathani, Ertmer, and Stark (2006); Woodward (1998); and Woodward and Hoyne (1999).

Although the vocalizations infants produce while they are babbling or using jargon may sound like short words or syllables, such vocalizations are not considered true words because they are not referential, nor do they convey meaning. Rather, at this stage, infants are still experimenting with the sounds of their native language.

Additional Milestones

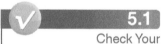

5.1
Check Your Understanding
Click here to gauge your understanding of the concepts in this section.

As you can see, infants reach many important milestones during the first year on their journey through language development. As we described in the sections on speech perception, awareness of actions and intentions, category formation, and early vocalizations, these milestones involve a series of *incremental* developments in the first year rather than all-or-nothing capabilities. See this chapter's Developmental Timeline for even more milestones infants reach with regard to phonology, semantics, and pragmatics.

WHAT ARE SOME OF THE EARLY FOUNDATIONS FOR LANGUAGE DEVELOPMENT?

During infancy, the quality and quantity of the input infants receive, as well as the types of social interactions in which they engage, form important early foundations for language development. Some of the foundations that pave the way for later language development are infant-directed speech, joint reference and attention, the daily routines of infancy, and caregiver responsiveness. As you read this section, consider the language-development theories you learned about in Chapter 4. Note that these early foundations for language development presuppose the importance of the environment in language development. They are also contingent on the linguistic input adults provide and the social interactions infants engage in with other people. As such, these factors are central to nurture-inspired and interactionist theories of language development.

Infant-Directed Speech

Infant-directed speech (IDS)—also called *motherese* and *baby talk*—is the speech adults use in communicative situations with young language learners. IDS falls within the broader umbrella of child-directed speech (CDS) that we discussed in Chapter 2, but it specifies that the recipient of speech is an infant. IDS has several distinctive paralinguistic, syntactic, and discourse characteristics. In fact, IDS is distinguishable from CDS, meaning adults talk differently to infants than they do to older children (Saxton, 2008). Paralinguistic features of IDS, or those that describe the manner of speech outside the linguistic information, include a high overall pitch, exaggerated pitch contours, and slower tempos than those of adult-directed speech (ADS; Snow 1972). *Syntactic* characteristics of IDS include a shorter mean length of utterance (MLU), or the number of morphemes in an utterance; fewer subordinate clauses; and more content words and fewer function words. *Discourse* features of IDS include more repetition and more questions than in ADS. See Table 5.1 for a comparison of the paralinguistic, syntactic, and discourse features of IDS and ADS.

Besides having distinctive characteristics, IDS appears to serve a host of special purposes. It attracts infants' attention, and infants, including those with hearing

TABLE 5.1

Comparison of infant-directed and adult-directed speech

FEATURES	INFANT-DIRECTED SPEECH (IDS) EXAMPLES	ADULT-DIRECTED SPEECH (ADS) EXAMPLES
Paralinguistic features High overall pitch Exaggerated pitch contours Slower tempos		
Syntactic features		
Shorter MLU	"You want potatoes?"	"Would you like mashed potatoes with your meal?"
Fewer subordinate clauses	"I brought you a gift. Grandmom brought you a gift. Grandpop brought you a gift."	"I brought you a gift and Grandmom and Grandpop did, too."
More content words and fewer function words	"See bike?"	"Do you see that bike on the sidewalk?"
Discourse features		
More repetition	"Let's look at the book. Should we open the book? You like books?"	"I'd like to read that book."
More questions	"Is that Daddy? Is that Daddy over there?"	"Hey, there's your friend from work."

loss, prefer it to ADS (Cooper & Aslin, 1990; Fernald & Kuhl, 1987; Robertson, von Hapsburg, & Hay, 2013). IDS also aids in communicating emotion and speakers' communicative intent (Fernald, 1989; Trainor & Desjardins, 2002). Researchers have documented paralinguistic modifications, thought to capture and maintain infants' attention, in several languages other than American English, including German (Fernald & Simon, 1984); French, Italian, Japanese, and British English (Fernald et al., 1989); and Mandarin Chinese (Papousek, Papousek, & Symmes, 1991). Examinations of these languages reveal that adults may universally modify the prosody (i.e., stress and rhythm) of their speech to infants (but see Bernstein Ratner & Pye, 1984).

With respect to language development, IDS contains exaggerated vowels, which may facilitate infants' processing of words containing these vowels in fluent speech (Burnham, Kitamura, & Vollmer-Conna, 2002). IDS also highlights content words, such as nouns and verbs, relative to function words, such as prepositions and articles (van de Weijer, 2001), and places these words on exaggerated pitch peaks at the ends of utterances, where infants are likely to remember them (Fernald & Mazzie, 1991). Moreover, IDS exaggerates pauses, which creates a salient cue to help infants detect major syntactic units in speech (Bernstein Ratner, 1986). The rhythm of IDS is marked by the presence of reliable acoustic correlates of both utterance and phrase boundaries in other languages as well (e.g., Japanese; Fisher & Tokura, 1996), and in the speech to infants who are profoundly deaf with a cochlear implant (Kondaurova & Bergeson, 2011). At the very least, using IDS to introduce new words and phrases should capture infants' attention and increase the chance that they will focus on the speech they hear.

Joint Reference and Attention

Recall from Chapter 4, Vygotsky's social interactionist perspective on language development. According to Vygotsky, language development is a dynamic process that occurs within children's zone of proximal development (ZPD) as they interact socially with more advanced peers and adults. Adamson and Chance's (1998) account of infants' language development through social interactions also takes a social interactionist approach. These researchers proposed that infancy comprises three major developmental phases with respect to joint reference and attention (Figure 5.4):

Phase 1: Attendance to social partners

Phase 2: Emergence and coordination of joint attention

Phase 3: Transition to language

In each phase, adults view infants' interactions as meaningful through the lens of their culture. Furthermore, adults support infants' expressions in each phase until infants can independently master components of the social exchange.

Phase 1: Attendance to Social Partners (Birth to Age 6 Months)

In the first phase, from birth to about age 6 months, infants develop patterns of attending to social partners. In these early months of life, infants value and participate in interpersonal interactions, learning how to maintain attention and be "organized" within sustained periods of engagement. Infants are especially interested in looking at people's faces during this phase, in particular their parents' faces. Caregiver responsiveness, which we discuss later in this chapter, is an important feature of this first phase.

From birth, infants demonstrate spontaneous expressiveness with their heads, body, and limbs to connect with other humans and over the first six months, they engage in rituals of body movement and joint intention with others. Infants also react to the emotional support others provide, as well as to others' reactions to their actions (Trevarthen, 2011; Trevarthen & Aitken, 2001).

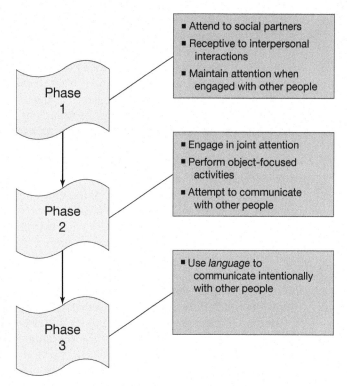

- Attend to social partners
- Receptive to interpersonal interactions
- Maintain attention when engaged with other people

Phase 1

- Engage in joint attention
- Perform object-focused activities
- Attempt to communicate with other people

Phase 2

- Use *language* to communicate intentionally with other people

Phase 3

FIGURE 5.4

Adamson and Chance's (1998) three phases of language development through social interactions.

Phase 2: Emergence and Coordination of Joint Attention (Age 6 Months to 1 Year)

In the second phase, from approximately 6 months of age to 1 year, infants begin to take more interest in looking at and manipulating the objects around them. During this phase, infants begin to shift their attention between an object of interest and another person (Adamson & Chance, 1998). This activity signals the emergence of joint attention, a concept we introduced in Chapter 2. To review, *joint attention* is the simultaneous engagement of two or more individuals in mental focus on a single external object of attention. For example, when a mother shakes a toy in front of her infant and he or she looks at it, mother and infant are engaging in joint attention with respect to the toy. When parents read storybooks to their children and they look at the pictures together, they are also engaging in joint attention. This seemingly simple activity provides a critical avenue for early communication development because periods of joint attention foster important communicative exchanges (Adamson, Bakeman, & Deckner, 2004). In fact, children who engage in longer periods of joint attention with their caregivers have relatively larger vocabularies at age 18 months than those of children with fewer such experiences (Tomasello & Todd, 1983).

Often, caregivers share much of the burden of sustaining the infant's participation throughout periods of joint attention. Adults may use such techniques as speaking with an animated voice or showing the infant novel objects as they engage in what is called supported joint engagement. The extent to which mothers use strategies to *maintain* their infant's attention is related to an infant's ability to engage in sustained attention at age 18 months. Conversely, the extent to which mothers consistently use strategies to *redirect* their infant's attention is negatively related to an infant's ability to engage in sustained attention (Bono & Stifter, 2003; J. L. Miller, Ables, King, & West, 2009). Caregivers have a greater likelihood of maintaining an infant's attention when they follow the infant's attentional focus as compared to when they redirect the infant's attentional focus. For example, if an infant is touching the family's pet dog, a caregiver following the infant's attentional focus might say something like "I like how you are petting the dog softly and gently," whereas a caregiver redirecting the infant's focus (away from the dog) might say something like "Look at this red toy car. Don't you want to play with the car?"

Why is joint attention so important? In the absence of joint attention, infants may miss out on word-learning opportunities as their parents and caregivers label objects and events for them. Imagine a scenario in which a mother is pushing her infant son in a stroller. As she points upward, she says, "Look at the birdie." Suppose the infant misses his mother's pointing gesture and hears the word *birdie* while he is carefully studying his new shoes. In this situation, the mother and her son are not jointly attending to the same entity in the world, so the baby boy will probably not learn what the word *birdie* refers to. In the worst-case scenario, the boy might associate the word *birdie* with his new shoes. However, infants soon become adept at using cues—including line of regard (the direction of a person's gaze, which indicates what the person is looking at), gestures (e.g., pointing), voice direction, and body posture—to support inferences about a speaker's referential intentions, and they learn not to associate the words they hear with the objects and events on which only they are focused (Baldwin, 1991).

Before infants can use cues to infer another person's intentions, they must possess intersubjective awareness, or the recognition of when one person shares a mental focus on some external object or action with another person (Note that intersubjective awareness differs from theory of mind (ToM), which describes the ability to understand one's own mental or emotional state, to understand that others also have mental or emotional states, and to realize that others' mental and emotional states, beliefs, intentions, and perspectives differ from one's own. We describe ToM and its relation to language development in more detail in subsequent chapters). Only after infants realize they can share a mental focus with other humans do they begin to interpret other people's referential actions as intentional and begin to use their own actions referentially. This skill is called *intentional communication*, or the infants' attempts to deliberately communicate with other people. Researchers who study intentional communication have devised some guidelines to determine whether infants' communicative behaviors are preintentional or intentional. Indicators of intentionality include the following: The infant alternates eye gaze between an object and a communicative partner; the infant uses ritualized gestures, such as pointing; and the infant persists toward goals by repeating or modifying his or her gestures when communicative attempts fail (Bates, Camaioni, & Volterra, 1975). Intentional communication begins to emerge around age 8–10 months. To illustrate, picture a mother bathing her infant daughter, Fumiyo, in the bathtub with several toys floating about. To show her mother she is interested in the rubber duck that is beyond her reach, Fumiyo might look at her mother, then at the duck, then back at her mother again. If Fumiyo's mother does not retrieve the duck, Fumiyo might then establish eye contact with her mother and then point at the duck. If Fumiyo's mother still does not retrieve the duck after she has tried alternating gaze between her mother and the duck and pointing at the duck, Fumiyo might then kick her feet while pointing at the duck as a way to make her request even clearer.

An interesting fact is that infants are skilled in using multiple forms of pointing. They use imperative pointing as requests to adults to retrieve objects for them. They begin to use this type of pointing at around age 10 months, for example, when they want someone to bring them a toy that is out of reach. Declarative pointing involves a social process between an infant and an adult. Infants use declarative pointing to call an adult's attention to objects and to comment on objects. Research results indicate that children produce and understand declarative pointing later than imperative pointing. Furthermore, infants' production of declarative pointing, but not imperative pointing, is linked to their understanding of other people's intentions (Camaioni, Perucchini, Bellagamba, & Colonnesi, 2004).

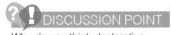
DISCUSSION POINT

Why do you think declarative pointing is more challenging for infants than imperative pointing is? How could declarative pointing relate to understanding other people's intentions?

Infants' production of declarative pointing to call attention to and comment on objects is linked to their understanding of other people's intentions.

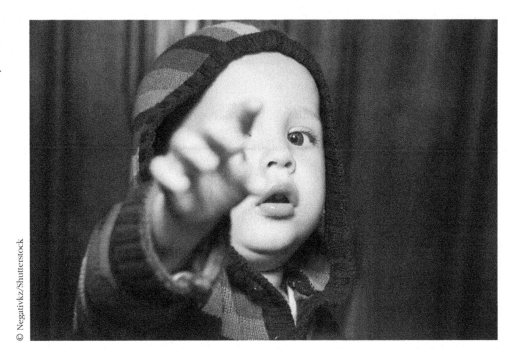

© Negativkz/Shutterstock

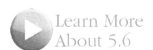

Learn More About 5.6

As you watch the video titled "The Still Face Experiment," consider what happens when the mother uses a still face and does not respond to her infant and what this indicates about an infant's expectations for social interaction.

https://www.youtube.com/watch?v=apzXGEbZht0

During this period between about six months and one year of age, infants demonstrate sensitivity to the identity and emotions of others who engage with them. For example, they may show a teasing happiness with familiar playmates, shyness toward strangers, and distress when others do not engage with them as expected (Trevarthen, 2011; Trevarthen & Aitken, 2001).

Phase 3: Transition to Language (Age 1 Year and Beyond)

In the third phase of the development of language through social interactions, children begin to incorporate language into their communicative interactions with other people. Having joint attention and an understanding of intentionality well established, infants in this phase shift to engage socially with other individuals and use language to represent events and objects within these interactions. The active involvement of parents and other adults is still important during this phase. Mothers' verbal encouragement of infants' attention at age 1 year is positively related to infants' language development at that age (Karrass, Braungart-Rieker, Mullins, & Lefever, 2002).

Given the importance of joint attention to infants' and young children's developing language abilities, more and more research is examining the implications of young children's interactions with electronic media, such as television and videos, smart phones and tablets. See Theory to Practice: *Language Development and Electronic Media* for a description of research investigating young children's experiences with electronic media.

Daily Routines of Infancy

Infants' daily lives consist of several routines that provide a sense of comfort and predictability. As a bonus, these seemingly dull routines, such as feeding, bathing, dressing, and diaper changing, provide many opportunities for language learning. Consider a scenario in which a father is feeding his infant. During this routine, caregivers often provide a commentary for their infants similar to that of sports commentators when they talk during baseball or football games. Babies hear such things as "Okay, open wide. Here comes your applesauce." "Oops, we got a little dribble

THEORY TO PRACTICE

Language Development and Electronic Media

Considering the ubiquitous nature of television and handheld electronic devices in our daily lives, it is important to consider the implications language-development theories and research pose concerning the potential effects of electronic media on infants and young children. Research findings to this effect have been making their way into national headlines, such as the following from the *Washington Post* on October 24, 2014, "Is you child under age 2? Keep them away from smartphones, tablets and computers" (Kucirkova, 2014), and the following from the *New York Times* on October 11, 2014, "Is e-reading to your toddler story time, or simply screen time?" (Quenqua, 2014).

In 1999, The American Academy of Pediatrics (AAP) published a policy statement discouraging electronic media use by children under the age of 2. At that time, media use included televisions, videos, and DVDs. The AAP warns against screen time, especially in households with children under the age of 2, because it can harm children's cognitive functioning and social play (American Academy of Pediatrics, 2012).

Since the AAP's 1999 press release, there is an even greater array of electronic media to which infants and young children might be exposed, including smart phones and tablets. Are these forms of media somehow different from televisions, videos, and DVDs when considering the risks and benefits to infants and young children? The AAP reports that children spend an average of 7 hours per day using entertainment media, including TVs, computers, phones, and other electronic devices, and recommend that television and other entertainment media be avoided for infants and children under age 2, as young children learn best by interacting with people, not screens (American Academy of Pediatrics, 2014). However, parents may wonder about using electronic media that appear or claim to have educational value, including electronic storybooks.

Research from Parish-Morris, Mahajan, Hirsh-Pasek, Golinkoff, and Collins (2013) revealed striking differences between young children's interactions with storybooks with and without electronic features. In the study, parents of children ages 3 to 5 years asked more story-related questions when reading books without electronic features, and both parents and children used more behavior-related speech and less story-related speech when reading books with electronic features. Moreover, 3-year-olds who read books without electronic features were significantly better at remembering the content and sequence of story events than their counterparts who read books with electronic features. Parish-Morris et al. suggest the types of interactions associated with better reading outcomes are more common with traditional books than books with electronic features. They also suggest that if parents have limited time for storybook reading, they can provide richer input by reading a book without electronic features.

there." "Wow, you ate the whole jar!" Although infants are too young to feed themselves, they benefit from hearing the same words and phrases repeated each day as their parents feed them. Infants are adept at identifying and making sense of the patterns they hear in speech. By hearing words and phrases repeatedly, infants become attuned to where pauses occur, which helps them to segment phrases, clauses, and eventually words from the speech stream. They also learn about phonotactics, or the combinations of sounds that are acceptable in their native language. Routines allow infants not only to encounter numerous linguistic patterns but also to have many opportunities to engage in episodes of joint attention with their caregivers.

Caregiver Responsiveness

Caregiver responsiveness describes caregivers' attention and sensitivity to infants' vocalizations and communicative attempts. Caregiver responsiveness helps teach infants that other people value their behaviors and communicative attempts. Caregivers who provide consistent, contingent, and appropriate responses to their infants' communicative attempts promote their children's ability and desire to sustain long periods of joint attention and increase their children's motivation to communicate. Research results show that mothers demonstrate remarkable consistency in identifying their infants' communicative acts during the second half of the first year (Meadows, Elias, & Bain, 2000), which may in turn promote even higher levels of responsiveness.

Both the quality and the quantity of responsiveness by caregivers play a large role in early language development. More responsive maternal language input is linked—even more so than infants' own early communicative behaviors, such as vocalizations—to the time at which infants reach important language milestones, including saying their first word and producing two-word utterances (Tamis-LeMonda, Bornstein, & Baumwell, 2001).

Weitzman and Greenberg (2002) described the following seven characteristics as key indicators of caregiver responsiveness. These indicators have been linked to improved rates of language development in young children (e.g., Girolametto & Weitzman, 2002):

1. *Waiting and listening.* Parents wait expectantly for initiations, use a slow pace to allow for initiations, and listen to allow the child to complete messages.

2. *Following the child's lead.* When a child initiates either verbally or nonverbally, parents follow the child's lead by responding verbally to the initiation, using animation, and avoiding vague acknowledgments.

3. *Joining in and playing.* Parents build on their child's focus of interest and play without dominating.

4. *Being face-to-face.* Parents adjust their physical level by sitting on the floor, leaning forward to facilitate face-to-face interaction, and bending toward the child when they are above the child's level.

5. *Using a variety of questions and labels.* Parents encourage conversation by asking a variety of *wh-* questions (e.g., "Who?" "Where?" "Why?"), by using yes–no questions only to clarify messages and obtain information, by avoiding test and rhetorical questions, and by waiting expectantly for responses.

6. *Encouraging turn taking.* Parents wait expectantly for responses, balance the number and length of adult-to-child turns, and complete their children's sentences only when they are not yet combining words.

7. *Expanding and extending.* Parents expand and extend by repeating their children's words and using correct grammar or by adding another idea, and use comments and questions to inform, predict, imagine, explain, and talk about feelings.

Research indicates a positive association between parents' and caregivers' use of responsive interaction strategies and children's own language development. As one example, in an intervention study involving toddlers with expressive vocabulary delays and their mothers, Girolametto, Weitzman, Wiigs, and Pearce (1999) found a positive association between mothers' use of responsive interaction strategies (such as expansion, described in #7 above) and toddlers' language abilities, as measured at a later point in time.

WHAT MAJOR ACHIEVEMENTS IN LANGUAGE FORM, CONTENT, AND USE CHARACTERIZE INFANCY?

Recall from Chapter 1 that language consists of three rule-governed domains that together reflect an integrated whole: form, content, and use. The five language components of phonology, morphology, syntax, semantics, and pragmatics provide a more specific and refined way to describe of each of the three language domains. As a reminder, language *form* is how people arrange sounds (phonology), words

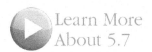

Learn More About 5.7

As you watch the video titled "Following the Child's Lead," notice how the mother responds to the 7-month-old's vocalizations by imitating them (which makes him laugh) and builds on the infant's interest by playing along with the game he is initiating.

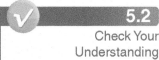

5.2

Check Your Understanding

Click here to gauge your understanding of the concepts in this section.

and parts of words (morphology), and sentences and phrases (syntax) to convey content. *Content* includes the words people use and the meanings behind them (semantics). People express content through their vocabulary system, or *lexicon*, as they retrieve and organize words to express ideas or to understand what other individuals are saying. *Use* is language pragmatics, or how people use language in interactions with other individuals to express personal and social needs.

Language Form

Recall that language form encompasses the components of phonology, morphology, and syntax. With regard to phonology, infants begin to produce sounds as soon as they are born. Recall from the discussion earlier in this chapter that infants produce sounds of distress, such as crying, from birth on. Interestingly, research suggests that the melody of cries tends to match the melody of a newborn's native language (Mampe, Friederici, Cristophe, & Wermke, 2009). For example, French newborns tend to exhibit rising melody contours, whereas German newborns tend to exhibit falling melody contours in their cries; both patterns match the predominant melody pattern of the newborns' native language.

Infants rapidly move to produce other nonspeech reflexive sounds, such as coughing, followed by speech-like vocalizations, over the first year. Speech-like vocalizations include primitive vowel-like sounds (emerging around age 2 months and lasting until age 6 or 8 months), vowel-like sounds that approximate mature adult vowels (emerging between ages 3 to 8 months), primitive consonant-vowel combinations (emerging before mature consonant-vowel combinations), and canonical syllables, or mature consonant-vowel combinations (emerging between ages 5 to 10 months) (Hsu, Iyer, & Fogel, 2014; Oller, 2000).

With regard to morphology and syntax, because infants do not produce their first word until about 1 year of age, infants' accomplishments in these areas are minimal, if not nonexistent. When infants do begin to use true words, they generally utter these words in isolation for several months (e.g., "Daddy") before they begin to combine words to make short phrases (e.g., "Daddy up"). However, although infants are not *producing* multiword utterances, they can typically *understand* some multiword utterances by age 1 year, particularly those they have heard many times (e.g., "Bye-bye, Mommy"; "More milk?").

First words usually refer to salient people and objects in infants' everyday lives, such as their mother, father, pets, and so forth.

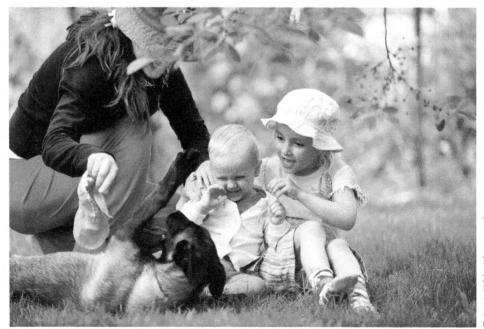

Although infants typically produce words in isolation before they produce multiword utterances, there is some debate about the "developmental ordering" of skills—whether infants actually develop lexical skills before they develop syntactic skills. Some theories propose that lexical development precedes and supports syntactic development (e.g., Marchman & Bates, 1994), whereas other theories claim syntax and vocabulary emerge synchronously (e.g., Dixon & Marchman, 2007). Because we don't witness syntactic development occurring over the first year of life, the way we witness lexical development happening, we might tend to agree with the former theory at first glance. However, Dixon and Marchman raise some interesting considerations, including how differences in how we measure and model early lexical and syntactic development might not adequately reflect the synchronicity between vocabulary and syntax development. As we discussed in Chapter 4, data from scientific experiments often prompt researchers to reexamine and reevaluate aspects of language-development theories. In the case of Dixon and Marchman's (2007) study, statistical models revealing that lexical development and grammatical development occur synchronously lend support to the notion that domain-general mechanisms (such as general cognitive processes or information processing abilities) rather than domain-specific processes, support language development.

Language Content

As you may remember, language content corresponds to semantics. Although infants reach a multitude of exciting milestones during their first year, none seems to be celebrated more than the first word. On average, infants produce their first true word around age 12 months. First words usually refer to salient people and objects in infants' everyday lives, such as *mama, dada, doggie*, and the like. Researchers consider an infant's vocalization to be a *true word* if it meets three important criteria.

First, infants must say true words with a clear intention. When a baby girl says the word *juice* while reaching for her cup of juice, she undoubtedly has the clear intention of referring to her drink. If the same baby says the word *juice* after her mother tells her "Say juice; tell me juice," researchers would consider the infant's utterance to be an imitation or a repetition rather than a true word.

Second, infants must produce true words with recognizable pronunciation that approximates the adult form. Twelve-month-olds cannot produce all sounds accurately, but their first word should sound like a close approximation of the adult form, and other people should be able to recognize it. Thus, a child's "mama" for *mommy* is a close enough approximation to be a true word. However, if a child produces *mommy* as "goo"—even consistently and while clearly referring to his or her mother—it would not meet the criteria for a true word because it does not closely approximate an adult form.

Third, a true word is a word a child uses consistently and generalizes beyond the original context to all appropriate exemplars. The baby girl who said "juice" could be expected to use this word not only with her apple juice but also with orange juice, grape juice, and pictures of juice in storybooks. As another example, a baby boy who knows the word "bike" should use it to refer to moving bikes, as well as bikes parked along the sidewalk. Because words name categories of objects, events, and activities—and not just single exemplars—infants must be able to generalize their words to several appropriate cases for their words to meet the criteria for true words.

Language Use

Language use corresponds to pragmatics. With regard to pragmatics, infancy is the calm before the language storm of toddlerhood, during which toddlers experiment (seemingly continuously) with all of their newly acquired language skills. Although

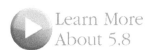

Learn More About 5.8

As you watch the video titled "Infant Pointing and Waving Bye-Bye," notice how the infant points to things in her environment in an effort to re-quest a label for those things. At the end of the video, the mother tells the infant to say "bye-bye" and she responds by waving. http://www.youtube.com/watch?v=xVDk_vd1fdA

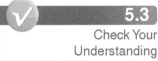

5.3
Check Your Understanding
Click here to gauge your understanding of the concepts in this section.

infants are not chatterboxes, they spend much of their time listening, observing, and learning how the people around them use language to communicate. Even before infants utter their first word, they are eager to communicate. Infants who are communicating intentionally (usually by age 8 months) use a variety of preverbal language functions, including the following (Kent, 1994):

- *Attention seeking to self.* Infants tug on an adult's clothing to gain his or her attention.
- *Attention seeking to events, objects, or other people.* Infants point to things in their environment to draw attention to them.
- *Requesting objects.* Infants use imperative pointing to indicate they would like to have an object.
- *Requesting action.* Infants hand objects to an adult when they would like the adult to do something with the objects.
- *Requesting information.* Infants may point to an object to have an adult provide a label for it or to give other information about the object.
- *Greeting.* Infants wave "hi" and "bye-bye" to other people.
- *Transferring.* Infants may give a toy they were playing with to another person.
- *Protesting or rejecting.* Infants may cry to protest when someone takes away a toy they were playing with or may push an object away to reject it.
- *Responding or acknowledging.* Infants may respond to other people and acknowledge their communicative attempts by smiling or laughing.
- *Informing.* Infants may inform other people when something is wrong—for example, by pointing to a broken wheel on a toy truck.

WHAT FACTORS CONTRIBUTE TO INFANTS' INDIVIDUAL ACHIEVEMENTS IN LANGUAGE?

Although infants develop language in a fairly predictable pattern because they meet certain milestones in the same order and at about the same age, some aspects of their language development vary. Next, we discuss one major *intraindividual* difference in language development and three major *interindividual* differences, along with factors that may account for such differences (Bates, Dale, & Thal, 1995).

Intraindividual Differences

If you observe an *individual* infant, you will most likely notice he or she does not develop all aspects of language at the same rate. In this section, we discuss how an infant's receptive and expressive language development differs and describe three factors that may account for this difference.

As mentioned previously in this text, at all stages of life, the amount of language an individual can produce spontaneously without imitating another person's verbalizations (expressive language) differs from the amount of language he or she can comprehend (receptive language). Infancy is no exception.

For example, although 1-year-olds comprehend an average of 80 words, they typically produce only about 10 words. Three factors account for the fact that language comprehension most often precedes language production (Golinkoff & Hirsh-Pasek, 1999). First, whereas language comprehension requires that people retrieve words from their lexicon, or mental dictionary, language production requires additional effort; namely, people must retrieve words and apply proper pronunciation as they utter the words. Second, with language comprehension, sentences are preorganized with lexical items, a syntactic structure, and intonation as people hear them. However, language production requires the speaker to search for words, organize them, and place stress where it is required. Third, and especially relevant to infants, language that adults use in communicative interactions with infants is usually highly contextualized, with many clues to assist comprehension. Children are generally at an advantage for comprehension because in many cases the words adults use when communicating with them have referents that are immediately available in the environment ("You want your bottle?" "Let's get your bib on"). However, in terms of production, children must construct a match between the intended referent and language to express meaning.

All of this is not to say that language comprehension is effortless; we know infants must use a whole host of abilities to comprehend even the simplest sentences. Still, language production requires that infants recruit an even greater number of abilities, which is why they tend to reach milestones in comprehension prior to those in production. The theme that language comprehension precedes language production resurfaces in Chapters 6–8. In those chapters, we discuss various language developments that occur during toddlerhood, the preschool years, and the school-age years and beyond.

Interindividual Differences

If you observe a *group* of infants, you will most likely notice language-development differences among them. First, some children develop language more quickly than others. Second, children express themselves for different communicative purposes. Third, certain children fall at either end of the continuum for language development and are late talkers or early talkers. We will now discuss these differences and some of the factors accounting for them.

When considering interindividual differences, it is important to keep in mind what it means to say an infant is above or below the median or mean with respect to a certain milestone. For example, to say an infant is above/below the median for using canonical babbling means he or she is among half of the infants of a representative sample whose onset time for canonical babbling is greater/lower than the median. As another example, to say the same infant is above/below the mean for using canonical babbling means the age at which he or she began to use canonical babbling is above/below the age of onset for all infants in a representative sample divided by the number of infants in that sample. It is important to recognize that as with other developmental phenomena, there is wide variation in when infants achieve language-development milestones, and that mean and median ages for achieving milestones are produced by statistical manipulations. There aren't real live infants who represent a true "average."

Variation in Language-Development Rate
The rate at which a group of children develop their receptive and expressive language abilities can vary considerably. One way to gauge the variability in infants' receptive and expressive vocabularies is by examining norm-referenced measures of language, such as the MacArthur–Bates Communicative Development Inventories (CDI; Fenson et al., 1993; Fenson, Pethick, et al., 2000). We describe the norming process for the CDI in Chapter 4, but what is important to note in this discussion is the variability among the more than 1,800 infants' expressive and receptive vocabularies in the sample (Bates et al., 1995). The number of words the infants understood at age 12 months ranged between 15 and 150, whereas the number of words the infants produced at the same age ranged between 0 and 30. As young children develop, differences between their receptive and expressive vocabularies becomes even more apparent. For example, the Bates et al. (1995) sample reveals that the number of words toddlers understood at age 16 months ranged between approximately 80 and 300, whereas the number of words toddlers produced at the

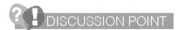

same age ranged between approximately 0 and 150. This means even toddlers who seem to say many words (compared to their same-age peers) might potentially understand twice as many words.

Variations in infants' receptive and expressive vocabularies can be accounted for only partly by age. Bates and colleagues (1995) reported that age accounts for only 22% of the variance in the number of words infants produce. Therefore, other factors explain the remaining 78% of the variance. Two variables of interest in interpreting variation in infants' vocabularies are socioeconomic status (SES), and the amount of talk parents engage in with their children. Researchers have determined that how much parents talk to their infants and young children is related to the parents' SES, but, regardless of SES, the more parents talk to their children, the more rapidly children's vocabulary grows and the better children perform on measures of verbal and cognitive competence at age 3 years (Hart & Risley, 1995, 1999).

Variation in Language-Learning Styles

Infants differ, too, in the ways they use language for communicative purposes. The main factor affecting this variation is the infants' predominant style for using language, which researchers describe as either expressive or referential (Nelson, 1973). *Expressive* language learners use language primarily for social exchanges. Their early vocabularies contain several words and phrases that allow them to express their needs and describe their feelings as they interact with other people. Common first words for expressive language learners include *hi* and *bye-bye*.

In contrast, *referential* language learners use language primarily to refer to people and objects. They enjoy labeling things they see, and they like when adults provide labels for them. Their early vocabularies contain a large proportion of object labels, including words such as *ball*, *doggie*, and *juice* (Nelson, 1973).

Variation at the Extremes of the Typical Range for Language Development

The final language-development difference among infants involves certain children who fall at either end of the language-development continuum: late talkers and early talkers. We describe more severe variations in language development in Chapter 10.

Expressive language learners use language primarily for social exchanges.

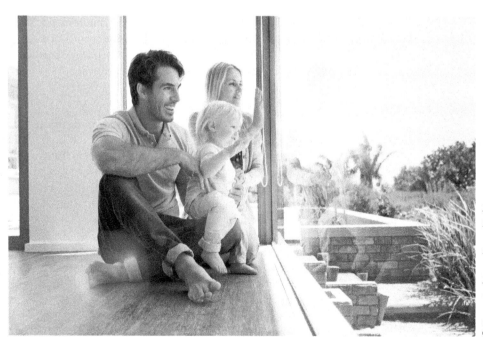

© Tomas Rodriguez/Fancy/Corbis

Late Talkers.   *Late talkers* are children who exhibit early delays in their expressive (rather than receptive) language development. Although there is no clinical diagnosis for being a late talker, one common definition considers children to be late talkers if they produce fewer than 50 words by age 2 (Rescorla, 1989). Zubrick, Taylor, Rice, and Slegers (2007) estimate that about 13.4% of the general population are late talkers (and they mention this figure is consistent with prior research estimating prevalence rates to be 10%–20%). These researchers also report that males are about three times more likely to be late talkers than females, and infants who are born earlier than 37 weeks' gestation, or who are less than 85% of their optimum birth weight are about twice as likely to be late talkers than infants without such neurobiological issues.

Late talkers are of concern to parents and clinicians. Being a late talker does not necessarily mean a child will have a language delay or impairment; however, it can be an important predictor of being diagnosed with a delay or impairment at a later age. Many late talkers can achieve normal language levels by age 3 or 4 years. However, they may still exhibit delays in subtle aspects of language development, and perform at significantly lower levels on measures of verbal short-term memory, sentence formulation, word retrieval, auditory processing of complex information, and elaborated verbal expression than their age-matched, typically developing peers at ages 6, 7, and 8 years (Rescorla, 1993b).

Early Talkers.   *Early talkers* are children who are ahead of their peers in expressive language use. Bates and colleagues (1995) defined early talkers as children between ages 11 and 21 months who score in the top 10% for vocabulary production for their age on the MacArthur–Bates CDI. Whereas children developing language typically produce an average of 200 words at 21 months, early talkers produce an average of 475 words (Thal, Bates, Goodman, & Jahn-Samilo, 1997). Although few studies on early talkers have been conducted, research results suggest these children have an advantage over their age-matched, typically developing peers on measures of vocabulary, grammar, and verbal reasoning throughout early childhood (Robinson, Dale, & Landesman, 1990).

5.4

Check Your Understanding

Click here to gauge your understanding of the concepts in this section.

HOW DO RESEARCHERS AND CLINICIANS MEASURE LANGUAGE DEVELOPMENT IN INFANCY?

Many methods are available for measuring language development. In this section, we discuss ways in which researchers measure language achievements as they strive to understand the course of language development. We also describe methods clinicians use to measure language development as they seek to determine whether children are progressing typically in their receptive and expressive achievements.

Researchers

People have likely been intrigued by how infants and young children develop language for thousands of years. One early "research study" involved a king in ancient Egypt who had two infants raised in silence to determine what language the infants would speak on their own. For the many centuries that followed, biographical and diary studies, such as Charles Darwin's 1877, "A Biographical Sketch of an Infant" were perhaps the only way to document infants' language achievements. It wasn't until the second half of the twentieth century that technology, such as the tape recorder, video recorder, and computer, began to change the study of language development in fundamental ways (Slobin, 2014). Beginning in the latter part of the 20th century and into the 21st century, researchers have been applying noninvasive neuroimaging technologies to the study of language development, changing the field further.

The fact that infants cannot tell adults what they know about language poses some interesting challenges with regard to measuring their language achievements. As a result, researchers who measure language achievements in infancy have devised an array of creative methods to shed light on infants' developing systems, including habituation–dishabituation tasks, the switch task variation on habituation–dishabituation tasks, the intermodal preferential looking paradigm, naturalistic observation, and neuroimaging technologies.

Habituation–Dishabituation Tasks

Habituation of an infant consists of presenting the same stimulus repeatedly (e.g., an image of a brown dog on a TV screen) until his or her attention to the stimulus decreases by a predetermined amount. For example, an infant might see a brown dog on the screen and he might initially look at the dog for about 8 out of 10 s and look away from the screen for about 2 out of 10 s. After he becomes bored with the image of the brown dog, his looking time will decrease; he might look at the screen for about 3 out of 10 s and look away from the screen for about 7 out of 10 s. Dishabituation describes the infant's renewed interest in a stimulus according to some predetermined threshold. For example, the infant who became habituated to the image of a brown dog might next see a brown cat on the screen and might again look at the screen for a longer period (e.g., for 8 out of 10 s). Researchers use habituation–dishabituation tasks to determine whether infants detect differences in prelinguistic and linguistic stimuli and how infants organize these stimuli categorically.

In a study by Pulverman and Golinkoff (2004), researchers were interested in determining the extent to which infants attend to potential verb referents (e.g., *bending*, *spinning*) as they watch motion events. These researchers habituated infants to one of nine stimulus events involving an animated starfish actor and a green ball, which serves as a point of reference (e.g., the starfish does jumping jacks over the ball). Infants were said to have *habituated* when the time of their visual fixation to the stimulus during three trials (Trials 4–6, Trials 7–9, etc.) decreased to less than 65% of their visual fixation time in the first three trials. Once the infants were habituated, researchers presented four test trials in a random order:

TEST TRIAL	DESCRIPTION	EXAMPLE
1. Control	Same event as in habituation trials	The starfish performs jumping jacks back and forth *over* the ball.
2. Path change	Same manner as in the habituation trials, but different path	The starfish performs jumping jacks back and forth *under* the ball.
3. Manner change	Same path as in the habituation trials, but different manner	The starfish *spins* back and forth over the ball.
4. Path and manner change	Different path and manner than in the habituation trials	The starfish *bends alongside* the ball back and forth.

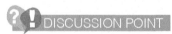
DISCUSSION POINT

The Spanish language contains more path verbs (*exit*, *descend*) than manner verbs (*slither*, *stagger*), whereas the opposite is true for English. How might Spanish- and English-learning infants show different habituation–dishabituation patterns in Pulverman and Golinkoff's (2004) task?

By measuring infants' dishabituation, researchers determined that young infants are sensitive to the nonlinguistic aspects of manner and path that potentially serve as verb labels in their native language. See Figure 5.5 for an illustration of the habituation–dishabituation stimuli from Pulverman and Golinkoff's (2004) study. Note, too, that in the study, the starfish enacted the motions in a continuous manner back and forth along the paths depicted at the bottom of the illustration.

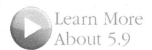

Learn More About 5.9

The video titled "Pulverman and Golinkoff's (2004) Habituation–Dishabituation Study" illustrates an 8-month-old participating in a habituation–dishabituation task in Dr. Roberta Golinkoff's research lab at the University of Delaware.

Learn More About 5.9 *(Continued)*

Pulverman and Golinkoff used this task to investigate infants' attention to specific aspects of motion events that languages label with verbs. For example, English verbs tend to label the manner of an action in motion events (how an action occurs—stagger, stroll, stumble) and place the path of an action (where an agent moves in relation to a point of reference—enter, exit) in a different part of the sentence outside of the verb ("He staggered out of the house"). By contrast, Spanish verbs tend to label the path of an action and place the manner of an action in a different part of the sentence outside of the verb (rough translation = "He exited the house in a staggering manner"). The aim of the study was to determine whether infants pay attention to the manner and/or the path of an action in motion events, and more specifically, whether infants pay particular attention to the aspects of motion events that verbs in their language label (manner for English).

In the habituation phase of the task, the computer presents a series of trials in which an animated starfish spins over a ball. The beginning of each new trial contains an attention-getter that is used to refocus the infant's attention to the screen. In this video, the attention-getter is a flashing blue and white shape accompanied by a sound. Note that as the infant loses interest with the presentation, he begins to look away from the screen more frequently. A researcher positioned out of the infant's view behind the video screen monitors the infant's attention to the presentation and presses a keyboard button to indicate when the infant is attending and when he is not attending to the presentation. Meanwhile, the computer uses specific criteria to determine when the infant is officially "bored" with the presentation. Once these criteria have been met, the dishabituation phase of the task begins.

The purpose of the dishabituation phase is to determine whether the infant notices subtle changes to the video presentation, based on assumption that he will demonstrate a renewed interest in the video when he detects something new. In this example, once the infant is habituated, he views a series of five test trials, three of which serve to measure his attention to novel changes, one of which serves as a familiar "control" to the test trials, and the last of which serves to verify that the infant is capable of increasing his looking time to a completely novel stimulus. In the first test trial, the animated starfish performs toe-touch actions over the ball; here, the manner of action is novel, but the path the starfish takes is familiar. If the infant was attending to the manner of action in the habituation phase of the task, he would be surprised by the new manner of action and his looking time to the screen should increase relative to the last few trials of the habituation phase. If he was not attending to the manner of action during the habituation phase, he should remain bored by the display as evidenced by a low level of attention to the screen.

Two important features of the experiment are worth mentioning here. First, the infant's mother must close her eyes throughout the presentation so that she cannot direct the infant's attention to the screen at any time (advertently or inadvertently). Second, the researcher is positioned behind the screen wearing headphones so that she is unaware of which display the infant is watching.

In the second test trial, the control trial, the infant sees the familiar action of the starfish spinning over the ball. The assumption of the control trial is that the infant will not demonstrate a renewed interest in this display.

In the third test trial, the infant sees the starfish perform jumping jacks under the ball. The infant should demonstrate interest in this display if he notices that either the manner of action or the path the starfish takes are different from those presented in the habituation trials.

In the fourth test trial, the infant sees the starfish spin next to the ball. Here, the infant should demonstrate interest in the display if he notices that the path the starfish takes is different from the path the starfish used in the habituation trial.

(Continued)

Finally, the infant sees a smiling baby in what is called the recovery trial. The purpose of the recovery trial is to indicate whether the infant renews his interest toward a completely novel stimulus. Infants who do not demonstrate an increased looking time in the recovery trial compared to the last few trials of the habituation phase may not have yielded reliable data during the dishabituation phase of the study. In such cases, researchers usually elect to disregard the individual's data.

In another version of the habituation–dishabituation paradigm, researchers use a newborn's sucking rate as a dependent measure instead of looking time. See Research Paradigms: *The High-Amplitude Nonnutritive Sucking Procedure* for more information on this method for measuring language development in young infants.

Switch Task

The switch task is a technique used in conjunction with habituation. During the habituation phase, infants see numerous pairings of different stimuli until their looking time decreases by a predetermined amount. For example, the infant might see an image of an apple paired with the spoken word *apple* and an orange paired with the spoken word *orange* multiple times in a randomized sequence. In the test phase, the infant sees either the same pairing as during the habituation phase (the "same trial") or a different pairing than he or she saw during the habituation phase (the "switch trial"). For example, in the switch trial, the infant might

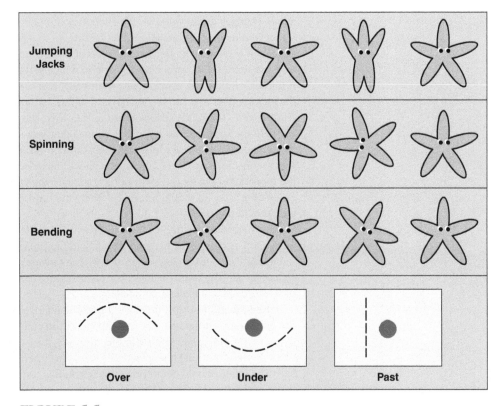

FIGURE 5.5

Sample stimuli for a habituation–dishabituation task.

Source: From *Seven-Month-Olds' Attention to Potential Verb Referents in Nonlinguistic Events*, by R. Pulverman and R. M. Golinkoff, 2004, in a paper presented at the proceedings of the 28th annual Boston University Conference on Language Development, Boston, MA. Copyright 2004 by Cascadilla Press. Reprinted with permission.

see an image of an apple paired with the spoken word *orange* or an image of an orange paired with the spoken word *apple*. Researchers presume that an infant who learned the original pairings during the habituation trials will look longer at the switch trial than at the same trial during the test phase. After the test phase, the infant watches a control trial that includes a novel stimulus he or she did not see during the habituation phase. Researchers expect an infant will look longer at the stimulus presented during the control trial than at stimuli he or she has already viewed.

Intermodal Preferential Looking Paradigm

In the *intermodal preferential looking paradigm* (IPLP), an infant sits on a blind-folded parent's lap approximately 3 feet from a television screen (parents are blindfolded so they cannot influence their infant's performance on the task; Hirsh-Pasek & Golinkoff, 1996; Spelke, 1979). The infant watches a split-screen presentation in which one stimulus is on the left side of the screen and another stimulus is on the right side. For example, the infant may see a person dancing on the left and a person jumping on the right. The audio stimulus accompanying the presentation matches the visual information on only one side of the screen (e.g., "Find dancing!" "Where's dancing?"). A hidden camera records infants' visual fixation throughout the presentation (See Figure 5.6 for an illustration of the setup for the IPLP). The premise behind the design is that infants will direct more visual attention to the matching side of the screen when they understand the language they hear; that is, they will find the link between the information presented in the auditory modality (that which they hear) and that in the visual modality (that which they see).

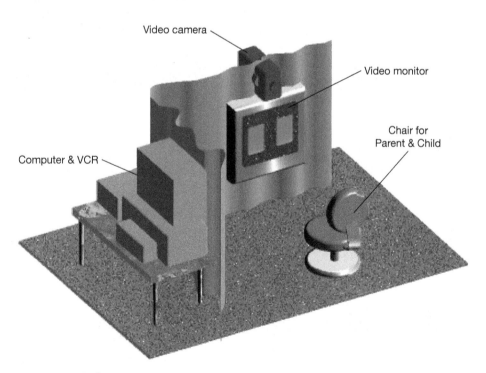

FIGURE 5.6

Intermodal preferential looking paradigm.

Source: From *Testing Language Comprehension in Infants: Introducing the Split-Screen Preferential Looking Paradigm*, by G. Hollich, C. Rocroi, K. Hirsh-Pasek, and R. Golinkoff, April 1999, in a poster session presented at the Society for Research in Child Development, Albuquerque, NM. Copyright 1999 by George Hollich. Reprinted with permission.

RESEARCH **PARADIGMS**

The High-Amplitude Nonnutritive Sucking Procedure

As you read about the high-amplitude nonnutritive sucking procedure, recall our discussion of behaviorism in Chapter 4.

Researchers use the high-amplitude nonnutritive sucking procedure to determine whether infants have a priori preferences for certain sound stimuli over others. Because young infants cannot speak, point, or otherwise directly indicate what they think about speech sounds, researchers use an infant's natural sucking reflex as an indirect way to learn about his or her speech-processing abilities.

In this procedure, a nonnutritive pacifier is connected to a computer. The infant sucks on the pacifier as he or she listens to audio stimuli played on a loudspeaker. The computer delivers a particular sound stimulus each time the infant sucks on the pacifier. This stimulus reinforces the infant's sucking behavior within the first 2 or 3 min of the study. As the audio stimulus reinforces the behavior, the infant becomes conditioned and sucks more frequently when he or she likes the sound and sucks less often when he or she does not like or is bored with the sound.

Some researchers have used this procedure to determine, for example, that 2-month-olds can distinguish between their native language and a foreign language (Mehler et al., 1988). Other researchers have determined that infants of the same age can retain information about speech sounds they hear for brief intervals (e.g., Jusczyk, Kennedy, & Jusczyk, 1995).

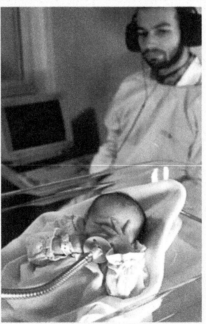

© Franck Ramus

High-amplitude nonnutritive sucking procedure

DISCUSSION POINT

The high-amplitude nonnutritive sucking procedure relies on behaviorist principles (which are empiricist, or nurture-inspired), yet researchers argue that children demonstrate innate (or nature-inspired) language abilities during such experiments. How do you explain this relationship or discrepancy?

Researchers have used the IPLP to explore a variety of linguistic and prelinguistic hypotheses. For example, Kuhl and Meltzoff (1982) used the IPLP to discover that 4-month-old infants prefer to look at a face whose mouth moves in concert with a speech sound than at a face whose mouth produces a different speech sound. More recently, researchers using the IPLP have found infants tend to associate novel labels with whole objects rather than object parts, even when one of the parts is interesting (Hollich, Golinkoff, & Hirsh-Pasek, 2007), for example.

There is also an interactive version of the IPLP, the *interactive intermodal preferential looking paradigm* (IIPLP), in which the infant is able to hold and explore objects before the experimenter affixes them to a board for the test trials. Rather than measuring the infant's attention to the matching side of a television screen, researchers measure attention to the target object as it appears alongside another object on a board.

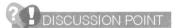

DISCUSSION POINT

What additional variables of interest could researchers manipulate in the IIPLP that are not possible to manipulate in the IPLP?

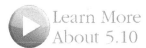

Learn More About 5.10

The video titled "Interactive Intermodal Preferential Looking Paradigm Task" illustrates a 1-year-old child participating in an interactive intermodal preferential looking paradigm (IIPLP) task in Dr. Roberta Golinkoff's research lab at the University of Delaware.

Learn More About 5.10 *(Continued)*

The purpose of the study is to determine the extent to which young children can utilize social cues (such as a speaker's eye gaze toward an object) to learn the name of a novel object.

In the beginning of the video, the experimenter presents two familiarization trials to ensure the child understands the task at hand; this requires that the child, Adam, direct his attention toward the object requested. After the experimenter allows Adam to play with the block and keys for a predetermined period of time, she places them onto a Fagan board and requests that he look at the keys. The premise is that he will look longer toward the keys if he understands the label.

Next, the experimenter allows the child to play with each of two novel objects (a wand with sparkles and a bottle opener). She then assesses whether he has a preference for either of these two objects in what is called a salience trial. In the salience trial, the experimenter asks Adam to look at the board using neutral requests. If he has an a priori preference for either of the two objects, he should look longer toward that object.

In the training phase, the experimenter provides several labels for one of the novel objects ("modi") and she looks at that object to provide a cue that she is labeling it.

The test phase of the experiment consists of four trials to assess whether the child has learned the new word. In the first two test trials, the experimenter asks Adam to "find the modi," assuming that he will devote a greater amount of attention to the labeled object than the nonlabeled object. In the third trial, the new label trial, the experimenter asks Adam to "find the danu." The assumption guiding this trial is that if Adam understands that the bottle opener is called "modi," he will look toward the unnamed object (the wand with sparkles) when the experimenter uses the word "danu." In the final trial, termed the recovery trial, the experimenter again asks Adam to "find the modi," with the assumption that Adam should redirect his attention to the labeled object.

Note that during the salience trial and the four test trials, the mother's eyes remain closed so she is unaware of which side of the board the target object will appear. The child's looking time toward objects during the salience trial and each of the four test trials is recorded using a video camera to be coded offline after he leaves the lab.

Naturalistic Observation

Naturalistic observation involves systematically observing and analyzing an infant's communicative behavior in everyday situations. Such observation usually takes place in the infant's home. Researchers may videotape, audiotape, and take notes as the infant interacts naturally with the people around him or her. The researchers may elect to gather information during specific activities, such as dinnertime or free play with a parent.

Researchers targeting specific language forms or prelinguistic behaviors may alternatively devise a semistructured or structured observation in a laboratory. During structured observations, researchers may provide infants with specific props or ask the same questions of all infants in the study as a point of comparison.

The Child Language Data Exchange System (CHILDES) database (available at http://childes.psy.cmu.edu) is an invaluable source for researchers interested in gaining access to naturalistic and structured language samples to answer questions about language development. The CHILDES system contains transcripts and audio files of naturalistic and structured observations in more than 30 languages as well as software for coding and analyzing these transcripts (CLAN).

According to the CHILDES Web site, CHILDES originated in 1984 in an effort to create a system to facilitate the exchange of child language data. Collecting and transcribing child language data is notoriously time-consuming, and the methods by which researchers collect and transcribe language samples can vary greatly (e.g., whether or not a researcher indicates grammatical omissions in a language sample; whether or not a researcher indicates phonological errors in a speech sample). CHILDES addresses these issues by providing a way for researchers to standardize their own language samples, using the CLAN transcription software, and to share their data with other researchers who might be interested in using those data to answer different questions.

Neuroimaging Technologies

There are a number of neuroimaging technologies available to study language development in infancy and throughout the lifespan. Researchers use two main types. First are methods that measure changes in the brain's electrical activity, such as event-related potential (ERP) and magnetoencephalography (MEG). Second are methods that measure changes in the brain's blood flow (hemodynamic response), such as functional magnetic resonance imaging (fMRI), or functional near infrared spectroscopy (fNIRS) (Kovelman, 2012).

Neuroimaging studies in infancy have focused largely on infants' perception of the phonemes that make up their native language or languages. Kovelman (2012) describes that researchers can use an "oddball" paradigm with any of the imaging methods. Using the oddball paradigm, researchers present a standard stimulus (e.g., the sound /ba/) about 80% of the time and an "oddball" stimulus (e.g., the sound /da/) about 20% of the time. They then analyze the infant's electric or hemodynamic brain response to the oddball versus the standard stimulus to determine the extent to which infants detect differences in the sounds. A number of studies using neuroimaging technologies to study infants' perception of phonemes have replicated the results of studies of research paradigms that do not measure brain activity (e.g., Petitto et al., 2012).

Clinicians

As we discussed, infants in their first year begin to establish many foundations for later language achievements. However, they are not true conversationalists at this age. In general, gauging whether children are lagging in their language skills is difficult before they reach toddlerhood, when their expressive language begins to emerge. However, in some instances, clinicians (including pediatricians, speech–language pathologists, and clinical psychologists) do examine infants' language skills. Such examinations may be necessary for infants born with developmental disabilities (e.g., cleft palate) or for infants who, for unknown reasons, seem to be lagging in meeting key milestones. Next, we discuss two informal measures of language development that clinicians use with infants: informal language screens and parent-report measures.

Informal Language Screens

Informal language screens for infants involve checklists of common early language milestones that clinicians and parents can use to check off whether or not an infant exhibits each behavior in question. The National Institute on Deafness and Other Communication Disorders (http://www.nidcd.nih.gov) offers a series of developmental

Milestones for speech and language development

BIRTH TO 3 MONTHS		
Reacts to loud sounds	YES ☐	NO ☐
Calms down or smiles when spoken to	YES ☐	NO ☐
Recognizes your voice and calms down if crying	YES ☐	NO ☐
When feeding, starts or stops sucking in response to sound	YES ☐	NO ☐
Coos and makes pleasure sounds	YES ☐	NO ☐
Has a special way of crying for different needs	YES ☐	NO ☐
Smiles when he or she sees you	YES ☐	NO ☐
4 TO 6 MONTHS		
Follows sounds with his or her eyes	YES ☐	NO ☐
Responds to changes in the tone of your voice	YES ☐	NO ☐
Notices toys that make sounds	YES ☐	NO ☐
Pays attention to music	YES ☐	NO ☐
Babbles in a speech-like way and uses many different sounds, including sounds that begin with p, b, and m	YES ☐	NO ☐
Laughs	YES ☐	NO ☐
Babbles when excited or unhappy	YES ☐	NO ☐
Makes gurgling sounds when alone or playing with you	YES ☐	NO ☐
7 MONTHS TO 1 YEAR		
Enjoys playing peek-a-boo and pat-a-cake	YES ☐	NO ☐
Turns and looks in the direction of sounds	YES ☐	NO ☐
Listens when spoken to	YES ☐	NO ☐
Understands words for common items such as "cup," "shoe," or "juice"	YES ☐	NO ☐
Responds to requests ("Come here")	YES ☐	NO ☐
Babbles using long and short groups of sounds ("tata, upup, bibibi")	YES ☐	NO ☐
Babbles to get and keep attention	YES ☐	NO ☐
Communicates using gestures such as waving or holding up arms	YES ☐	NO ☐
Has one or two words ("Hi," "dog," "Dada," or "Mama") by first birthday	YES ☐	NO ☐

FIGURE 5.7

Language screens for infants from birth to age 3 months, from age 4 months to age 6 months, and from age 7 months to 1 year of age.

Source: From *Speech and Language Developmental Milestones*, by National Institute on Deafness and Other Communication Disorders (2014) (NIH Publication No. 13-4781). Bethesda, MD: Author. http://www.nidcd.nih.gov/staticresources/health/voice/NIDCD-Speech-Language-Dev-Milestones.pdf

language screens that parents and clinicians can use informally. See Figure 5.7 for an example of a screen for infants from birth to age 3 months, a screen for infants age 4 months to age 6 months, and a screen for infants age 7 months to 1 year of age.

Parent-Report Measures

Not only is having parents report directly on their infant's development a quick way to gauge an infant's progress, but researchers believe such reporting to be a reliable and valid measure of language ability when compared with other direct assessments (P. Dale, 1991, 1996). Parents report on specific language behaviors, using checklists and questionnaires. Common self-report measures for infants include the Language Development Survey (LDS; Rescorla, 1993a), and the MacArthur–Bates CDI (Fenson et al., 1993; Fenson, Pethick, et al., 2000). To expand on just one of these measures, we provide some detail on the CDI next.

Bates and Carnevale (1993) explain that the CDI grew out of an interest in capturing the most valid and reliable data possible on children's language. Because parents presumably spend more time with their own children than does any other person, they are well positioned to report on infrequent, new, and unpredictable language behaviors as those behaviors emerge. For centuries, researchers, such as Charles Darwin, have captured rich information about their own children's language development in *diary studies*. The developers of the CDI, realizing that diary studies are time-consuming and do not generalize to larger populations of children, aimed to "bottle" the diary studies and administer them on a larger scale (p. 440). As researchers were developing the CDI, they created three rules to strengthen the reliability and validity of the instrument. First, they decided to ask only about current behaviors, as retrospective reports tend not to be accurate. Second, they decided to ask only about salient behaviors that are just starting to emerge and that parents can reasonably keep track of. Third, they decided to rely on parents' recognition rather than recall. For example, the CDI asks whether a child says certain words, such as *dog*, *cat*, or *bird*, rather than ask the parent to list the animal names the child produces (e.g., "What animal names does your child say?"). As we mentioned in Chapter 4, the CDI was originally normed in English on a sample of more than 1,800 infants and toddlers. According to the CDI Web site (http://mb-cdi.stanford.edu/), the CDI is available in 63 languages as of 2015.

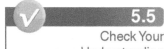

5.5

Check Your Understanding

Click here to gauge your understanding of the concepts in this section.

SUMMARY

This chapter begins with a discussion of the major language-development milestones infants achieve, including the ability to perceive speech sounds and to use speech sounds as a way to break into the continuous streams of speech they hear. Other milestones include being aware of and attending to actions and the intentions underlying actions; categorizing objects, actions, and events according to perceptual and conceptual features; and producing early vocalizations that are precursors to language.

Some early foundations for language development that follow from infants' social interactions with other people include infant-directed speech, joint reference and attention, the daily routines of infancy, and caregiver responsiveness. Infants' major achievements in language form, content, and use during the first year

include various types of vocal development (moving from sounds of distress, such as crying, to advanced forms, such as multisyllabic strings) to producing their first word and using several new pragmatic functions after about age 8 months, when they are communicating intentionally.

Although infants follow a fairly predictable pattern of language development during the first year, some aspects of this development vary. An individual infant's expressive and receptive vocabularies differ in size and, among a group of infants, there are differences in the language-development rate, language-learning style, communicative purpose, and starting time for producing speech. Various factors account for such differences.

Researchers and clinicians measure language development in infancy using a variety of creative methods.

Some major research paradigms include habituation–dishabituation tasks, the switch task (which incorporates habituation), the intermodal preferential looking paradigm, the interactive intermodal preferential looking paradigm, naturalistic observation, and neuroimaging technologies. Two clinical methods for gathering information about infants' language progress include informal language screens and parent-report measures.

 Apply Your Knowledge

Click here to apply your knowledge to practical scenarios.

BEYOND THE BOOK

1. Take a look at an alphabet book for young children and classify the pictures corresponding to each letter (e.g., *A* = apple, *B* = ball) as referring to either a superordinate-level term, a basic-level term, or a subordinate-level term. What type of category has the largest representation in the alphabet book? Is this consistent with the types of words infants generally learn first?

2. Using the Web, search for a video of an infant vocalizing. Analyze the vocalizations using the Stark Assessment of Early Vocal Development—Revised (summarized earlier in this chapter) and decide which stage of vocal development best characterizes the infant's vocalizations.

3. Compile a list of your own first words (with help from your parents or caregivers) as well as the first words of your own children or your friends' children. Discuss the extent to which the words are typical first words.

4. Using the CHILDES Web site (http://childes.psy.cmu.edu/), listen to an audio file from the database that features an adult interacting with an infant (for some examples of infants age 1 year, 1 month, see http://childes.psy.cmu.edu/browser/index.php?url=Eng-NA-MOR/Bernstein/Children/Alice/alice1.cha and http://childes.psy.cmu.edu/browser/index.php?url=Eng-NA-MOR/Bernstein/Children/Kay/kay1.cha) and document the paralinguistic, syntactic, and discourse features of infant-directed speech you hear.

5. Search for one video of an infant using declarative pointing and another video of an infant using imperative pointing. How can you tell the difference between the two forms of pointing? Are the infants vocalizing in any way while they point? How do the two kinds of communicative situations play out?

 Check Your Understanding

Gauge your understanding of the chapter concepts by taking this self-check quiz.

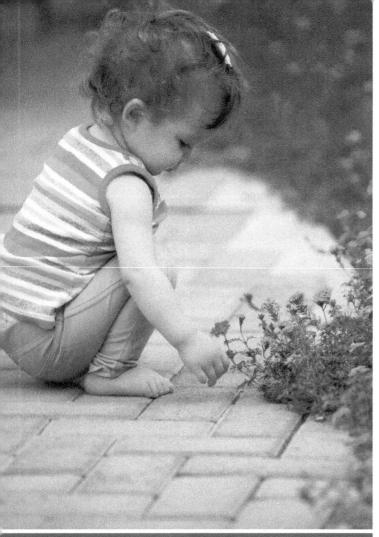

6

Toddlerhood

Exploring the World and Experimenting with Language

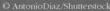

LEARNING OUTCOMES

After completion of this chapter, the reader will be able to:

1. Identify major language-development milestones that occur in toddlerhood.

2. Describe major achievements in language form, content, and use that characterize toddlerhood.

3. Explain factors that contribute to toddlers' individual language achievements.

4. Describe how researchers and clinicians measure language development in toddlerhood.

Toddlerhood, or the period between about age 1 and age 3 years, is a time of exploration for children. Toddlers can move around by crawling or walking, and this newfound mobility heralds many new opportunities to explore the world that had not previously been available without the assistance of other people. Toddlers are inherently curious about the objects, people, and actions around them and are likewise, inquisitive about the language they hear other individuals using. During toddlerhood, children begin to consciously attempt to create matches between objects and actions in the world and the language that describes them. For example, you have probably heard toddlers ask "Wha-dat?" in their attempts to link language to concepts of interest to them. In this chapter, we first provide an overview of the major language-development milestones of toddlerhood, including the use of first words and gestures. Second, we explore toddlers' achievements in language form, content, and use. Such achievements involve phonological, morphological, syntactic, semantic, and pragmatic developments. We also discuss word-use errors typical of toddlers. Third, we investigate factors that contribute to intraindividual and interindividual differences among toddlers. These factors include variation in language-development rate, and the effects of gender, birth order, and familial socioeconomic status on language development. Fourth, and finally, we detail ways in which researchers and clinicians measure language development in toddlerhood. Among these measures are various production, comprehension, and judgment tasks, as well as evaluation and assessment tools.

WHAT MAJOR LANGUAGE-DEVELOPMENT MILESTONES OCCUR IN TODDLERHOOD?

First Words

A baby's first word marks the beginning of a transition from preverbal to verbal communication, and ushers in a new and exciting period of language development. Parents may record their child's first word along with the age at which the child spoke the word and the context in which he or she said it. Partly because of the excitement about this achievement, researchers know that, on average, babies produce their first word around age 12 months.

Words are different from prelinguistic vocalizations infants make when they babble. Although words are composed of meaningful sounds, they are also symbolic and arbitrary. They are symbolic because they represent something in the world. They are arbitrary because the sound sequences of words do not directly stand for the concepts the words represent (one exception is onomatopoeic words, such as *whoosh* and *gurgle*, which do sound like the concepts they represent). For each word babies learn, they create an entry in their *lexicon*, or mental dictionary. A lexical entry contains a series of symbols that compose the word, the sound of the word, the meaning of the word, and its part of speech (Pinker, 1999). Figure 6.1 illustrates how the word *sun* might appear in the lexicon.

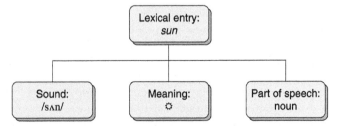

FIGURE 6.1
Lexical entry for the word *sun*.

First words usually refer to salient people and objects in babies' everyday lives, such as *mama, dada, doggie, kitty,* and the like. For a vocalization to be a *true word,* it must meet three important criteria. First, the baby must produce the word with a clear purpose. For example, when baby Zander holds up a book while saying the word *book,* he has the clear purpose of referring to the book. However, when his mom, Lori, wants to show her son's feat to a group of friends by prompting Zander, "Say book," the resulting utterance would be considered a direct imitation or repetition rather than a true word.

Second, a true word must have recognizable pronunciation similar to the adult form of the word. According to some estimates, even 18-month-old children's pronunciations are only 25% intelligible (e.g., Weiss, Gordon, & Lillywhite, 1987); however, a true word should be a close approximation of the adult form, and other people should be able to recognize it as such. Thus, a baby girl's "wawa" for *water* is close enough to the adult form of the word that it would meet one of the criteria for a true word. In contrast, if a child produces the word *water* as "aaaah"—even consistently and while clearly using this sound to request a drink—this vocalization would not be a true word because it does not closely approximate the adult form.

The term phonetically consistent forms (PCFs) describes the idiosyncratic wordlike productions children use consistently and meaningfully but that do not approximate adult forms. As the term suggests, PCFs have a consistent sound structure, but children may use them to refer to more than a single referent. For example, the baby girl who uses the PCF "aaaah" to refer to *water* might also use this sound when requesting other objects or actions, such as when asking someone to pick her up or give her a toy. The first author's oldest son used the PCF "dah-dah" initially when he did not know a word or phrase he wanted to use. He later used this PCF in place of the phrase "I don't know" and then stopped using the PCF altogether around age 2.5 years, when he started using the phrase "I don't know" consistently. Although PCFs are not true words, they are important aspects of children's language development because, by using them, children learn the value of adopting a stable pronunciation for communicating in a particular situation (McEachern & Haynes, 2004).

Third, a true word is a word a child uses consistently and extends beyond the original context. The baby girl who said "wawa" could be expected to use this word not only when asking for a drink of water but also when seeing her dog drinking from his water dish—and possibly even when splashing around in the bathtub.

Subsequently in this chapter, we discuss how children extend words beyond their original context. Next, however, we investigate the role of gesture use in language development. For even more milestones, see the Developmental Timeline: Toddlerhood.

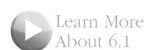

Learn More About 6.1

As you watch the video titled "Phonetically Consistent Forms (PCFs)," notice how the 20-month-old boy uses the PCF "dah-dah" when the word or phrase he wants to use is not part of his vocabulary. In one instance, he uses the word "orange" to request the cup with the orange egg inside.

Gestures

In Chapter 5, we discuss the emergence of gestures, such as imperative and declarative pointing, in episodes of joint attention between prelinguistic infants and other people. In this section, we examine the important role gestures continue to play in language development in the second and third years of life.

Over the second year, toddlers continue to rely on others' gestures as an important source of information as they learn language, although there appears to be a significant developmental shift during this time. Specifically, toddlers come to rely less on gestures and more on words when making inferences about how to categorize or label new objects. One study showed that 14-month-olds are able to interpret *both* words and gestures (other than pointing, such as those a parent might use when teaching "baby signs") to determine what new words refer to, whereas 22-month-olds rely on others' words, but not gestures alone, to learn what new words refer to (Graham & Kilbreath, 2007). Thus, as (hearing) toddlers develop, they seem to move from using a more generalized symbolic system (that equally accepts others' use of words and gestures) to a more narrow and restricted symbolic system that privileges words. When considering gesture *use*, a similar pattern is evident. As we discuss next, younger toddlers use more gestures than older toddlers as they attempt to fill in verbal gaps by using a more generalized symbolic system that incorporates both words and gestures.

Gesture Use

Gesture use precedes spoken language as children transition from the prelinguistic stage to the one-word stage of language development and then from the one-word stage to the two-word stage. As an illustration, children who are beginning to transition from the prelinguistic stage to the one-word stage use referential gestures, such as holding a fist to the ear to indicate *telephone*, pretending to go *to sleep*, or waving the hand to indicate *bye-bye* (Caselli, 1983, as cited in Volterra, Caselli, Capirci, & Pizzuto, 2005). A referential gesture is one that indicates a precise referent and has stable meaning across different contexts. These gestures are different from the *deictic gestures* (e.g., pointing, showing, giving) that characterize infancy, as deictic gestures are gestures whose meanings change depending on the context. As an example of a deictic gesture, an infant might point to a bottle and make a grabbing motion with his hand when he would like to drink his milk, and he might later point to a toy that he dropped from his high chair while making the same grabbing motion; the same gesture has two different meanings in these two contexts. The more advanced gestural form, referential gestures, shares some of the properties of first true words, and their use signals an impending transition from prelinguistic to linguistic communication.

Furthermore, as children are preparing to transition from the one-word stage to the two-word stage, they begin to exhibit gesture–word combinations. For instance, a 24-month-old child might point to a chair while saying "Mommy" as a way to request that her mother sit in a chair. Or, a child at this age might use two-gesture combinations, such as pointing to a banana while pretending to eat it to request to be fed (Capirci, Iverson, Pizzuto, & Volterra, 1996; Caselli, Volterra, & Pizzuto, 1984, as cited in Volterra et al., 2005). Toddlers who use more gesture + speech combinations (particularly those conveying sentence-like ideas) at 18 months also demonstrate greater sentence complexity at 42 months of age (Rowe & Goldin-Meadow, 2009).

Interestingly, when children begin to use two-word utterances, they stop combining two referential gestures. The reason may be that toddlers fill in gaps with gestures before they develop the competence to combine words but then allow their words to dominate when they can combine them successfully. The importance of gesture use to children's developing spoken language holds not only for children who are developing typically, but also for children who have developmental disabilities (Brady, Marquis, Fleming, & McLean, 2004) such as Down syndrome (Iverson, Longobardi, & Caselli, 2003).

Research has found that children's gesture use at 14 months is a significant predictor of their vocabulary size at 42 months, above and beyond the effects of parent and child word use at 14 months (Rowe, Özçalışkan, & Goldin-Meadow, 2008). Parents' gesture use at 14 months is also related to children's gesture use at 14 months. Although parents' gesture use at 14 months is not directly related to children's vocabulary size at 42 months, children whose parents use more gestures at 14 months also gesture more themselves, which is related to larger vocabulary sizes at 42 months. These research findings suggest that when it comes to predicting children's language development, it is important to pay attention not only to the words parents and children use during toddlerhood, but also to how they communicate using gestures.

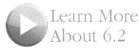

Learn More About 6.2

As you watch the video titled "Lights," notice how the 18-month-old boy uses gestures to point toward the lights he sees and wants his mother to look at. Notice also how he uses the phonological process of liquid gliding as he pronounces the word "lights" as "yights." Finally, notice how he combines words to form the sentence "Bye-bye lights" when he is finished looking at the lights and begins to walk away.

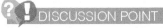

DISCUSSION POINT

What types of gestures would you expect to see toddlers who are more advanced in their language-development use? What about toddlers who are less advanced in their language development?

The earliest humans might have communicated with one another primarily by using hand gestures.

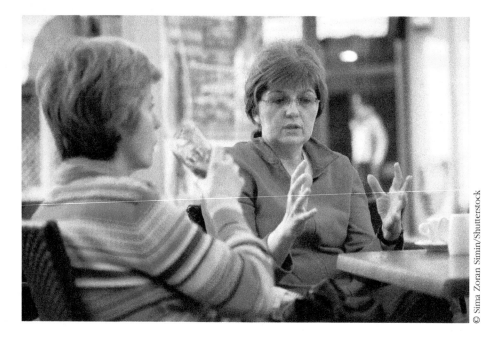

© Sima Zoran Simin/Shutterstock

Mirror Neurons and Gestures

Mirror neurons, a type of *visuomotor neurons* (related both to vision and to muscular movement), activate when people *perform* actions (including communicative actions) and when they *observe* other people perform actions. Evidence for a mirror neuron system in humans comes from neurophysiological and brain-imaging studies such as those discussed in Chapter 3. Some researchers have proposed mirror neurons are responsible for the evolution of gestures and language in humans. For example, Rizzolatti and Craighero (2004) proposed that hand–arm gestures and speech share a common neural substrate. They cited evidence from transcranial magnetic stimulation (TMS) studies—which involve noninvasive electrical stimulation of the nervous system—showing that when adults read and produce spontaneous speech, the excitability of the hand motor cortex increases in the left hemisphere of the brain. Furthermore, this activation is absent in the leg motor area and in the right hemisphere of the brain. So, could humans' earliest ancestors have communicated primarily through hand gestures, and does evidence of this system remain with people today? If so, a good reason may exist for why gesture use (either alone or accompanying speech) continues throughout the preschool years, the school-age years, and adulthood as a means of communication and a way to enhance communication. Future advances in neuroscience will undoubtedly continue to shed light on this theory.

Theory of Mind

In Chapter 5, we defined theory of mind (ToM) as the ability to understand one's own mental or emotional state, to understand that others also have mental or emotional states, and to realize that others' mental and emotional states, beliefs, intentions, and perspectives differ from one's own. In toddlerhood, the connection between ToM and language development becomes increasingly evident. Before explaining more about the connection, it is important to have some background about how researchers measure ToM development.

One common measure of ToM development is a false-belief task (of which there are a number of variations). False-belief tasks assess whether children demonstrate understanding that another's beliefs can differ from one's own beliefs. As one example, an experimenter hides an object in front of the child being assessed and

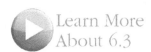

Learn More About 6.3

As you watch the video titled "False-Belief Task," notice how theory of mind develops and how researchers measure it with false belief tasks. https://www.youtube.com/watch?v=8hLubgpY2_w.

another observer (e.g., the experimenter hides a toy in a box in plain sight of the child and the observer). After the observer leaves the room, the experimenter moves the object to a different location that the child knows about but the original observer does not know about (e.g., the experimenter removes the toy from inside the box and places it under a couch). The experimenter then asks the child where the observer will think the object is. Children who have developed ToM indicate the observer will think the object is in its original hiding place (e.g., inside the box), whereas children who have not yet developed ToM indicate the observer will think the object is in the new hiding place (e.g., under the couch), demonstrating they are unable to take the perspective of the observer who presumably would not know the object had been moved.

A meta-analysis of 104 studies and nearly 9,000 children demonstrated a significant relation between children's language and theory of mind, as measured by false-belief tasks (Millington, Astington, & Dack, 2007). Results indicated a bidirectional relation between language and false-belief understanding (earlier performance on language measures predicts later performance on false-belief measures, as well as the reverse). However, results were stronger when predicting later false-belief understanding from earlier language measures, providing evidence that language appears to play a vital role in children's false-belief understanding and theory of mind development.

Some research (particularly research supportive of interactionist perspectives of development) suggests theory of mind develops from birth, and is evident by 18 months of age as toddlers are adept at reading the goals and intentions in other people's actions (Meltzoff, 1999). Recalling our discussion of joint engagement in Chapter 5, research indicates that toddlers (18 to 21 months of age) who spend more time in coordinated joint engagement (active coordination of attention between objects and social partners) and toddlers (27 to 30 months of age) who spend more time in symbol-infused joint engagement, including conversations and pretend play, demonstrate higher scores on false-belief tasks in the preschool years (between 42 and 66 months of age) (Nelson, Adamson, & Bakeman, 2008). This research suggests that as toddlers observe a social partner's actions and reactions to shared objects during periods of coordinated joint engagement and as they talk about shared objects during symbol-infused joint engagement, they learn vital information about other's mental states, which is crucial for theory of mind development.

The relation between theory of mind and language development becomes even more evident in the preschool years and the school-age years and beyond and is also relevant when considering specific disorders, such as autism.

✓ 6.1 Check Your Understanding

Click here to gauge your understanding of the concepts in this section.

WHAT MAJOR ACHIEVEMENTS IN LANGUAGE FORM, CONTENT, AND USE CHARACTERIZE TODDLERHOOD?

Recall the three rule-governed domains we first introduced in Chapter 1, that compose language: *form*, or how we organize sounds, words, and sentences to convey content; *content*, or words and their meanings; and *use*, or how we use language in interactions with other people to express personal and social needs. Toddlerhood heralds important achievements in each of these three areas. In the span of just a year or two, toddlers begin to use new speech sounds and acquire new phonological processes as they combine sounds in fluent speech. Toddlers begin to use morphology to change the form of words and they move from using single-word utterances to combining words. Toddlers also acquire their first word, their fiftieth word, and even their hundredth word and they are able to articulate many more communicative functions than they could in infancy.

DEVELOPMENTAL TIMELINE

PHONOLOGY

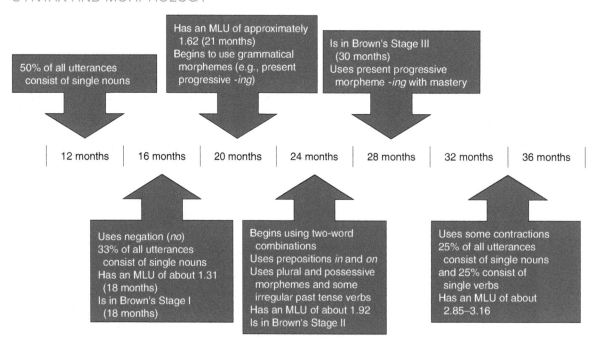

Pronounces about 70% of all words intelligibly — Demonstrates phonological processes (e.g., final-consonant omission, substitution of consonants)

Has mostly unintelligible speech, except for a few words

Processes spoken words incrementally

| 12 months | 16 months | 20 months | 24 months | 28 months | 32 months | 36 months |

Pronounces about 25% of all words intelligibly

Asks questions with rising intonation — Pronounces about 65% of all words intelligibly

Suppresses most common phonological processes by this age — Pronounces about 80% of all words intelligibly

SYNTAX AND MORPHOLOGY

Has an MLU of approximately 1.62 (21 months) — Begins to use grammatical morphemes (e.g., present progressive -ing)

Is in Brown's Stage III (30 months) — Uses present progressive morpheme -ing with mastery

50% of all utterances consist of single nouns

| 12 months | 16 months | 20 months | 24 months | 28 months | 32 months | 36 months |

Uses negation (no) — 33% of all utterances consist of single nouns — Has an MLU of about 1.31 (18 months) — Is in Brown's Stage I (18 months)

Begins using two-word combinations — Uses prepositions in and on — Uses plural and possessive morphemes and some irregular past tense verbs — Has an MLU of about 1.92 — Is in Brown's Stage II

Uses some contractions — 25% of all utterances consist of single nouns and 25% consist of single verbs — Has an MLU of about 2.85–3.16

(continued)

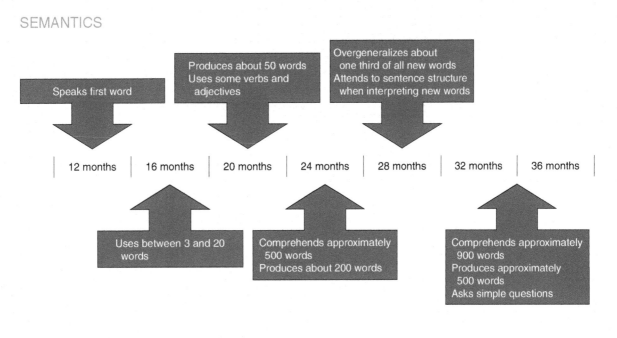

SEMANTICS

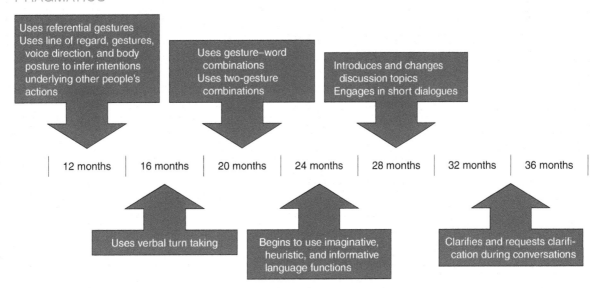

PRAGMATICS

Sources: Baldwin and Baird (1999); R. Brown (1973); Capirici et al. (1996); Fernald, Swingley, and Pinto (2001); Fisher (2002); Gard, Gilman, and Gorman (1993); Halliday (1978); Rescorla (1980); Volterra et al. (2005); and Weiss et al. (1987).

Language Form

Achievements in Phonology

Recall from Chapter 5, that the human phonological system begins to solidify from early infancy as babies take in the speech sounds they hear, categorize these sounds in meaningful ways, and use their implicit knowledge of speech sounds to begin to segment fluent speech into increasingly smaller units of meaning (clauses, words, morphemes). Phonological achievements in toddlerhood are much more noticeable than those that occur in infancy because people can *hear* these achievements. Toddlers begin to acquire and refine their repertoire of speech sounds, or phonemes, and, as they do so, adults witness their phonological processes or those arguably cute rule-governed errors children make when pronouncing certain words.

Norms for Phoneme Attainment.

Recall from our discussion of norms in Chapter 4, that the ages by which children can produce consonantal phonemes in English vary widely among research reports. Perhaps the most popular set of norms for phoneme attainment are Sander's (1972) customary ages of production (Figure 4.1), and ages of mastery of speech sounds (see Table 4.2, fifth column). The term customary age of production describes the age by which 50% of children can produce a given sound in multiple positions in words in an adultlike way. The term age of mastery describes the age by which most children produce a sound in an adultlike manner.

When attempting to assess toddlers' sound production abilities, practitioners must consider that phonemes are not typically produced in isolation. Neighboring sounds and combinations of sounds may affect children's production of particular sounds. Thus, to obtain an accurate picture of children's abilities, practitioners usually ask children to produce speech sounds in various positions (e.g., initial position of words and final position of words) and with a variety of neighboring sounds (e.g., followed by a vowel, after certain consonants). For instance, to understand whether a child can accurately use the speech sound /s/, we might entice a child to use this sound not only in the initial position of a word (*soft, soap, Sam*) but also in the medial (*castle, possum*) and final position (*yes, toss, bus*). Also, some consonants occur often in clusters with other consonants (e.g., *S + P* in *speech* and *spot*). Producing sounds within a cluster can be more challenging than producing sounds in isolation.

Phonological Processes.

As toddlers begin to gain more control over their articulators, adults witness developments in their phonology. Some people may view toddlerhood as a period during which young children talk in cute or funny ways. Cartoons even have characters, such as Tweety Bird, that emulate the phonological patterns of early childhood ("I tawt I taw a puddy tat"). However, what adults may not realize is that children who appear to make errors are in fact using systematic, rule-governed processes as they speak and are not simply making haphazard sound substitutions. The systematic, rule-governed patterns that characterize toddlers' speech are called phonological processes. Many researchers believe young children use phonological processes in an effort to simplify their inventory of phonetic elements and strings (e.g., Oller, 2006). Phonological process categories include syllable structure changes, assimilation, place-of-articulation changes, and manner-of-articulation changes. More specific types of phonological processes compose each category.

Syllable structure changes are simply changes to syllables in words. A common type of syllable structure change in child phonology is to repeat, or *reduplicate*, a stressed syllable in a word (*water* becomes "wa-wa" and *Daddy* becomes "Da-Da"). Another type of syllable structure change involves removing a portion of a cluster of consonants so it has fewer sounds, such as when a child says "stong" instead of "strong."

Assimilation is the process by which children change one sound in a syllable so it takes on the features of another sound in the same syllable. For example, in *velar assimilation*, the sound /d/ in *dog* takes on the velar sound (produced at the velum near the back of the mouth) of the /g/ that follows it, and *dog* becomes "gog." Assimilation is a context-dependent change, which means children make changes to certain sounds on the basis of influential neighboring sounds. In the example in which *dog* becomes "gog," the syllable-final /g/ exerts an influence on the syllable-initial /d/, so /d/ changes to /g/.

Children also make changes to sounds that are not context dependent, including place-of-articulation changes and manner-of-articulation changes. *Place-of-articulation changes* occur when children replace a sound produced at

With fronting, toddlers replace sounds produced farther back in the mouth (/k/) with sounds produced farther forward in the mouth (/t/), so that *cake* becomes "take."

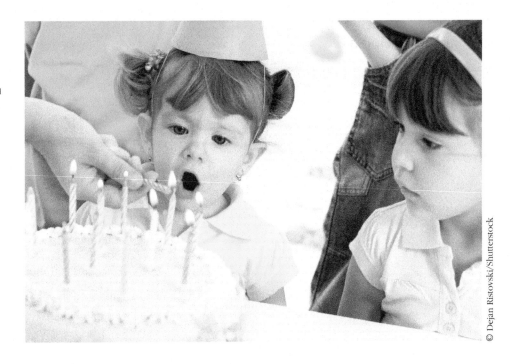

© Dejan Ristovski/Shutterstock

one location in the mouth with a sound produced at a different location in the mouth. For instance, children often replace sounds produced farther back in the mouth (e.g., /k/) with sounds produced farther forward in the mouth (e.g., /t/), so a child's pronunciation of *cake* becomes "take" in this process, which is called fronting. Place-of-articulation changes are not context dependent because children make these changes in the absence of influential neighboring sounds. In the example in which *cake* becomes "take," notice that /k/ does not change to /t/ because of the influence of any neighboring sounds that are produced closer to the front of the mouth; hence, this change is not context dependent.

Manner-of-articulation changes occur when children replace a sound produced in a particular manner with a sound produced in a different manner. A common substitution—called *stopping*—is to replace an affricate sound with a stop sound. In a *stop sound*, the airflow stops temporarily (e.g., the first and last sounds in the word *dot*). An *affricate sound* consists of a stop sound followed by a *fricative* (a sound produced by forcing air through a constricted passage; e.g., the consonant *s*). Thus, an affricate sound is a sound in which the airflow stops temporarily and then passes through a constricted space in the mouth—for example, the first sound in the word *jeep* or the first and last sounds in the word *church*. Consequently, when children replace the affricate *j* in *jeep* with the stop sound *d*, they say "deep" instead of "jeep" in a manner-of-articulation change.

Examples of common phonological processes appear in Table 6.1. Children typically suppress (i.e., eliminate) several of these processes by age 3 years, including final-consonant deletion, reduplication, consonant harmony, and weak-syllable deletion (Stoel-Gammon & Dunn, 1985). For instance, by 3 years of age, children will say "banana" instead of "nana" and "doggie" instead of "doddie." Other phonological processes, including cluster reduction and gliding, are often not suppressed until later, although few processes persist past 5 years of age.

Phonological Perception. As toddlers impress adults with their productive phonological achievements, such as their ability to combine sounds to produce words and phrases, they continue to make progress behind the scenes as well. Toddlers who are expanding their lexicons must possess skills to integrate incoming speech sounds with their existing linguistic and conceptual knowledge if they

? ! DISCUSSION POINT
Do you think toddlers would notice anything strange if an adult were to use childlike phonology? Why might they or might they not notice?

TABLE 6.1
Common phonological processes

CATEGORY	TYPE	DESCRIPTION	EXAMPLE
Syllable structure changes	Weak-syllable deletion	Child deletes an unstressed syllable	*banana* = "nana"
	Final-consonant deletion	Child deletes the last consonant in a syllable	*cat* = "ca"
	Reduplication	Child repeats an entire syllable or part of a syllable	*water* = "wa-wa"
	Cluster reduction	Child reduces a cluster of consonants to include fewer consonant sounds	*splash* = "spash"
Assimilation	Consonant harmony	Child uses consonants with like features in a word	*doggie* = "doddie"
	Velar assimilation	Child produces a nonvelar consonant as a velar consonant because of a nearby velar sound	*dog* = "gog"
	Nasal assimilation	Child produces a nonnasal sound as a nasal sound because of a nearby nasal sound	*candy* = "nanny"
Place-of-articulation changes	Fronting	Child replaces a sound produced farther back in the mouth with a sound produced farther forward	*corn* = "dorn"
	Backing	Child replaces a sound produced farther forward in the mouth with a sound produced farther back	*daddy* = "gaggy"
Manner-of-articulation changes	Stopping	Child replaces a fricative or an affricate sound with a stop sound	*jeep* = "deep"
	Gliding	Child replaces a liquid sound with a glide	*love* = "wove"

are to continue to acquire new words rapidly. One such skill involves becoming familiar with the differences in speech that do and do not signal a difference in meaning (Swingley, 2008). Toddlers, unlike their younger infant counterparts, recognize that that when different speakers say two identical words, they are the same word. This achievement provides evidence that toddlers have developed the ability to recognize that vocal characteristics of a speaker are not properties of the words themselves. A toddler with this ability can safely assume when his or her mother says the word "water" and his or her father says the word "water," both parents are referring to the same thing.

The time at around 18 months of age, or approximately when many toddlers show evidence of a vocabulary spurt, seems to mark a transitional period in phonological development (see Swingley, 2008). A *transitional period* is a developmental time frame during which language abilities are emerging and changing. During a transitional period, it may sometimes appear that a toddler has mastered a certain ability, such as word learning, and at other times, it may appear that the same toddler has not mastered the same ability. The transitional period in phonological perception is evidenced, in part, by toddlers' successful learning of *novel nonneighbors* (new words that are not phonologically similar to known words) and difficulty in learning *novel neighbors* (new words that are phonologically similar to known words). For example, in a word-learning study, Swingley and Aslin (2007) found that toddlers experience difficulty learning the novel neighbors "tog" and "gall" when they are familiar with the words "dog" and "ball." Because we know from other research on word learning that toddlers are indeed capable of learning novel nonneighbors, and that older children and adults are capable of learning novel neighbors, it appears that toddlers' difficulty in learning novel neighbors reflects a transition in their phonological perception abilities.

In terms of other developments in phonological perception in toddlerhood, research indicates that toddlers become increasingly adept at recognizing words after hearing only parts of the words, or what is called *partial phonetic information*. For example, in one study, 18- and 21-month-olds could approximately associate the first two phonemes of a word with its corresponding picture, which indicates toddlers process spoken words incrementally before speakers even finish uttering the words (Fernald et al., 2001). Researchers have further found that they can use spoken word recognition speed and vocabulary size at 25 months to make

LANGUAGE DIVERSITY AND DIFFERENCES

Multiple Language Exposure and Toddler Language Development

Parents sometimes express concern that exposing their children to multiple languages might have negative effects on the rate at which their children develop language, decrease the level of linguistic competency the children will be able to attain, and potentially confuse the children. In a study examining native language phonetic representations in bilingual and monolingual infants and toddlers, Burns, Yoshida, Hill, and Werker (2007) found that the development of phonetic representation in toddlers learning two languages is not delayed. Burns and colleagues (2007) tested infants and toddlers in three age groups (6–8 months, 10–12 months, and 14–20 months) from English-only environments and English–French environments to determine whether they could discriminate between French and English speech sounds. The French speech sounds included /pa/ and /ba/, and the English speech sounds included /pa/ and /pʰa/ (where /pʰ/ is pronounced with additional aspiration or breath, which slightly delays the voicing of the vowel sound as compared to /pa/). Consistent with the phonetic representation research described in Chapter 5, researchers found that the younger infants (both monolingual and bilingual) were able to discriminate between the subtle differences in all the speech sounds they heard. However, the results were different for the older infants and toddlers. The 10- to 12-month-olds and the 14- to 20-month-olds from English-only environments could only distinguish between the two sounds that are phonemic, or meaningful, in English (/ba/ and /pʰa/), whereas the 10- to 12-month-olds and the 14- to 20-month-olds from English–French environments could distinguish between the sounds corresponding to the French and English representations (/ba/ and /pa/ for French and /pa/ and /pʰa/ for English). Because the monolingual and bilingual older infants and toddlers demonstrated different discrimination patterns, the researchers concluded bilingual infants and toddlers establish phonetic representations for each of their languages in the same way and at the same time as monolingual infants and toddlers. This suggests that when infants are exposed to two languages from the time they are born, they are equipped to process the phonology of both languages in a nativelike manner.

predictions about children's linguistic and cognitive skills at 8 years (Marchman & Fernald, 2008). It thus appears that speech-perception abilities are important not only to word learning that occurs in toddlerhood, but also to speech processing and language abilities throughout the life span.

One question that sometimes arises at this stage of language development is whether exposure to multiple languages might delay aspects of toddlers' phonological perception. See Language Diversity and Differences: *Multiple Language Exposure and Toddler Language Development* for a discussion of this topic.

Achievements in Morphology

The 50-word mark for productive vocabulary, which toddlers reach between about ages 18 months and 2 years, signals some important changes, including the vocabulary spurt. The 50-word mark also usually co-occurs with the appearance of children's first grammatical morphemes.

Grammatical Morphemes. A *morpheme* is a meaningful linguistic unit that cannot be divided into smaller meaningful parts. *Grammatical morphemes* are inflections we add to words to indicate aspects of grammar, such as the plural *-s* (*two dogs*), the possessive *'s* (*the dog's bone*), the past tense *-ed* (*The dog barked*), and the present progressive *-ing* (*The dog is still barking*). We add morphemes to a word to change its form, and they are an important aspect of grammatical development.

Grammatical morphemes begin to appear in children's speech between ages 18 and 24 months—at about the time when they have learned their first 50 words. Roger Brown (1973), a pioneer in studying early morphological development, documented the order in which and the ages by which children master 14 grammatical morphemes (see Table 6.2). These grammatical morphemes develop in roughly the

TABLE 6.2
Grammatical morphemes acquired in early childhood

GRAMMATICAL MORPHEME	AGE OF APPEARANCE (MONTHS)	EXAMPLE
Present progressive *-ing*	19–28	"Baby eat<u>ing</u>"
Plural *-s*	27–30	"Doggie<u>s</u>"
Preposition *in*	27–30	"Toy <u>in</u> there"
Preposition *on*	31–34	"Food <u>on</u> table"
Possessive *'s*	31–34	"Mommy<u>'s</u> book"
Regular past tense *-ed*	43–46	"We paint<u>ed</u>."
Irregular past tense	43–46	"I <u>ate</u> lunch."
Regular third person singular *-s*	43–46	"He run<u>s</u> fast."
Articles *a, the, an*	43–46	"I want <u>the</u> blocks."
Contractible copula *be*	43–46	"She<u>'s</u> my friend."
Contractible auxiliary	47–50	"He'<u>s</u> playing."
Uncontractible copula *be*	47–50	"He <u>was</u> sick."
Uncontractible auxiliary	47–50	"He <u>was</u> playing."
Irregular third person	47–50	"She <u>has</u> one."

Source: Information from *A First Language: The Early Stages*, by R. Brown, 1973, Cambridge, MA: Harvard University Press.

same order for English-speaking children; children do not generally master all of these morphemes until about preschool age.

Researchers have devised some creative methods to learn when toddlers begin to comprehend certain morphemes. As an example, we describe one such study that incorporated a manual search method to explore toddlers' comprehension of the singular–plural morphology distinction in English (Wood, Kouider, & Carey, 2009). Using the manual search method, an experimenter placed a familiar object (e.g., a car) inside a box so the toddler could not see it. After a few practice trials, during which the toddler learned how to reach inside the box to retrieve objects, the experimenter performed a series of test trials. Each test trial incorporated different morphology and other markers that signified whether the box contained one or more objects. The experimenter requested that the child retrieve the object or objects in one of four ways: (a) singular search trials with multiple marking (e.g., "Now I'm going to put <u>a car</u> in my box. … Wow! There's a car in my box. … Could you get <u>the car</u> for me?"); (b) plural search trials with multiple marking (e.g., "Now I'm going to put <u>some cars</u> in my box. … Wow! There are <u>some cars</u> in my box. … Could you get <u>some cars</u> for me?"); (c) singular search trials with noun marking only (e.g., "Now I'm going to put my car in the box. … Wow! I see my car in my box. … Could you get my car for me?"); and (d) plural search trials with noun marking only (e.g., "Now I'm going to put my cars in the box. … Wow! I see my cars in my box. … Could you get my cars for me?"). In all cases, there was actually only one object in the box as the infants began to search, and researchers measured the amount of time toddlers spent searching inside the box with their hand. They hypothesized that toddlers who understood plural morphology and the associated markers would search longer when the experimenter made a request using plural morphology and markers than when the experimenter used singular morphology and markers. Findings revealed that at 24 months of age, but not at 20 months, toddlers searched the box longer when they heard plural morphology with multiple markers (example b) but not when they heard plural morphology with noun marking only (example d). This study indicates toddlers begin to understand verbal morphology sometime between 20 and 24 months of age; furthermore, they seem to require extra cues (markers such as *a*, *the*, *some*) to support their comprehension of English singular–plural morphology.

In terms of production, the first grammatical morpheme children tend to produce is the present progressive *-ing*, as in *Baby sleeping*. Children begin to use this morpheme at around age 18 months and use it with mastery by age 28 months. Additional morphemes that appear during toddlerhood include the prepositions *in* and *on*, which children start to use at about age 2 years (*<u>in</u> cup*, *<u>on</u> table*). At this time, toddlers also start to use the regular plural *-s*, as in *two dog<u>s</u>*; the possessive *'s*, as in *kitty<u>'s</u> bowl*; and irregular past tense verbs, as in *eat–<u>ate</u>* and *break–<u>broke</u>*.

Irregular past tense verbs do not conform to the regular verb pattern, which is to add *-ed*. Therefore, toddlers must memorize them. The English language has between 150 and 180 irregular verbs. When you talk with toddlers, you will likely notice they tend to *overgeneralize* the rule for regular past tense verbs ("Add *-ed*") by applying it to irregular verbs. As a result, toddlers often say things such as "I maked it" and "Mommy goed to the store." Pinker (1999) explained that children who have acquired the regular past tense rule often overgeneralize its use to irregular verbs until they have had sufficient exposure to and practice with words (e.g., the irregular form of a verb) and rules (e.g., applying the past tense ending of a regular verb, *-ed*).

Children learn words and rules in other morphological cases as well. For example, when learning contractions, children sometimes apply a rule (e.g., "Add *n't* to change *have* to *have<u>n't</u>* and add *n't* to change *has* to *has<u>n't</u>*"). Other times, children learn contractions as a unit or a word (e.g., *won't*), most likely because the sound of the root (*will*) is not the same in the contracted form (*won't*). So, just as children memorize irregular past tense verbs, they must also memorize contractions that do not conform to the typical pattern.

Achievements in Syntax

In addition to inflecting words with grammatical morphemes, toddlers begin to combine words to create multiword utterances. Instead of requesting a favorite ball by saying "ball," as an infant in the one-word stage might do, toddlers might instead say "Mommy ball." This stage (sometimes called the *two-word stage*), in which toddlers begin to combine words to make utterances, marks the true beginning of *syntax*, or the rules that govern the order of words in a child's language. Toddlers recognize the value that combining words has over using single words and can use language for many more communicative functions than they did in the one-word stage. Some simple functions toddlers can express during the two-word stage include commenting ("Baby cry"), negating ("No juice"), requesting ("More juice"), and questioning ("What that?").

Child language researchers credit Roger Brown not only with documenting the order and ages by which children acquire grammatical morphemes, but also with creating *Brown's Stages of Language Development* (see Chapter 2 for an introduction to Brown's work). Brown's stages characterize children's language achievements according to the ability to produce utterances of varying syntactic complexity (see Table 6.3). One measure of the complexity of children's language is their mean length of utterance (MLU). MLU is the average length, in morphemes, of children's

TABLE 6.3
Roger Brown's (1973) stages of language development

BROWN'S STAGE	AGE (UPPER LIMIT IN MONTHS)	MLU	MLU RANGE	MAJOR ACHIEVEMENTS
I	18	1.31	0.99–1.64	Single-word sentences are used. Nouns and uninflected verbs are used ("Mommy"; "eat")
II	24	1.92	1.47–2.37	Two-element sentences are used. True clauses that are not evident are used ("Mommy up"; "Eat cookie")
III	30	2.54	1.97–3.11	Three-element sentences are used. Independent clauses emerge ("Baby want cookie").
IV	36	3.16	2.47–3.85	Four-element sentences are used. Independent clauses continue to emerge ("The teacher gave it to me").
V	42	3.78	2.96–4.60	Recursive elements predominate. Connecting devices emerge ("and"; "because").
Post-V	54	5.02	3.96–6.08	Complex syntactic patterns appear. Subordination and coordination continue to emerge. Complement clauses are used ("She's not feeling well").

MLU = mean length of utterance.

Source: Information based on *Guide to Analysis of Language Transcript*, 3rd Ed. (pp. 111–112), by K. S. Retherford, 2000, Austin, TX: PRO-ED. Copyright 2000, by PRO-ED, Inc.; and from *Reference Manual for Communicative Sciences and Disorders: Speech and Language* (pp. 285–286), by R. D. Kent, 1994, Austin, TX: PRO-ED. Copyright 1994 by PRO-ED, Inc. Adapted with permission.

utterances. We can calculate MLU by counting the total number of morphemes in a sample of 50–100 spontaneous utterances and then dividing that number by the total number of utterances:

$$\text{MLU} = \frac{\text{Total number of morphemes}}{\text{Total number of utterances}}$$

There are additional conventions for counting morphemes (see Brown, 1973 for the complete set of rules), including the following: Do not count fillers, such as umm or oh; count proper names, compound words (e.g., birthday) and ritualized reduplications (e.g., choo choo) as a single word; count catenatives (e.g., gonna, wanna) as a single word, but count auxiliaries (e.g., is, have) as separate morphemes.

As children's language develops, their MLU increases systematically, as Table 6.4 illustrates. Researchers and clinicians alike use MLU regularly to evaluate children's language skills against the expectations, or norms, for children of the same age. As a general standard, we calculate MLU using a language sample of 50 utterances or more to obtain a representative sample of what the child can produce. For the sake of explanation, however, we present a short sample to demonstrate how you might calculate the MLU for a 3-year-old:

UTTERANCE NUMBER	UTTERANCE	NUMBER OF MORPHEMES
1	"I want the ball."	4
2	"Make it go."	3
3	"No!"	1
4	"Up there."	2
5	"I want turn."	3
6	"Going over there."	4
7	"Look at that one."	4
8	"Mommy's turn."	3

In this brief sample, the child produced eight utterances and 24 morphemes, which resulted in an MLU of 3.0. The norms appearing in Table 6.4 indicate the predicted MLU for a child who is 3 years old is 3.16. Sixty-eight percent of children have scores within one standard deviation of 3.16, or between 2.47 and 3.85. If our sample is accurate, this child's MLU is within normal limits.

Sentence Forms. When grammatical morphemes first emerge and children begin to combine words, language exhibits a telegraphic quality that results when children omit key grammatical markers. We describe toddlers' speech as telegraphic because persons sending telegrams would omit function words (e.g., *a, the*) to save money on the transmission. A toddler's "Mommy no go" and "Fishy swimming" are telegraphic reductions of "Mommy, don't go" and "The fish is swimming." Toddlers also tend to omit or misuse pronouns in their sentences ("Me do it"; "Her going"). Despite these awkward constructions, toddlers begin to use more adultlike forms for a variety of sentence types, including the yes–no question ("Are we going, Mommy?"), *wh-* questions ("What's that?"), commands ("You do it"), and negatives ("Me no want that").

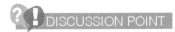
DISCUSSION POINT

Do you think speaking to toddlers at their own level—for example, by using telegraphic speech—would be beneficial? Why or why not?

TABLE 6.4

Normative references for interpreting MLU

AGE (MONTHS)	PREDICTED MLU	PREDICTED MLU ± 1 STANDARD DEVIATION (68% OF POPULATION)
18	1.31	0.99–1.64
21	1.62	1.23–2.01
24	1.92	1.47–2.37
27	2.23	1.72–2.74
30	2.54	1.97–3.11
33	2.85	2.22–3.48
36	3.16	2.47–3.85
39	3.47	2.71–4.23
42	3.78	2.96–4.60
45	4.09	3.21–4.97
48	4.40	3.46–5.34
51	4.71	3.71–5.71
54	5.02	3.96–6.08
57	5.32	4.20–6.45
60	5.63	4.44–6.82

Source: From "The Relation Between Age and Mean Length of Utterance in Morphemes," by J. F. Miller and R. Chapman, 1981, *Journal of Speech and Hearing Research, 24,* p. 157. Copyright 1981 by American Speech-Language-Hearing Association. Adapted with permission.

Language Content

Toddlerhood is witness to tremendous growth in language content. During this time, toddlers progress from novice to expert word learners and make large gains in both their receptive and expressive lexicons. In the sections that follow, we discuss the process of word learning, including strategies toddlers use to acquire words rapidly. We also discuss how toddlers learn to link meaning in the events they see with their syntactic correlates in sentences.

Acquisition of New Words: The Quinean Conundrum

For a toddler to learn a new word—or create a new lexical entry—he or she must minimally do the following: segment the word from continuous speech; find objects, events, actions, and concepts in the world; and map the new word to its corresponding object, event, action, or concept. The final task, *mapping*, is the key to learning a new word successfully and may require more than meets the eye. Imagine, as philosopher W. V. O. Quine proposed, that you encounter a native speaker of a foreign language who utters the word *gavagai* in the presence of a rabbit. Should you infer the word *gavagai* means "rabbit," "food," "undetached rabbit part," or something else? This dilemma—the uncertainty surrounding the mapping of a word to its referent in the face of seemingly endless interpretations—is called the *mapping problem, induction problem*, or *Quinean conundrum*. The mapping problem poses challenges for all people learning a new language, but especially for infants and toddlers learning their first language. Just as theories of language learning differ, so do explanations for how children overcome the Quinean conundrum as they learn new words.

Lexical Principles Framework for Acquiring New Words

Recall from Chapter 4 that language-development theories have implications for how people view various language achievements. Word learning is no exception. The fact is that children rapidly learn new words in a very short period of time, and we know far less about how they do this than we want to admit. Because we cannot look into the child's brain and see exactly what is happening when he or she acquires a new word, we have to rely on theories, of which there are many. Some language-learning theories presuppose that children arrive at the task of word learning with predispositions or biases that help them eliminate some of the nearly infinite number of referents a novel word could describe (the Quinean conundrum). Golinkoff, Mervis, and Hirsh-Pasek (1994) organized a series of word-learning biases proposed by other researchers into what they termed the *lexical principles framework* for early object labels. This framework consists of two tiers: The first tier includes the principles of reference, extendibility, and object scope; the second tier includes the principles of conventionality, categorical scope, and novel name–nameless category (N3C; Figure 6.2).

First-Tier Principles.   The three principles that compose the first tier of the lexical principles framework do not require much linguistic sophistication. Children can use Tier 1 principles as soon as they begin to acquire words because these principles rely on cognitive-perceptual abilities (Hollich, Hirsh-Pasek, & Golinkoff, 2000). The principle of reference states that words symbolize objects, actions, events, and concepts. For example, the word *Daddy* stands for or symbolizes someone's father; a child can use this word in the presence of his or her father, or the child can refer to his or her father who exists in a different place ("Daddy is at work") or time ("Daddy wore a red hat yesterday").

The principle of extendibility conveys that words label categories of objects and not just the original exemplar. Therefore, the word *ball* can describe multiple objects that fall under the basic-level category *ball* (baseball, basketball, soccer ball, tennis ball). Children commonly extend words to include objects of similar shape,

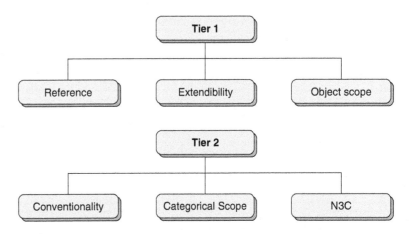

FIGURE 6.2

Lexical principles framework.

N3C = novel name–nameless category.

Source: Golinkoff, R. M., Mervis, C. B., & Hirsh-Pasek, K. (1994). Early object labels: The case for a developmental lexical principles framework. *Journal of child language, 21*(01), 125-155. Copyright © 1994 by Cambridge University Press. Reprinted by permission.

size, color, smell, and material makeup; shape is the most common feature that children extend early in language development (Landau, Smith, & Jones, 1998; Smith, Jones, & Landau, 1992).

The principle of object scope states that words map to whole objects. First, children using the principle of object scope assume novel words label objects rather than actions. When children hear a novel label, they prefer to attach the label to an object instead of an action (e.g., Meyer et al., 2003). Second, object scope presupposes the whole object assumption, which means words label whole objects and not object parts (Markman, 1990, 1991). Therefore, a toddler who witnesses a bird flying in the sky as his or her mother exclaims "A bird!" will likely assume the word *bird* refers to the bird rather than the action of flying and, more specifically, to the whole bird rather than to the bird's wings, beak, or feet.

Second-Tier Principles.   The three principles that compose the second tier of the lexical principles framework are more sophisticated and become available to children as they refine their hypotheses about the nature of words. The principle of conventionality states that for children to communicate successfully, they must adopt the terms that people in their language community understand (see Clark, 1993). Children begin to refine their vocabulary and the Tier 1 principle of reference by using the principle of conventionality when they recognize that some of their "baby" words, such as *blankie* for *blanket*, are not conventional among other speakers in their culture.

The principle of categorical scope builds on the Tier 1 principle of extendibility by limiting the basis for extension to words in the same category. Consider the following scenario: An experimenter shows a toddler a picture of a banana then asks the child to "find another dax." The experimenter then allows the child to choose between three pictures: a bunch of grapes (an item in the same superordinate category as the banana—fruit), a monkey (an item thematically related to the banana), and a crescent-shaped moon (an item perceptually similar to the banana). Children who honor the categorical scope constraint would choose the grapes instead of the thematically similar item (the monkey) or the perceptually similar item (the crescent moon). This particular word-learning constraint may thus help toddlers narrow the correct interpretation for new superordinate-level terms they encounter (Golinkoff, Shuff-Bailey, Olguin, & Ruan, 1995).

The principle of novel name–nameless category (N3C) supports the Tier 1 principle of object scope by helping children select a nameless object as the recipient of a novel label. The N3C principle rests on the principle of *mutual exclusivity*, which states that objects have only one label (Markman, 1989; Merriman & Bowman, 1989). The principle of mutual exclusivity comes into play in situations where children hear a novel label and see a series of objects in the environment for which they already have labels. For example, suppose you present a toddler with a box containing a ball, a book, and a thermometer. Suppose further that the toddler knows the words *book* and *ball* but does not know the word *thermometer*. If you then requested the thermometer, the toddler would likely select the thermometer because he or she knows the ball is not called "thermometer" and the book is not called "thermometer." The N3C principle operates similarly to mutual exclusivity, with one exception: N3C does not presuppose children avoid attaching more than one label to an object.

Social-Pragmatic Framework for Acquiring New Words

Proponents of the social-pragmatic view of word learning believe children do not require domain-specific mechanisms, including the lexical principles just mentioned, to acquire new words. Rather, these theorists propose young children are adept at using social cues to determine what a speaker is referring to, and that understanding speakers' referential intentions assists children in learning language (Sabbagh & Baldwin, 2005) and overcoming the Quinean conundrum. According

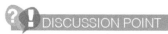
DISCUSSION POINT
How might toddlers, preschoolers, school-age children, and adults differ in how they determine the meanings of unfamiliar words?

to social-pragmatic theorists, as adults interact with children, they offer many social cues to the meanings of words, which makes lexical principles unnecessary. Infants and toddlers can understand an array of sophisticated social cues at an early age. They can follow another person's gaze and pointing gestures, engage in joint attention, and imitate actions by age 9–12 months (Baldwin, 1995). As early as age 12 months, infants can use social cues—including line of regard (the direction of a person's gaze, which indicates what the person is looking at), gestures, voice direction, and body posture—to infer the intentions underlying other people's actions (Baldwin & Baird, 1999). Research results indicate toddlers are adept at using social-pragmatic cues to word meanings, even in seemingly difficult circumstances. Such circumstances include when the referent of the word is not physically present (Akhtar & Tomasello, 1996), when an adult uses an *imperative* statement ("Put the toma down") rather than an explicit labeling statement ("That is a toma"; Callanan, Akhtar, Sussman, & Sabbagh, 2003), and when the child overhears a word by monitoring other people's conversations (Akhtar, 2005; Akhtar, Jipson, & Callanan, 2001).

Fast Mapping

Have you ever used a fairly complex word in front of a toddler and later, to your amazement, heard the toddler use that word? As you undoubtedly know, toddlers' ability to pick up words after only a few incidental exposures, or even a single exposure, is remarkable. This ability is termed fast mapping because of the brief exposure to the novel word and its referent, for which children form a lexical representation (Carey & Bartlett, 1978). As one example, a toddler might quickly learn that his parents exclaim "uh oh!" when he drops something on the floor from his high chair. After just a few exposures to that word, the toddler might himself exclaim "uh oh!" when he drops a toy or a piece of food on the floor.

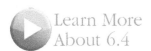

Learn More About 6.4

As you watch the video titled "Fast Mapping Task Using the IPLP," you will see a 33-month-old child participating in an Intermodal Preferential Looking Paradigm (IPLP) task in Dr. Roberta Golinkoff's University of Delaware research lab.

Learn More About 6.4 *(Continued)*

This method is similar to that of the Interactive Intermodal Preferential Looking Paradigm (IIPLP) we introduced in Chapter 5, with one difference being the training phase is not interactive. Instead, participants watch a video that presents novel labels for the child to learn. In this case, the novel labels describe attributes of an animated starfish and a tin-man.

Like the IIPLP, the IPLP begins with two familiarization trials that help the child understand her role in the task. In the first familiarization trial, the experimenter asks Abby to point to the ball (which is on the left side of the screen); in the second familiarization trial, the experimenter requests that Abby point to the hat (which is on the right side of the screen).

During the training phase of the study, the experimenter introduces the two characters in the video, Starry and Tin-man. We then see Starry performing jumping jacks as the experimenter describes Starry as "blickish." This word ends with the morpheme *ish*, which in English denotes a characteristic of something (e.g., childish = characteristic of a child, greenish = characteristic of the color green). In this case, Starry is a solid green color.

A salience trial follows, during which the experimenter directs the child's attention to the screen using a neutral request. A brown, textured Starry performs jumping jacks on the left side of the screen and a solid green Starry spins in a circle on the right side of the screen. The purpose of this trial is to introduce the child to two different versions of Starry side-by-side, each performing a different action, to determine whether she has an a priori preference for one of the two versions of the character.

(Continued)

During the test trials, the child again sees a brown, textured Starry performing jumping jacks on the left side of the screen and a solid green Starry spinning in a circle on the right side of the screen. The experimenter then says, "Starry is blickish. Can you point and show me?" If the child understands that "blickish" describes a characteristic, she should point to the solid green Starry on the right side of the screen. To make the task more difficult, the child must realize that "blickish" does not describe the action Starry is performing. If she understood "blickish" to mean the jumping jacks action, she might instead point to the brown, textured Starry on the left side of the screen. Following this trial is a second, identical test trial, a new label trial, during which the experimenter requests that the child indicate where "Starry is fepish," and a recovery trial identical to the first two test trials. The video clip of the IIPLP (associated with Chapter 5) provides a description of the purpose of the new label trial and recovery trial.

The next portion of the video illustrates the camera's point of view during a similar task that assesses children's understanding of the morpheme *ing*. The camera records the child's pointing responses throughout the study. Coding is performed offline by an observer who is blind to the study condition, meaning he or she does not know on which side of the screen the target responses appear.

There is evidence that although young children can fast map new words, fast mapping is not an ability specific to word learning. For example, researchers have discovered that 3-year-olds, 4-year-olds, and adults can learn and retain a fact about an object (such as who gave the object to the experimenter as a gift) as easily as they can learn and retain a new object name (Markson & Bloom, 1997). Markson and Bloom suggested that because fast mapping is not restricted to word learning, there is evidence for a *domain-general* word-learning mechanism. This claim spurred an interesting interchange between Waxman and Booth (2000, 2001) and P. Bloom and Markson (2001) about whether word learning is a result of domain-specific or domain-general mechanisms. Waxman and Booth disagreed with Bloom and Markson's findings and countered that although fast mapping need not be specific to word learning, no evidence exists that word learning and fact learning rest on the same set of underlying principles. This exchange demonstrates how contention may exist with regard to the mechanisms that drive language development and whether these mechanisms are domain general or domain specific.

Thematic Roles Toddlers Acquire

A *thematic role* is the part a word plays in an event, and such roles include agent, theme, source, goal, and location (O'Grady, 1997). An agent is the entity that performs the action (*Nicole ate pasta*). The theme is the entity undergoing an action or a movement (*Tamika flew a kite*). A source is the starting point for movement and a goal is the ending point for movement (*Maurie drove from Richmond to Charlottesville*). Location is the place where an action occurs (*Ryan hiked through the park*).

Toddlers begin to understand thematic roles from an early age and, more important, they learn how thematic roles link to corresponding syntactic elements. For example, 2.5-year-old toddlers attend to the overall structure of sentences when interpreting new words. Moreover, they use syntactic bootstrapping (as we discussed in Chapter 4) to interpret the meanings of novel verbs when they are familiar with the nouns that surround an unfamiliar verb in a sentence. As illustrated in a study by Fisher (2002), young children who know some nouns can correctly interpret the meaning of a novel verb by counting the number of nouns they hear in a sentence. The children in the study correctly inferred that in the sentence "She's pilking over there," the word *pilking* refers to an intransitive verb (one that does not have a direct object), and that in the sentence "She's pilking her over there," the word *pilking* refers to a transitive verb (one that requires a direct object). Fisher reached this conclusion when she found children more often picked the agent (the girl performing the pilking action) as the subject of transitive verbs than intransitive verbs. Because the children performed differently depending on the type of sentence they heard, it means they noticed the sentences differed by only one noun: Both the intransitive and transitive verbs had the noun *she* as the subject of the sentence, and the transitive verbs additionally had the noun *her* as the direct object of the sentence. The toddlers in the study used this seemingly small piece of information to interpret the meaning of the new verbs correctly. Having an implicit understanding of thematic roles and how thematic roles correspond to syntactic elements thus seems to assist toddlers in narrowing the number of possible interpretations for new words they hear.

Receptive and Expressive Lexicons

Recall that the *receptive lexicon* is the words children comprehend, and the *expressive lexicon* is the words children produce. Although young children begin acquiring new words relatively slowly, some researchers contend that toddlers' word learning enters an explosive period between approximately 18 and 24 months of age, or at around the time they can produce 50 words. This period has been aptly termed the *vocabulary spurt*, *word spurt*, or *naming explosion*. During this time, children may learn up to seven to nine new words per day. Parents who have begun to record their toddler's words in a diary remark that they begin to lose track of the child's new words during this period of accelerated growth. However, although children learn about seven to nine new words per day between ages 18 and 24 months, they do not always use these words the way adults do. Rather, they often overextend, underextend, and overlap words.

Overextension. Overextension, or *overgeneralization*, is the process by which children use words in an overly general manner. Toddlers make three major kinds of overextensions: categorical, analogical, and relational. Toddlers make *categorical overextensions* when they extend a word they know to other words in the same category. For example, if a child learns the word *dog* and then calls all four-legged animals "dog," he or she is making a categorical overextension. Another example would be if a child learned the word *milk* and called all liquids "milk."

Toddlers make *analogical overextensions* when they extend a word they know to other words that are perceptually similar. For example, a child may learn the word *ball* and then call other round objects (e.g., the moon, an orange) "ball" as well. The second author (L. J.) witnessed another example of this type of overextension as used by her then 2-year-old son Griffin. He picked up a hanger from the floor of her closet, held it up, and exclaimed "umbrella!" At first blush, this seems a bit strange (as are many things toddlers do), but it makes perfect sense from a word-learning perspective, because hangers do look a bit like umbrellas from a perceptual perspective.

Toddlers make *relational overextensions* when they extend a word they know to other words that are semantically or thematically related. For instance, Dillon may use the word *flower* to refer to a watering can that he sees his mother use to water flowers. He may use the same word to refer to flowerpots his mother uses to house the flowers.

Toddlers overgeneralize about one-third of all new words on the basis of categorical, analogical, and relational similarities (Rescorla, 1980). However, even more common than overextensions are underextensions.

Underextension. When toddlers learn new words, they use these words cautiously and conservatively at first. This process, whereby toddlers use words to refer to only a subset of possible referents, is called underextension. When a toddler girl uses the word *book* only when referring to the hardcover books in her collection (and not to her parents' paperback books), or when she uses the word *bottle* to

Toddlers engaging in under-extension might, for example, fail to label multiple exemplars of cups as "cup."

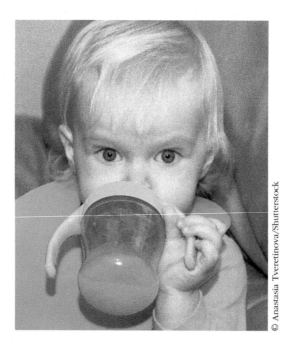

© Anastasia Tveretinova/Shutterstock

refer only to her baby bottle (and not to glass bottles or plastic water bottles), she is engaging in underextension.

Overlap.   When toddlers overextend a word in certain circumstances and under-extend the same word in other circumstances, this process is called overlap. For example, when a toddler boy uses the word *candy* to refer to jelly beans *and* his grandmother's pills (overextension) but *not* to chocolate bars (underextension), he is engaging in overlap.

Reasons for Word-Use Errors.   Toddlers' overextensions, underextensions, and overlaps might be viewed as types of errors in their early word use. These errors are often very cute (as when a toddler yells "mama" to a stranger), but they also present the opportunity to learn a great deal about young children's language acquisition and the way in which they learn new words. Why do children make such errors? At least three possible explanations have been offered as to why children use words in different ways than adults (see Gershkoff-Stowe, 2001). First, children may make *category membership errors*. For instance, they may truly think a horse and a cow are the same kind of animal and thus use the word *horse* to label a cow because they know the word *horse*.

Second, children may make *pragmatic errors*. Children make such errors when they know two objects are conceptually different but do not yet have a name for one of the objects and intentionally substitute a semantically related word. For example, a young boy may know a horse and a dog are different animals, but because he does not know the word *horse*, he uses the word *dog* instead *to refer to the horse*.

Third, children may make a *retrieval error* when they know a certain word but for some reason cannot retrieve the word and unintentionally select a different word. For example, a child may know the word *horse* but accidentally utter the word *dog* when describing the horse.

Language Use

In addition to acquiring new grammatical constructions and words as they transition from the one-word stage to combining two or more words, toddlers obtain important new language, or discourse, functions and conversational skills.

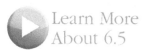

DISCUSSION POINT

What are some ways in which a parent can determine whether his or her toddler overgeneralizes and undergeneralizes new words?

Learn More
About 6.5

As you watch the video titled "Word-Use Error," notice how the 27-month-old boy retrieves a pumpkin carving tool with a red handle and makes a word-use error by repeatedly calling the handle a "hamburger." Even after his mother and father correct the error by using the word "handle," he continues to call it a "hamburger."

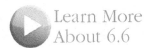

Learn More About 6.6

As you watch the video titled "Discourse Functions," notice how the 26-month-old boy uses at least two different discourse functions as he converses with his mother. For example, he uses a personal function to express that he is walking carefully. He uses informative functions to let his mother know he sees a lot of apples on the ground in the grass.

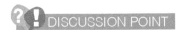

DISCUSSION POINT

Talking about an activity or object of interest to a toddler is one way adults might promote conversation. Can you think of other strategies adults might use to sustain conversation with a toddler?

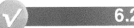

6.2
Check Your Understanding
Click here to gauge your understanding of the concepts in this section.

Discourse Functions

By the time children begin to combine words, they can use a variety of language functions. These functions include instrumental, regulatory, interactional, personal, heuristic, imaginative, and informative functions, terms we introduced in Chapter 1 (Halliday, 1978; see Table 1.1). Children can use *instrumental* functions, including requests, to satisfy their needs. They can also use *regulatory* functions, such as imperatives (commands), to control other people's behavior, *interactional* functions to interact with others in a social way, and *personal* functions to express their feelings about something. In addition, children can use *heuristic* functions by requesting information from other people to learn about the world, *imaginative* functions by telling stories to pretend, and *informative* functions to provide information to other people. Children's success in using communication for a variety of purposes is one of the most important aspects of communicative development during toddlerhood.

Conversational Skills

One area in which toddlers *do not* display much skill is conversation. Conversational skill requires the ability to initiate a conversational topic, sustain the topic for several turns, then appropriately take leave of the conversation. In Chapter 2, we discuss the concept of a *conversational schema*, which is a model specifying the organization of conversations. Toddlers are beginning to develop this schema, but they are relatively poor conversationalists. Anyone who has attempted to have a conversation with a young child knows it is not usually sophisticated, as in the following examples:

Conversation 1:

PARENT: What did you do at Grandma's house?

TODDLER: Played.

Conversation 2 (a bit later):

PARENT: Why do you love going to Grandma's house?

TODDLER: Because I love it.

Toddlers may demonstrate some skill in starting a conversation, but they cannot usually sustain it for more than one or two turns. Typically, the adult bears the burden of maintaining the conversation on a particular topic. Toddlers also have difficulty keeping their audience's needs in mind: They may use pronouns without appropriately defining to whom they refer ("He is cheating!"), and they may discuss topics without ensuring the listener has a sufficient frame of reference to understand the context ("I want to read my favorite book, not this book"). You may also notice that in conversations, when you ask a toddler a specific question or give him or her an explicit opportunity to take a turn, the child will not always take the opportunity. The toddler may simply not respond or may respond *noncontingently* (off the topic). Toddlers are not yet proficient at realizing when they are not following along in a conversation and are thus not likely to seek clarification.

WHAT FACTORS CONTRIBUTE TO TODDLERS' INDIVIDUAL ACHIEVEMENTS IN LANGUAGE?

Like infants, toddlers develop language in a fairly predictable pattern because they meet certain milestones in the same order and at about the same age. However, certain aspects of their language development vary. In the next section, we discuss both *intraindividual* and *interindividual* language differences among toddlers, along with factors that may account for such differences. As you read this section, please keep in mind our discussion of averages and medians in Chapter 5. As was true for infancy, there is no such living person who represents the "average toddler." When we describe averages and medians, we are referring to descriptive statistical manipulations, not to real children.

Intraindividual Differences

If you observe an *individual* toddler for any length of time, you will most likely notice that his or her language development is not linear. For example, a toddler might learn several new words within a week and then not learn any new words for the next few weeks. In fact, children individually experience a series of spurts and plateaus in their language abilities as they develop (Fenson, Bates, et al., 2000).

Likewise, as we mentioned in Chapter 5, comprehension of language generally precedes production. This fact makes sense on many levels. Consider, for example, your personal abilities to comprehend and produce foreign languages. Most likely, you can understand significantly more than you can say. The idea that comprehension precedes production holds true for the size of toddlers' receptive and expressive lexicons as well. In fact, this intraindividual difference continues throughout the preschool and school-age years and even into adulthood.

Interindividual Differences

If you observe a *group* of toddlers, you will most likely note language-development differences among them. Interindividual differences in toddlers' language development relate to a number of factors, including gender, birth order, and socioeconomic status. Next, we discuss interindividual differences and some of the factors accounting for them.

Effects of Gender

Several studies have revealed some effects of gender on language development in terms of both the pace at which children acquire language and the communication styles they use. For example, Fenson, Bates, and colleagues (2000) determined that boys both comprehend and produce fewer words than girls. Specifically, they found that 18-month-old girls understand an average of 65 words and produce about 27 words, whereas boys of the same age understand an average of 56 words and produce about 18 words. Bauer, Goldfield, and Reznick (2002) similarly reported that boys lag behind girls in lexical development. Likewise, a study of 386 pairs of toddler twins, revealed that girls produce more words and more two-word combinations than boys (Van Hulle, Goldsmith, & Lemery, 2004).

What factors underlie these gender differences? Bauer and colleagues (2002) posited that differences in boys' and girls' maturation rates, particularly with respect to neurological development, may contribute to gender differences in language acquisition. In addition, parents may interact differently with boys and girls, and these different interaction styles may affect language-development patterns. For example, parents of 3-year-old boys tend to initiate more conversation in play settings, whereas parents of 3-year-old girls typically initiate more conversation in nonplay settings. Girls may thus acquire more complex language constructions as their parents talk about objects and events outside the here and now. By contrast, boys may acquire less complex language as their parents comment on perceptually available objects and actions in the context of toy-play activities (Apel & Masterson, 2001a).

Effects of Birth Order

In addition to gender, researchers have discovered associations between birth order and language development. For example, for toddlers between the ages of 18 and 29 months, firstborn children exhibit more advanced lexical and grammatical development than their later-born counterparts, whereas later-born children exhibit more advanced conversational skills (Hoff-Ginsberg, 1998). Why might the order in which children are born relate to language development? One suggestion is that firstborn children (and only children, who are firstborn by default) receive much more one-on-one attention than do children who are not firstborn, and thus receive a greater quantity of child-directed speech.

In a review of the literature, Hoff (2006) noted that younger siblings receive input from their older siblings and such input likely affects their language development as well. For example, the speech older siblings use with their younger siblings tends to serve social-regulatory functions (e.g., "Give me my book back"; "Let's play over there"), and tends to be structurally less complex and uses a smaller vocabulary than the speech adults use with young children. Hoff also summarizes results of a study suggesting that the functions of mothers' speech differ, depending on whether they are interacting with one child or two children. When mothers are interacting with two children, their speech tends to center on activities and social exchanges, whereas when they are interacting with one child, their speech tends to include more talk about language itself (i.e., it tends to be more metalinguistic). Such research suggests that the language firstborn children experience is qualitatively different from input second-born children experience and that these differences may be related to children's own language development.

In considering the relation between birth order and language development, it is important to note some important limitations. One limitation is that because children are nested within families, there is a lack of independence in the data analyses. To be independent, each unique set of child's data would need to correspond to a unique set of parent data. This is not possible when investigating birth order, because parents who have more than one child are necessarily linked to multiple children. Thus, parents with more than one child would have their data represented

THEORY TO PRACTICE

Child Care Selection and Toddler Language Development

As we described in Chapter 4, theoretical perspectives concerning language development influence many areas of people's lives, including some of the choices parents and caregivers make. One particularly important decision is the selection of child care providers for developing toddlers. Although when we, the authors, were young, relatively few children participated in child care in the years prior to formal schooling, this situation has changed drastically in the last few decades. Today, the vast majority of children participate in child care (or preschool), largely because of shifts in family structure (e.g., more single-parent homes) and employment patterns (e.g., women's participation in the workforce). In 1991, the National Institute of Child Health and Human Development (NICHD) began a longitudinal study—the Study of Early Child Care and Youth Development (SECCYD). In Phase I, researchers enrolled 1,364 children from 10 locations across the United States and followed these children to gather data on their cognitive, social, emotional, and language development (among other factors) from birth through age 3 years. The study did not end there, however. Data on the study children are available through age 15 years to researchers who apply for permission to use them. The information available on these children's developmental experiences has substantially

bolstered our understanding of how child care experiences affect children both early in life and into adolescence.

As one result of this intensive study, researchers concluded that a number of important indicators are consistently associated with positive caregiving behaviors within each of the five types of nonmaternal child care they examined. The indicators include a small group size, low child–adult ratios, nonauthoritarian child-rearing beliefs, and safe, clean, and stimulating physical environments (National Institute of Child Health and Human Development Early Child Care Research Network, 1996). Furthermore, researchers concluded that the overall quality of child care—and *language stimulation* in particular—is consistently but modestly related to toddlers' cognitive and language outcomes at ages 15, 24, and 36 months (National Institute of Child Health and Human Development Early Child Care Research Network, 2000). Researchers measured child care providers' use of language stimulation by examining the extent to which providers asked questions, responded to children's vocalizations, and talked to children. These research results have significant implications for the selection of quality child care, considering the impact child care experiences may have on children's developing language competencies throughout toddlerhood.

more than one time in a given analysis, which violates the independence of the data. A second limitation is that it is not possible to draw causal conclusions about birth order. In other words, researchers cannot say for certain that birth order *causes* language outcomes in children. In order to draw a causal conclusion about something of interest, researchers must use a rigorous experimental design that randomly assigns children to study conditions. Random assignment to conditions is important because it helps eliminate potential sources of bias in study findings. In the case of birth order and language development, it is possible that firstborn children exhibit more advanced lexical and grammatical development for reasons other than birth order per se. Because it is not possible to randomly assign children to be first born, second born, and so on, it is not possible to know for certain whether birth order *causes* certain language outcomes.

Effects of Socioeconomic Status and Parental Education

Socioeconomic status (SES), which usually includes some measure of family income, parental education, or occupational status, is associated with a variety of health, cognitive, and socioemotional outcomes in children; these effects begin before birth and continue into adulthood (Bradley & Corwyn, 2002). As is true for infants, SES is associated with toddlers' receptive and expressive language development. For example, typically developing African American toddlers from low SES backgrounds perform more poorly on standardized measures of receptive and expressive language than do their counterparts from middle SES backgrounds (Horton-Ikard and Ellis Weismer, 2005). Analyses of spontaneous language samples reveal similar effects of SES. Even after adjusting for ethnicity, toddlers from lower SES backgrounds (as measured by maternal education) have shorter MLUs and use fewer words than toddlers from higher SES backgrounds (Dollaghan et al.,1999). Although family income and education levels are highly related, a longitudinal study examining caregivers' speech to toddlers between 14 and 30 months of age found that parents' education level is more closely associated with the complexity of parents' language than family income (Huttenlocher et al., 2007).

Why does SES make a difference? Recall our discussion in the Language Diversity and Differences box of Chapter 2 about the strong negative relationship between poverty and language achievement. Researchers suspect parents' SES is related to the amount and complexity of speech parents use with their children, which in turn is related to children's own language outcomes (e.g., Raviv, Kessenich, & Morrison, 2004). Although many characteristics related to interindividual differences in language development are beyond a parent's control (e.g., gender, birth order), parents are able to make choices about some of the environmental factors that may contribute to interindividual differences. See Theory to Practice: *Child Care Selection and Toddler Language Development* for a discussion of the importance of child care experiences for toddler language development.

HOW DO RESEARCHERS AND CLINICIANS MEASURE LANGUAGE DEVELOPMENT IN TODDLERHOOD?

Researchers

When studying language development in toddlerhood, researchers have a broader range of language data to consider than do researchers studying language development in infancy. The reason is that toddlers not only comprehend language but also produce it. As language researchers, we, the authors, have used a variety of measures to assess children's language development. Here we review several methods, in three categories: production tasks, comprehension tasks, and judgment tasks.

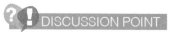

DISCUSSION POINT

Toddlers from low-SES backgrounds tend to perform more poorly on both standardized and naturalistic language measures than their mid- and high-SES counterparts. Why is knowing this fact important?

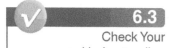

6.3

Check Your Understanding

Click here to gauge your understanding of the concepts in this section.

Production Tasks

Production tasks allow toddlers to demonstrate their competence in various areas of language development. In these tasks, researchers ask children to produce, or say, the language targets under investigation. Some production tasks are unstructured or semistructured, such as naturalistic observation; other production tasks are structured and systematic, such as elicited imitation and elicited production tasks.

Naturalistic Observation. We introduced naturalistic observations in Chapter 5 when we described methods researchers use to study language development in infancy. Naturalistic observations of children's spontaneous productions are of great value in toddlerhood as well, when researchers can analyze children's morphology and syntax for the first time. Probably the most famous naturalistic observations are Roger Brown's (1973) longitudinal observations of children with the pseudonyms Adam, Eve, and Sarah. As a result of Brown's analysis, we know, for example, that children's earliest utterances containing forms of the verb *to be* (*am, is, are, was, were*) include contractions (e.g., *it's*). Recall from our earlier discussion that toddlers may learn some contractions as a "word," or whole unit, rather than as two separate words to which they apply a contraction rule.

Researchers must consider several factors when they collect, transcribe, and analyze naturalistic language samples. Such factors include the number of children to analyze, the number of recordings to collect from each child, and the variety of contexts in which to collect samples. See Rowe (2012) for additional background information and practical suggestions concerning how to record, transcribe, and code language samples.

Elicited Imitation Tasks. To gauge children's underlying linguistic competence, researchers can use elicited imitation tasks, which take advantage of children's natural ability to imitate other people's movements and speech sounds. In elicited imitation tasks, the experimenter produces a target phrase and then requests that the child repeat it exactly as he or she heard it. The experimenter carefully selects sentences that vary only by the grammatical structure under investigation. Researchers have used elicited imitation tasks to explore children's competence with word order and *anaphora*, which are linguistic units (such as pronouns) that refer to a previous linguistic unit. (For example, in the sentence "Doug prefers to cook for *himself*," the word *himself* refers to *Doug*.)

In elicited imitation tasks, researchers assume that for a child to successfully imitate a target, it must be a part of the child's grammatical repertoire (Lust, Flynn, & Foley, 1996). The following two examples illustrate how an elicited imitation task might play out for one child who has acquired the rule for forming *wh-* questions in English and for a second child who has not yet acquired the rule:

ADULT 1: What is your favorite color?

CHILD 1: What is your favorite color?

ADULT 2: What is your favorite color?

CHILD 2: What your favorite color <u>is</u>?

In a true elicited imitation task, the experimenter would have the child repeat several phrases containing the target linguistic skill under investigation and compare the child's utterances with adultlike forms.

Elicited Production Tasks. Elicited production tasks are designed to reveal aspects of children's language abilities (e.g., syntax, morphology, pragmatics) as they produce specific sentence structures. Researchers elicit sentence structures in the context of a game, during which the child must ask questions or make statements in response to an experimenter's prompt. Perhaps the most famous elicited production task is Jean Berko's (1958) Wug Test (Figure 6.3). Berko (now Berko Gleason) designed the Wug Test to investigate children's acquisition of English morphemes, including the plural marker. English plural nouns are marked by adding one of three *allomorphs* (variants of a morpheme with the same meaning but different sounds) of the morpheme *-s*. These allomorphs are as follows:

ALLOMORPH OF -*S*	USE	EXAMPLE
/z/	Added to nouns that end in voiced consonants	*pig—pigs*
/s/	Added to nouns that end in voiceless consonants	*pit—pits*
/ɪz/	Added to nouns that end in /s/, /z/, the "sh" sound, or the "ch" sound	*kiss—kisses* *quiz—quizzes* *wish—wishes* *lunch—lunches*

Berko elicited these three allomorphs by presenting children with a pseudoword and then prompting them to say what two of the same word would be called. Consider the following examples of how the Wug Test might play out with a child who is already producing the plural morpheme:

ADULT: This is a wug. (*points to picture of single object*)

ADULT: Now there are two of them. (*points to picture of two objects*) There are two _____.

CHILD: Wugs! [/wʌgz/]

As you can see, the adult elicits the target word with a prompt but does not provide a target for the child to repeat, as in elicited imitation tasks.

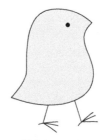

This is a wug.

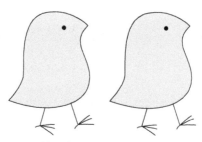

Now there is another one.
There are two of them.
There are two __.

FIGURE 6.3

Wug Test.

Source: From "The Child's Learning of English Morphology," by J. Berko, 1958, *Word*, *14*, p. 154. Copyright by Jean Berko Gleason. Reprinted with permission.

Comprehension Tasks

Comprehension tasks reveal toddlers' language competencies not by asking them to produce language targets, but by having them either match or point to pictures of target words and phrases or act out phrases they hear an experimenter say.

The Picture Selection Task.   In a picture selection task, an experimenter presents a language target and asks the child to choose the picture corresponding to the target. For example, an experimenter who wants to determine whether a child can differentiate between the /l/ and /r/ sounds might ask the child to select the picture of *glass* from between a picture of *glass* and a picture of *grass*. Researchers frequently use picture selection tasks to investigate children's understanding of lexical items and syntactic constructions, including the distinction between active and passive voice (e.g., *John wrote the book* = active voice; *The book was written by John* = passive voice). For examples of morphosyntactic contrasts that can be assessed with the picture selection task, see Table 6.5.

Although researchers can measure a toddler's language abilities using the relatively inexpensive procedures described here, they can also use neuroimaging techniques (such as those described in Chapter 5) to answer research questions about specific aspects of a toddler's language development. See Research Paradigms: *Neuroimaging and Toddler Language Development* for a discussion of how neuroimaging studies can help researchers assess the responses of the toddler brain to known and unknown words.

The Act-Out Task.   Researchers can use an act-out task to investigate a child's competence with various language constructions. To administer the task, an experimenter presents a child with a series of props and instructs the child to act out the sentences he or she hears. For instance, if you are interested in assessing a 3-year-old's ability to comprehend agent and recipient relations, you might say something such as "The dog tickled the cat", and then ask the child to act out that particular sequence with a toy dog and cat.

Judgment Tasks

In judgment tasks, researchers ask children to decide whether certain language constructions are appropriate as a way to assess their level of grammatical competence. Researchers can infer that children possess adultlike levels of grammatical competence when they judge adultlike constructions to be correct and nonadultlike sentences to be incorrect. Two types of judgment tasks researchers routinely use are truth value judgment tasks and grammaticality judgment tasks.

Truth Value Judgment Tasks.   In truth value judgment tasks, children must judge certain language constructions to be correct or incorrect. These tasks take two forms: yes–no tasks and reward–punishment tasks. In a yes–no task, an experimenter presents a scenario and asks the child a question. For example, an experimenter who wants to gauge a child's comprehension of quantifiers might present a picture and ask, "Is every mother holding a baby?" or "Is a mother holding every baby?" and note the child's response. In a reward–punishment task, an experimenter introduces a puppet and explains to a child that he or she should reward the puppet with a cookie (or some other treat) when the puppet says something "right", and should punish the puppet by withholding a treat when the puppet says something "wrong." The experimenter uses sentences containing the target linguistic construction, but such sentences are declarative rather than yes–no questions. For example, a puppet might say, "Every mother is holding a baby," and if the puppet's sentence describes a photo correctly, the child would reward the puppet with a treat.

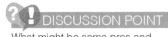
DISCUSSION POINT

What might be some pros and cons of using truth value judgment tasks with toddlers?

Grammaticality Judgment Tasks.   Grammaticality judgment tasks are generally suited for preschoolers, older children, and adults, so we discuss them in Chapter 7.

TABLE 6.5
Examples of morphosyntactic contrasts that can be assessed with the picture selection task

CONTRAST	EXAMPLE SENTENCE PAIR	EXAMPLE PICTURES FOR EACH CONTRAST
Affirmative vs. negative	*The girl is jumping.* *The girl is not jumping.*	
Subject vs. object (active voice)	*The boy kisses the baby.* *The baby kisses the boy.*	
Present progressive tense vs. future tense	*The man is snoring.* *The man will snore.*	
Singular pronoun vs. plural possessive pronoun	*That's his house.* *That's their house.*	
Present progressive tense vs. past tense	*The fire is burning.* *The fire burned.*	

(Continued)

TABLE 6.5 *(Continued)*

CONTRAST	EXAMPLE SENTENCE PAIR	EXAMPLE PICTURES FOR EACH CONTRAST
Mass noun vs. count noun	*There's some glub.* *There's a blop.*	
Singular vs. plural auxiliary *be*	*The sheep is sleeping.* *The sheep are sleeping.*	
Singular vs. plural inflections	*The car races.* *The cars race.*	
Subject vs. object (passive voice)	*The baby is kissed by the boy.* *The boy is kissed by the baby.*	
Indirect object vs. direct object	*The woman shows the girl the doctor.* *The woman shows the doctor the girl.*	

⌕ RESEARCH **PARADIGMS**

Neuroimaging and Toddler Language Development

Neuroimaging techniques are fast becoming an important method for gaining deeper understanding about language development. Some neuroimaging techniques are even appropriate for investigating the language development of infants and toddlers. One such technique involves event-related potentials (ERPs). In ERP studies, participants wear a cap that attaches to the head with several suction cups and contains several electrodes that measure the brain's electrical responses to particular linguistic stimuli. In one such study, researchers demonstrated that 14-month-olds detect differences between known words (e.g., *bear*) and phonetically similar nonsense words (e.g., *gare*) or phonetically dissimilar nonsense words (e.g., *kobe*). However, the same study found that 20-month-olds only detect differences between known words and phonetically dissimilar nonsense words (i.e., they detect the difference between *bear* and *kobe*, but they do not detect the difference between *bear* and *gare*; Mills et al., 2004). This research, using ERPs, complements research using other methodologies showing that as young children age, their ability to detect fine phonetic contrasts diminishes in the context of word comprehension tasks. See Conboy, Rivera-Gaxiola, Silva-Pereyra, and Kuhl (2008) for an extensive discussion of ERP studies of early language processing.

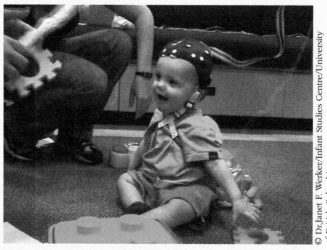

© Dr. Janet F. Werker/Infant Studies Centre/University of British Columbia

An event-related potentials (ERP) study.

Clinicians

Clinicians have a wide array of measures at their disposal, ranging from parent-completed checklists to comprehensive direct assessments that cost hundreds of dollars. Even though toddlers are prone to acting according to their own agendas, measuring the language development of toddlers is arguably easier than measuring that of infants. The reason is that toddlers can follow simple instructions during an assessment and are generally eager to play along when the clinician structures the assessment to resemble a game rather than a test. It is crucial that the assessment used to document children's language abilities be matched to the purpose of the assessment. For example, a clinician who wants to evaluate the syntax and morphology abilities of a young boy with a suspected language impairment would select a different assessment than a clinician who wants to screen the vocabulary of multiple toddlers in a child care program for potential indicators of risk. Here, we describe three assessment purposes: (a) screening, (b) comprehensive evaluation, and (c) progress monitoring, and we provide an example of an assessment for each of the three purposes.

Screening

Clinicians may screen a child's language skills to determine whether the child is experiencing difficulty with particular aspects of language and whether the child might need a more comprehensive language evaluation. Screening measures in toddlerhood, like those in infancy, use common early language milestones, against which the clinician or a parent can compare the child's own language abilities. Screening measures generally use an informal approach, such as a checklist format, to quickly and efficiently assess a child's language abilities. As one example of a screening measure available online, the National Institute on Deafness and Other Communication Disorders (http://www.nidcd.nih.gov) distributes a series of developmental language screens that parents and clinicians can use to screen a child informally. See Figure 6.4 for an example of a screening measure for toddlers ages 1 to 2 years and 2 to 3 years.

Another popular screening tool is the MacArthur–Bates Communicative Development Inventories (CDI; Fenson et al., 2003). You may recall that the CDI is a parent-report checklist and is available in more than 60 languages. The CDI Toddler short form (Fenson et al., 2000) is a 100-item checklist (in two parallel forms)

Milestones for speech and language development

1 TO 2 YEARS		
Knows a few parts of the body and can point to them when asked	YES ☐	NO ☐
Follows simple commands ("Roll the ball") and understands simple questions ("Where's your shoe?")	YES ☐	NO ☐
Enjoys simple stories, songs, and rhymes	YES ☐	NO ☐
Points to pictures, when named, in books	YES ☐	NO ☐
Acquires new words on a regular basis	YES ☐	NO ☐
Uses some one- or two-word questions ("Where kitty?" or "Go bye-bye?")	YES ☐	NO ☐
Puts two words together ("More cookie")	YES ☐	NO ☐
Uses many different consonant sounds at the beginning of words	YES ☐	NO ☐
2 TO 3 YEARS		
Has a word for almost everything	YES ☐	NO ☐
Uses two- or three-word phrases to talk about and ask for things	YES ☐	NO ☐
Uses k, g, f, t, d, and n sounds	YES ☐	NO ☐
Speaks in a way that is understood by family members and friends	YES ☐	NO ☐
Names objects to ask for them or to direct attention to them	YES ☐	NO ☐

FIGURE 6.4

Language screens for toddlers from 1 to 2 years of age and from 2 to 3 years of age.
Source: From *Speech and Language Developmental Milestones*, by National Institute on Deafness and Other Communication Disorders (2014) (NIH Publication No. 13-4781). Bethesda, MD: Author.
http://www.nidcd.nih.gov/staticresources/health/voice/NIDCD-Speech-Language-Dev-Milestones.pdf.

designed to assess expressive vocabulary in toddlers ages 16–30 months. The measure also includes one item that asks whether children are combining words. The Web site for the MacArthur–Bates CDI (http://mb-cdi.stanford.edu/) contains information on how to order the CDI forms and how to score the measure, as well as information on how to generate screening reports and letters to parents that explain how their child's language abilities compare to those of their same-age peers. The Web site also includes lexical norms in English and Spanish, where you can learn about the percentage of children whose parents reported that they produced certain CDI words. For example, the English norms reveal that whereas 10.3% of toddlers' parents in the norming sample reported that their child said the word *brother* by 16 months of age, 62.9% of parents reported that their child said the word by 30 months of age. As another example, parents of toddlers in the norming sample reported that 5.1% of toddlers said the word *build* by 16 months of age and 75.7% of parents reported that their child said the word by age 30 months. In general, the CDI Toddler short form is relatively inexpensive, and is quick and easy for clinicians to administer as a language screening measure.

Comprehensive Evaluation

Clinicians may use a comprehensive language evaluation to determine whether a child has a language disorder and, if so, to learn more about the nature of the disorder. Unlike screening measures, evaluations are generally structured, standardized, norm-referenced (see Chapter 4 for a discussion of norm-referenced measures), and limited in duration rather than ongoing (i.e., they are not designed to be administered repeatedly to the same child). When administering a comprehensive evaluation, clinicians should always consider ecological validity, or the extent to which the data resulting from these tools can be extended to multiple contexts, including the child's home and child care settings. It is also important that clinicians verify the results of a comprehensive evaluation with parents to determine whether the child's results are representative of his or her abilities before drawing any conclusions about the child (e.g., "The evaluation revealed that Neil tends to confuse the pronouns *him* and *he*, *us* and *we*, *me* and *I*, and *her* and *she*. Do you notice the same problems at home or when he's talking to you or when he's playing with his brothers?")

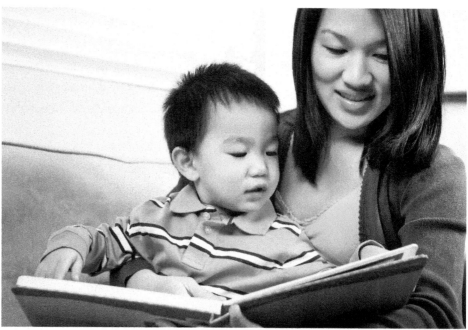

Using informal language screens, parents can complete a checklist to assess their toddler's language abilities.

© 123rf

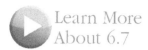

Learn More About 6.7

In the video titled "Sample Administration of the CELF–Preschool 2," an adult administers three subtests of the CELF–Preschool 2 to another adult: Sentence Structure, Word Structure, and Expressive Vocabulary, demonstrating how a clinician might administer the instrument to a child https://www.youtube.com/watch?v=nv1Gco7GeGo

One example of a comprehensive language evaluation appropriate for toddlers (and preschoolers) is the Clinical Evaluation of Language Fundamentals—Preschool, Second Edition (CELF–Preschool 2; Wiig, Secord, & Semel, 2004). The CELF–Preschool 2 is designed for children ages 3–6 years and can identify whether a child has a language disorder, to determine his or her eligibility for language services, or to identify the child's relative strengths and weaknesses in language. The CELF–Preschool 2 includes three subtests that together allow the clinician to calculate a *Core Language Score*—Sentence Structure, Word Structure, and Expressive Vocabulary. To determine whether a child has a language disorder, a clinician would first administer these three subtests before administering additional subtests.

The Sentence Structure subtest measures a child's ability to understand spoken sentences of increasing length and complexity. To administer the subtest, the clinician reads a sentence aloud and asks the child to point to a picture in the assessment manual that corresponds to that sentence. The sentences assess various aspects of language form, including prepositional phrases (*in the box*, *under the tree*), copula (*is sleepy*, *is ready*), and passive voice (*is being followed*, *is being pushed*), among others.

The Word Structure subtest measures a child's ability to apply morphology to words (e.g., to inflect nouns with the plural marker, to inflect regular verbs with the past tense marker) and to use pronouns appropriately. To administer this subtest, the clinician asks the child to complete sentences with the targeted structure. For example, to assess a child's ability to make nouns plural, the clinician might point to a series of pictures and say, "This boy has one dog. This boy has two ____" (answer: dogs). To assess a child's ability to inflect regular verbs with the past tense marker, the clinician might point to a series of pictures and say, "This lady is baking cookies. Here are the cookies she _____" (answer: baked).

The Expressive Vocabulary subtest measures a child's ability to label drawings of people, objects, and actions. To conduct this subtest, the clinician points to a picture and asks the child to name the item, person, or action depicted. Items for each of the three core language subtests are arranged in order of difficulty so the child is able to attempt answering easier items before proceeding to more difficult items. The clinician discontinues the subtest after the child has incorrectly answered a certain number of items or when the child completes the last item in the subtest. After administering the three Core Language subtests and calculating a Core Language score, the clinician may decide to analyze the items for each subtest to better understand the child's specific strengths and weaknesses or to administer additional CELF–Preschool 2 subtests.

Progress Monitoring

As the name implies, progress monitoring tools measure and monitor a child's progress in a certain area of language development (e.g., expressive vocabulary). Clinicians can administer progress monitoring instruments multiple times and they are generally quick and easy to administer.

An example of a progress monitoring instrument appropriate for toddlers is the Individual Growth and Development for Infants and Toddlers (IGDIs; http://www.igdi.ku.edu/index.htm). According to the Web site, the IGDIs have been designed and validated for use by early childhood practitioners to monitor infant and toddler growth and progress. Practitioners may use them repeatedly to estimate a child's progress acquiring key skills over time in the same way a pediatrician measures growth in a child's height and weight during each well-child visit. To assess a toddler's early communication using an IGDI, the adult engages the child in a 6-minute play session using a specific toy (i.e., a Fisher Price house or barn) and records and counts the number of communicative behaviors the child produces. The assessor may compare a toddler's results to normative expectations, predict future performance, or develop interventions for children whose growth and development are not as expected.

6.4
Check Your Understanding
Click here to gauge your understanding of the concepts in this section.

SUMMARY

In this chapter, we open with a discussion of the major language milestones toddlers achieve. These milestones include not only the transition from prelinguistic to linguistic communication as toddlers utter their first word, but also toddlers' increasingly sophisticated use of gestures. We also discuss the relation between theory of mind (ToM) and language development, as this relation starts to become evident in toddlerhood and strengthens as children age.

In the second section, we describe toddlers' achievements in language form, content, and use during the second and third years—which are numerous. With respect to language form, we explore major achievements in phonology, including acquiring new phonemes, phonological processes, and phonological perception. We define grammatical morphemes and explain how toddlers transition from using one-word utterances to using two-word utterances.

With respect to language content, toddlers' receptive and expressive lexicons continue to grow, and children use overextension, underextension, and overlap as they learn new words. In our discussion of these achievements, we describe the Quinean conundrum and explore two possible ways children overcome this conundrum as they attempt to narrow the nearly infinite number of referents for novel words: the lexical principles framework for acquiring new words and the social-pragmatic framework for acquiring new words. We also examine toddlers' ability to fast map new words.

With respect to language use, we explore some of the new discourse functions and conversational skills that become available to toddlers.

In the third section, we explain that intraindividual and interindividual differences in language achievements continue throughout toddlerhood. *Individual* toddlers vary in their language acquisition rate and in their expressive and receptive lexical development. Three major factors that may contribute to differences in language development *among a group* of toddlers are gender, birth order, and SES and parental education.

In the final section, we describe how researchers and clinicians measure language development in toddlerhood. We detail six specific paradigms researchers use to measure language development—naturalistic observation, elicited imitation tasks, elicited production tasks, the picture selection task, the act-out task, and truth value judgment tasks—and three ways clinicians measure language development—screening, comprehensive evaluation, and progress monitoring.

 Apply Your Knowledge

Click here to apply your knowledge to practical scenarios.

BEYOND THE BOOK

1. Record and transcribe a short (2 min) language sample from a toddler between 1 and 3 years of age. Using Brown's rules for counting morphemes, calculate the toddler's mean length of utterance (MLU) using the formula appearing earlier in this chapter. Does the toddler's MLU correspond to what you would expect for his or her age range according to the norms presented in Table 6.4?

2. Observe a toddler communicating with another individual. What phonetically consistent forms (PCFs) do you hear? What phonological processes does the toddler use?

3. Watch a group of toddlers together at a party, play group, or the like. Describe some of the differences you see in their language skills and communication abilities. Do the boys and girls seem to differ with regard to these skills and abilities? How so?

4. Observe a toddler communicating with a parent or another individual and note which discourse functions the toddler uses. Does the toddler incorporate gestures to express any of these functions? If so, which ones?

5. Talk with a parent who has used "baby signs" with his or her toddler. Ask the parent to recall when he or she noticed the toddler had stopped using these signs. Determine whether the toddler used specific signs less often once he or she could use the corresponding words, or whether the toddler continued to use signs while speaking the corresponding words. Is the information consistent with our earlier discussion of gesture use in toddlerhood?

Check Your Understanding

Gauge your understanding of the chapter concepts by taking this self-check quiz.

7

Preschool

Building Literacy on Language

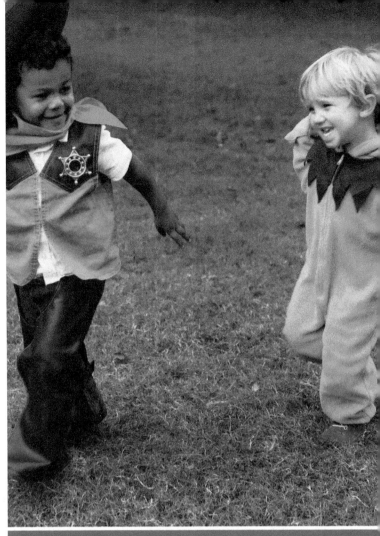

© Blend Images/Getty Images

LEARNING OUTCOMES

After completion of this chapter, the reader will be able to:

1. Identify major language-development milestones that occur in the preschool period.

2. Describe major achievements in language form, content, and use that characterize the preschool period.

3. Explain factors that contribute to preschoolers' individual language achievements.

4. Describe how researchers and clinicians measure language development in the preschool period.

In the United States, the preschool period typically includes the 2 years before a child enters elementary school, or between about ages 3 and 5 years. Children experience many remarkable "firsts" during the preschool period. For example, they begin to use language to talk about objects, events, and thoughts outside the immediate context. Preschoolers also begin to gain important abilities in emergent literacy, which marks their transition to comprehending and expressing language in multiple modalities: oral and written. In the preschool years, children's language becomes even more sophisticated than in the toddler years as children begin to master form, content, and use in new ways. In this chapter, we begin with an overview of some major language-development milestones for preschoolers, including decontextualized language, complex language associated with developing theory of mind, and emergent literacy. Next, we explore achievements in language form, content, and use. We also discuss aspects of language development that differ within individual preschoolers and ways in which preschoolers differ from one another in their language development. Finally, we detail how researchers and clinicians measure preschool-age children's language development.

WHAT MAJOR LANGUAGE-DEVELOPMENT MILESTONES OCCUR IN THE PRESCHOOL PERIOD?

Compared with their younger toddler counterparts, preschoolers accomplish a lot in a day. No longer having to concentrate on keeping their footing, preschoolers have plenty of time for building towers out of blocks (and knocking them down), drawing and coloring, engaging in pretend play, riding bikes, and digging in the dirt. With exposure to so many different objects and activities, preschoolers (even those who do not attend preschool programs) have many opportunities to hear new words, grammatical constructions, and language functions. One significant milestone of the preschool period is the acquisition of a specific type of language that does not rely on the immediate context for interpretation: decontextualized language (recall that we introduced this concept, also called *displacement*, in Chapter 1). Preschool-age children who are reared in literate households, or who attend preschool are also exposed to written language and begin to acquire important emergent literacy skills, which is probably the crowning achievement of the preschool period.

Decontextualized Language

As preschoolers continue to add to the *quantity* of words they understand and produce, there is a noticeable shift as well in the *quality* of words they understand and use. During the preschool years, children begin to incorporate *decontextualized language* in their conversations in addition to the *contextualized language* they began using in infancy and toddlerhood. Contextualized language is grounded in the immediate context, or the here and now. Such language relies on the background knowledge a speaker and a listener share, and on gestures, intonation, and immediately present situational cues. A child using contextualized language might say "Gimme that" while pointing to something in the listener's hands, or might describe a lion as "that big and furry one" while standing in front of the lion's cage at the zoo.

In contrast, when a child wants to discuss people, places, objects, and events that are not immediately present, decontextualized language becomes appropriate and necessary. Decontextualized language relies heavily on the language itself in the construction of meaning. Such language may not contain context cues and does not assume a speaker and a listener share background knowledge or context.

A boy who uses decontextualized language might call for his mother in the kitchen when he is in the living room, remembering that they do not share the same physical context ("Mom, I spilled milk on the couch!"), or might describe an event to someone after it occurs ("We watched fireworks on the Fourth of July"). In both situations, the child realizes he cannot rely on the immediate physical context to help him communicate to the listener. As with all types of decontextualized discourse, the child must use highly precise syntax and vocabulary to represent events beyond the here and now.

The ability to use decontextualized language is fundamental to academic success because nearly all the learning that occurs in schools focuses on events and concepts beyond the classroom walls. For example, when teaching about the life cycle of a plant, a teacher might use the words *seed, dirt, water, sunlight, sprout,* and *grow,* even though he or she and the students cannot witness all these components and processes of the cycle simultaneously in the context of their conversation.

Theory of Mind

In Chapter 5, we defined theory of mind (ToM) as the ability to understand one's own mental or emotional state, to understand that others also have mental or emotional states, and to realize that others' mental and emotional states, beliefs, intentions, and perspectives differ from one's own. In Chapter 6, we reviewed some research illustrating the connection between ToM and language development. As you may have guessed, the relation between language development and ToM continues throughout the preschool years and beyond, and it helps explain some of the social and communicative challenges certain persons, such as children with autism and Asperger's syndrome, experience.

Theory of mind follows a fairly reliable progression (Wellman, Fuxi, & Peterson, 2011; Peterson, Wellman, & Slaughter, 2012). First, children demonstrate sensitivity to diverse desires, or the understanding that people can have different desires for the same thing. Second, they demonstrate sensitivity to diverse beliefs, or the understanding that people can have different beliefs about the same situation. Third, children show sensitivity to knowledge access, or the understanding that something can be true but someone might not know it to be true. Fourth, they understand false belief, which we described in Chapter 6 to involve knowing that something can be true but another person might believe something different. Fifth, children understand hidden emotion, or the notion that someone can feel a certain way while displaying a different emotion. Sixth, children understand sarcasm—a nonliteral type of language in which the meaning of a speaker's words is the opposite of the literal interpretation.

During the preschool years, children typically develop an understanding of false belief, which is the fourth achievement in the progression. As with other aspects of ToM, language is related to this developmental change. More specifically, research indicates that children's knowledge of sentential complements facilitates ToM development. Sentential complements are structures that represent a person's speech or mental state. They contain a main clause with a verb of communication (e.g., to say; to exclaim) or a mental state verb (e.g., to think; to believe), and an embedded clause that may or may not be true. For example, in the sentence, *Murray thought that his brother ate the last donut*, the embedded clause *that his brother ate the last donut* may or may not represent the truth. In one study, researchers demonstrated that direct training in sentential complements (using verbs of communication) can facilitate false belief understanding in 4-year-old children (Hale & Tager-Flusberg, 2003). The researchers interpret this finding to mean the structural knowledge of specific language constructions fosters children's ability to attribute mental states to themselves and to others. Such results illustrate the important contribution of language to children's conception of mind.

Of course, the study occurred under controlled conditions and preschoolers outside of lab settings would not typically receive training in sentential complements. Instead, most language development occurs implicitly rather than as a result of explicit teaching or training. Peterson and colleagues (2012) explain that conversations and social interactions contribute to social-cognitive advances, including theory of mind development. For this reason, as children develop, conversational exchanges tend to pose particular challenges for atypically developing children (such as children with autism, Asperger's syndrome, and deaf children from hearing families) because of their greater reliance on complex features, such as opinion exchange and concealment, shared fantasizing, teasing, joking, sarcasm, and other affectively laden nonliteral uses of language.

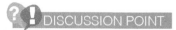

DISCUSSION POINT

What kind of task might a researcher design to determine whether a preschooler is using decontextualized language?

Emergent Literacy

During the preschool period, children develop several important literacy skills that allow them to begin to comprehend and use written language. They learn how print works, they begin to play with the sound units that compose syllables and words, and they develop an interest in reading and writing. Researchers refer to the earliest period of learning about reading and writing as emergent literacy. Although at this time children are not yet reading and writing in a conventional sense, their emerging knowledge about print and sounds forms an important foundation for the reading instruction that begins when they enter formal schooling (Justice & Pullen, 2003). The evidence base to support building an early foundation for literacy is so compelling that the American Academy of Pediatrics issued a policy statement recommending that pediatricians promote early literacy development for children beginning in infancy and continuing at least until the age of kindergarten entry (American Academy of Pediatrics, 2014).

Children's literacy abilities depend heavily on the oral language skills they began to acquire in infancy and toddlerhood—those skills necessary for comprehending language and using language expressively. For example, children need not only well-developed phonological systems before they can make sense of grapheme-to-phoneme (letter-to-sound) correspondences, but also well-developed vocabularies to derive meaning from text. For this reason, preschoolers are said to "build literacy on language."

Emergent literacy achievements depend largely on children's metalinguistic ability, or the ability to view language as an object of attention. Preschoolers may view language as an object of scrutiny as they pretend to write, look at words in a storybook, or make up rhyming patterns (Chaney, 1998). This ability to engage with language at a metalinguistic level is an important achievement of the preschool period that correlates well with children's success with writing and reading instruction, both of which depend on the ability to focus on language as an object of attention (Justice & Ezell, 2004).

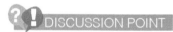

DISCUSSION POINT

Adults rely on metalinguistic abilities in certain circumstances as well. Can you think of some occasions when you had to focus on language as an object of attention?

Three important achievements in emergent literacy for preschoolers are alphabet knowledge, print awareness, and phonological awareness. Alphabet knowledge is children's knowledge about the letters of the alphabet. Print awareness is children's understanding of the forms and functions of written language, and phonological awareness is children's sensitivity to the sound units that make up speech (phonemes, syllables, words).

Alphabet Knowledge

Children who grow up in households where book reading is common begin to show emerging knowledge of the alphabet during the first 3 years of life. Some children even know a letter or two before their second birthday. During the preschool years, children typically recognize some of the letters in their names, show interest in specific letters occurring in the environment on signs or labels, and begin to write some letters with which they are especially familiar (Chaney, 1994). By age 5 years, children are often familiar with the letters that make up their names, a phenomenon referred to as the *own-name advantage* (Treiman & Broderick, 1998). In an informative study, Treiman and Broderick showed that 79% of preschoolers from middle-class homes were able to identify the first letter in their name. Also interesting is that the letter names children know appear to be related to the order of the alphabet, such that children tend to learn letters at the beginning of the alphabet (e.g., *A*, *B*, *C*) before they learn letters at the end of the alphabet (e.g., *X*, *Y*, *Z*; McBride-Chang, 1999). This phenomenon is likely related to children's increased exposure to the beginning letters of the alphabet. Results of a separate study confirmed that the order in which children learn alphabet letters is not random and that multiple forces interact to contribute to this order. Specifically, researchers found that four complementary hypotheses aptly characterize the order in which preschool children learn the names of individual alphabet letters. These hypotheses are as follows (Justice, Pence, Bowles, & Wiggins, 2006):

1. *Own-name advantage:* Children learn the letters of their names earlier than other letters.

2. *Letter-name pronunciation effect:* Children learn alphabet letters with the name of the letter in its pronunciation earlier than letters for which this is not the case (e.g., letter *B* is pronounced /**bi**/, but letter *X* is pronounced /ɛks/).

3. *Letter-order hypothesis:* Children learn letters occurring earlier in the alphabet string (e.g., *A*, *B*, *C*) before letters occurring later in the alphabet string (e.g., *X*, *Y*, *Z*).

4. *Consonant-order hypothesis:* Children learn letters for which corresponding consonantal phonemes are learned early in development (e.g., *B*, *M*) before letters for which corresponding consonantal phonemes are learned later (e.g., *J*, *V*).

Print Awareness

Print awareness describes a number of specific achievements children generally acquire along a developmental continuum (Justice & Ezell, 2004): developing *print interest*, recognizing *print functions*, understanding *print conventions*, understanding *print forms*, and recognizing *print part-to-whole relationships* (see Figure 7.1). First, young children develop interest in and appreciation for print. They recognize

Preschool-age children show interest in specific letters occurring in the environment.

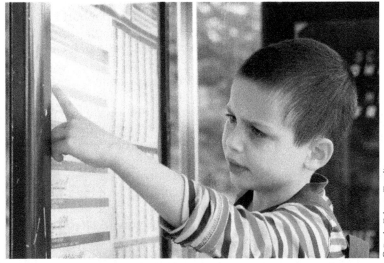

© Pavla Zakova/Fotolia

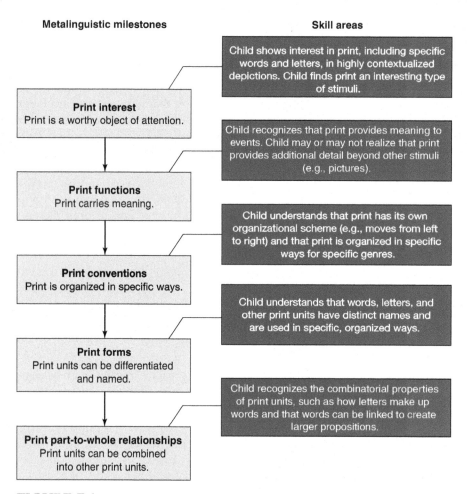

Metalinguistic milestones

Print interest
Print is a worthy object of attention.

Print functions
Print carries meaning.

Print conventions
Print is organized in specific ways.

Print forms
Print units can be differentiated and named.

Print part-to-whole relationships
Print units can be combined into other print units.

Skill areas

Child shows interest in print, including specific words and letters, in highly contextualized depictions. Child finds print an interesting type of stimuli.

Child recognizes that print provides meaning to events. Child may or may not realize that print provides additional detail beyond other stimuli (e.g., pictures).

Child understands that print has its own organizational scheme (e.g., moves from left to right) and that print is organized in specific ways for specific genres.

Child understands that words, letters, and other print units have distinct names and are used in specific, organized ways.

Child recognizes the combinatorial properties of print units, such as how letters make up words and that words can be linked to create larger propositions.

FIGURE 7.1

Achievements in print awareness.

Source: From "Print Referencing: An Emergent Literacy Enhancement Technique and Its Clinical Applications," by L. M. Justice and H. K. Ezell, 2004, *Language, Speech, and Hearing Services in Schools, 35,* p. 188. Copyright 2004 by American Speech-Language-Hearing Association. Reprinted with permission.

that print exists in the environment and in books. Second, they begin to understand print conveys meaning and has a specific function. Third, children develop an understanding of specific print conventions, including reading print from left to right and from top to bottom. Fourth, children learn the language that describes specific print units, including *words* and *letters*. Fifth, children learn the relationship among different print units, including how letters combine to form words.

Children's oral language abilities and the interactions they have with print contribute to children's development of print awareness. Some research indicates preschoolers do not, on their own, focus on print; they seem to need prompting from adults to pay attention to print. For example, one research study revealed that in the absence of explicit verbal references to print or gestures toward print, preschoolers looked at print only about 5%–6% of the time when reading a storybook. However, when adults made explicit references to print, either nonverbally (by pointing or tracking the print with their finger) or verbally (by calling children's attention to words or letters on the pages), children looked at print more often. More specifically, they looked at print in the storybook about 12.5 times when an adult read the book verbatim, 17.7 times when an adult made nonverbal references to print, and 21.2 times when an adult made verbal references to print (Justice, Pullen, & Pence, 2008). Other research indicates that when adults refer to print during storybook-reading sessions ("I see the letter *D*, like in your name"), children ask more questions and make more comments about print (Ezell & Justice, 2000). Research also shows that children show marked improvement in important early literacy abilities when adults question about and point to print during book-reading sessions (Justice & Ezell, 2002b).

Phonological Awareness

Phonological awareness, another important metalinguistic skill, is children's sensitivity to the sound structure of words. This awareness emerges incrementally, beginning at around age 2 years and moves from a "shallow" level to a "deep" level of awareness (see Table 7.1; Stanovich, 2000). Children with a shallow level of phonological awareness show an implicit and rudimentary sensitivity to large units of sound structure. They can segment sentences into words and multisyllabic words into syllables. They can also detect and produce rhymes, combine syllable onsets with the remainder of the syllable to produce a word (e.g., /b/ + /ɪt/ = *bit*), and detect beginning sound similarities among words (e.g., *sing, sack, sun*). Children develop shallow sensitivities during the preschool years, from about 3 to 5 years of age. In contrast,

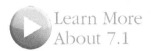

Learn More About 7.1

As you watch the video titled "Print Interest," notice how the 3-year-old demonstrates interest in print by lifting the flaps in the book to find hidden words and phrases. Although he misreads the word "Hello" as "Hellen," he exhibits an understanding of the combinatorial properties of print units, such as how letters combine to form words.

TABLE 7.1
Achievements in phonological awareness

PHONOLOGICAL AWARENESS SKILL	DESCRIPTION	LEVEL	DEVELOPMENTAL EXPECTATION
Word awareness	Segments sentences into words	Shallow	Early to middle preschool
Syllable awareness	Segments multisyllable words into syllables	Shallow	Early to middle preschool
Rhyme awareness	Recognizes when two words rhyme; produces pairs of words that rhyme	Shallow	Early to middle preschool
Onset awareness	Segments the beginning sound (onset) from the rest of a syllable; blends the beginning sound (onset) with the rest of a syllable	Shallow	Late preschool
Phoneme identity	Identifies sounds at the beginning and end of the word; identifies words that start with the same sound	Shallow	Late preschool, early kindergarten
Phoneme blending	Blends phonemes to make a word	Deep	Early kindergarten
Phoneme segmentation	Segments a word into its phonemes	Deep	Middle to late kindergarten
Phoneme counting	Identifies the number of phonemes in a word	Deep	Late kindergarten to end of first grade
Phoneme manipulation	Deletes, adds, and rearranges phonemes in a word	Deep	Elementary grades

Source: From "Embedded-Explicit Emergent Literacy. II: Goal Selection and Implementation in the Early Childhood Classroom," by J. N. Kaderavek and L. M. Justice, 2004, *Language, Speech, and Hearing Services in Schools, 35*, p. 218. Copyright 2004 by American Speech-Language-Hearing Association. Reprinted with permission.

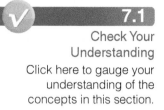

7.1

Check Your
Understanding
Click here to gauge your
understanding of the
concepts in this section.

children with a deep level of phonological awareness demonstrate an explicit and analytical knowledge of the smallest phonological segments of speech (phonemes). They can count the number of phonemes in words (e.g., *bit* has three sounds, and *spit* has four sounds), can segment words into their constituent phonemes (e.g., can break *bit* into /b/ + /ɪ/ + /t/), and can manipulate the phonological segments within words (e.g., delete the first sound in *spit* and move it to the end of the word to make *pits*; Justice & Schuele, 2004). See Developmental Timeline: Preschool for an overview of more milestones children achieve during the preschool years.

DEVELOPMENTAL TIMELINE

PHONOLOGY

36 months	40 months	44 months	48 months	52 months	56 months	60 months

Begins to develop shallow phonological awareness abilities (36 months)

Has mastered most consonants (44 months)

Is very intelligible in connected speech / Has mastered almost all consonant sounds, but they may not be mastered in all contexts (52 months)

Continues to refine articulatory skills (40 months)

Decreases use of phonological processes (e.g., weak-syllable deletion, cluster reduction) (48 months)

Knows letters that make up own name / Shows only languishing difficulties with the later-developing sounds / Has some persisting phonological processes (e.g., liquid gliding, substitution) (56 months)

SYNTAX AND MORPHOLOGY

36 months	40 months	44 months	48 months	52 months	56 months	60 months

Uses four to five words in sentences / Uses compound sentences with *and* (36 months)

Uses articles / Uses past tense consistently / Uses contractions consistently (44 months)

Uses subordination and coordination in sentences / Uses irregular plural forms consistently (52 months)

Uses pronouns consistently / Uses adverbs of time (40 months)

Combines four to seven words in sentences / Uses contractible auxiliaries and uncontractible auxiliaries / Uses irregular third person verbs (e.g., *has*) (48 months)

Combines five to eight words in sentences (56 months)

SEMANTICS

Uses pronouns such as *they, them, us*
Continues to use fast mapping to learn new words

Understands some kinship terms
Uses syntactic information to narrow the possible meanings of new words

Uses "what do, what does, what did" questions

| 36 months | 40 months | 44 months | 48 months | 52 months | 56 months | 60 months |

Uses 1,000–1,500 words
Comprehends 1,500–2,000 words
Understands some relational terms such as *hard–soft*

Overextends new words on the basis of object function
Uses animacy information to infer the meanings of new words
Uses reflexive pronouns such as *himself, herself, itself*

Uses 1,500–2,000 words
Comprehends 2,500–2,800 words
Uses deictic terms *this, that, here, there*

PRAGMATICS

Begins to engage in longer dialogues

Understands indirect requests accompanied by nonverbal pointing

Uses indirect requests

| 36 months | 40 months | 44 months | 48 months | 52 months | 56 months | 60 months |

Begins to use primitive narratives
Begins to make conversational repairs

Uses interpretive, logical, participatory, and organizing functions
Constructs true narratives

Uses narrative with a sequence of events but no main character or theme

Sources: Gard, Gilman, and Gorman (1993); Haelsig and Madison (1986); Hall, Burns, and Pawluski (2003); Halliday (1975, 1977, 1978); Jaswal and Markman (2001a); Kaderavek and Sulzby (2000); Kelly (2001); Kemler Nelson, Herron, and Holt (2003); and Treiman and Broderick (1998).

WHAT MAJOR ACHIEVEMENTS IN LANGUAGE FORM, CONTENT, AND USE CHARACTERIZE THE PRESCHOOL PERIOD?

As we first mentioned in Chapter 1, and then reviewed in Chapters 5 and 6, the three rule-governed domains that together compose language are *form*, or how people organize sounds, words, and sentences to convey content; *content*, or the words people use and their meanings; and *use*, or how people use language in interactions with other individuals to express personal and social needs. As you may suspect, the preschool period ushers in even more achievements in each of these three areas.

Language Form

During the preschool years, children refine their phonology, morphology, and syntax in significant ways. Preschoolers make noteworthy advances in speech production abilities, grammatical and derivational morphology, and sentence forms.

Achievements in Speech Production

During the preschool years, children continue to refine their speech sound repertoires. By the end of the preschool period, most children have mastered nearly all the phonemes of their native language. Four- and 5-year-old children generally show only minimal difficulties with a few of the later-developing phonemes, including /r/ (_row_), /l/ (_low_), /s/ (_sew_), /tʃ/ (_cheese_), /ʃ/ (_show_), /z/ (_zoo_), /θ/ (_think_), and /ð/ (_though_). Children may also exhibit persistent difficulties with some of the earlier-acquired phonemes when they appear in complex multisyllabic words (e.g., /s/ in _spaghetti_), or in words with consonant clusters (such as the first three sounds in _split_). Despite a few ongoing challenges, preschoolers are highly intelligible and have an adultlike expressive phonemic repertoire.

The _phonological processes_ (or systematic errors children make in their speech) continue to diminish during the preschool years as children's phonological systems stabilize; in the age 3–4 period, children have the fastest suppression rate (Haelsig & Madison, 1986). Four-year-olds may still exhibit weak-syllable deletion (e.g., _banana_ becomes "nana") and cluster reduction (e.g., _street_ becomes "treet"), but these processes usually disappear by age 5 years. Two patterns that may persist past the fifth birthday are as follows:

Pattern	Description	Examples
1. **Liquid gliding**	When a liquid consonant (/r/ or /l/) is replaced by a glide consonant (/w/ or /j/—the first sound in _yellow_)	_rabbit_ = "wabbit" _land_ = "yand"
2. **Stopping**	When a fricative (such as /θ/—the "th" sound in _think_—or /ð/—the "th" sound in _though_) or an affricate (such as the first sound in _jeep_) is replaced by a stop consonant (such as /t/ or /d/)	_think_ = "tink" or "dink" _though_ = "dough" or "tow" _jeep_ = "deep"

Receptive phonology also continues to develop during the preschool years, which becomes important to children's early reading development. As we discussed previously, reading requires a child to have robust phonological representations to make sense of the alphabetic principle, or the relationship between letters or combinations of letters (graphemes) and sounds (phonemes). Environmental and biological factors can affect children's development of adequate phonological representations. For instance, children who receive little linguistic stimulation, and those who have ongoing middle ear infections are at risk for having delays in the development of phonological representations (Nittrouer, 1996).

Grammatical and Derivational Morphology

We introduced grammatical morphemes in Chapter 1; they are the units of meaning we add to a word to provide additional grammatical precision, such as the plural morpheme (_bird–birds_) and the verb inflection for present progressive actions (_it can fly–it is flying_). _Derivational_ morphology is similar to grammatical morphology in that it modifies the structure of words. However, derivational morphemes are the prefixes and suffixes we add to a word to change its meaning and sometimes its part of speech. For instance, the suffix _-er_ can be added to _write_ to change its meaning and its part of speech from a verb to a noun (*writer*). The prefix *re-* can be added to *write* to change its meaning (*rewrite*). Additional common derivational morphemes include *pre-* (*preschool*), *-est* (*smallest*), *-ness* (*sweetness*), and *-ly* (*slowly*). As children learn new morphemes, they can manipulate word structure to become more precise and specific in their communication. Children can increase their possibilities for communicating exponentially once they master a few important morphemes. For example, a child who knows the word *read* can use the variations *reading*, *reread*, *reader*, and so forth.

As we discussed in Chapter 6, children acquire grammatical and derivational morphemes in about the same order, even among different languages. Six factors contribute to the order in which children acquire these types of morphemes (O'Grady, Dobrovolsky, & Arnoff, 1997):

1. *Frequent occurrence in utterance-final position:* Infants and children are most sensitive to sounds and words at the ends of utterances. Children first learn morphemes occurring as suffixes.

2. *Syllabicity:* Children first learn morphemes that constitute their own syllables (e.g., present progressive *-ing*) and later learn morphemes that contain only a single sound (e.g., third-person singular *-s*).

3. *Single relation between morpheme and meaning:* Children first learn morphemes with only one meaning (e.g., the morpheme *the* functions only as a definite article) before they learn morphemes that express multiple meanings (e.g., *-s* denotes present tense, third person, and plural number).

4. *Consistency in use:* Children learn the names of morphemes that are used consistently (e.g., possessive nouns always end in *'s*) more easily than morphemes that vary in their use (e.g., past tense verbs sometimes end in *-ed* but at other times take an irregular form).

5. *Allomorphic variation:* Children learn morphemes that have a consistent pronunciation (e.g., *-ing*) before they learn morphemes that have allomorphic variation (e.g., the plural morpheme has three variations: /s/, /z/, and /ɪz/).

6. *Clear semantic function:* Children first learn morphemes that have a clear meaning (e.g., plural morpheme) before they learn morphemes with less clear meaning (e.g., third-person singular morpheme such as "he *runs*").

The most significant area of morpheme development in the preschool period is *verb morphology*. One way English speakers inflect verbs is with tense (e.g., past, present, future) to provide information about time. Often, the verb *to be* is an important marker of time. When the verb *to be* or any of its derivatives (*am, is, are, was, were*) is the main verb in a sentence—as in *I am Doug*—it is called a *copula*. When the verb *to be* or one of its derivatives is a helping verb in a sentence—as in *I am hugging Doug*—it is called an *auxiliary*. The *to be* copula and auxiliary forms can be made into contractions (*Doug's funny; I'm bouncing the ball*) or left in their uncontracted forms (*Doug is funny; I am bouncing the ball*). Preschoolers master the verb *to be* in its copula and auxiliary forms, representing a major syntactic achievement of these years.

Sentence Forms

In addition to these major morphological achievements, preschoolers make significant advances in using complex sentences. Preschoolers move from simple declarative subject–verb–object constructions ("Daddy drives a truck") and subject–verb–complement constructions ("Truck is big") to more elaborate sentence patterns, such as the following three (Justice & Ezell, 2002a):

1. *Subject–verb–object–adverb:* "Daddy's hitting the hammer outside."

2. *Subject–verb–complement–adverb:* "Daddy is hungry now."

3. *Subject–auxiliary–verb–adverb:* "Daddy is eating now."

Children also begin to embed multiple phrases and clauses into their utterances to create complex and compound sentences and to use coordinating conjunctions (e.g., *and, or, but*) and subordinating conjunctions (e.g., *then, when, because*) to connect clauses. By the end of the preschool period, children produce compound sentences, such as *I told Daddy and Daddy told Mommy,* as well as complex sentences with embedded clauses, such as *I told Daddy, who told Mommy* (Justice & Ezell, 2002a).

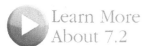

Learn More About 7.2

In the video titled "Preschool-Age Boy Language Sample," the 3-year-old demonstrates the ability to respond contingently to questions and to provide elaborate answers.

Learn More About 7.2 *(Continued)*

At the beginning of the video, he explains that he and his classmates couldn't go swimming that day because the water was "too wet," "too cold," and "bad." Although the pH level might actually have been to blame, this young child makes some very reasonable guesses as to why he and his friends could not enter the pool and uses an informative discourse function to provide this information to another person.

Next, he uses a multiclause cause-and-effect statement that incorporates the word because to describe why the children got so wet when jumping over the sprinkler ("We got very wet because we were jumping over the sprinkler where all the water comes out"). Next, the boy demonstrates proper yes/no question formation when he asks, "Is there a picture of me?" Finally, the boy uses a multiclause utterance in the future tense to make a prediction "When Katrin takes a picture I think I'm gonna see hers and I think hers is gonna be better." It is important to remember that children demonstrate great variability in their language production abilities. Although this child produced a sentence containing nearly 20 morphemes, many children the same age tend to produce sentences containing fewer morphemes.

Language Content

Even before children enter formal schooling, they acquire skills that ease their transition into the academic realm and the language that accompanies this transition. For example, preschoolers continue to acquire new words at a lightning pace—about 860 words per year—averaging about two new words per day during this period (Biemiller, 2005). However, the strategies preschoolers use for acquiring new words and the kinds of words they learn are different from those in the infancy and toddler periods. We next discuss how preschoolers use fast mapping to add words to their lexicons, use their knowledge of semantics and syntax to infer the meanings of new words, and learn new words through shared storybook reading. We also describe some specific types of new language content preschoolers acquire, including various types of relational terms.

Fast Mapping

Many researchers view word learning as a gradual process in which word representations progressively develop from immature, incomplete representations to mature, accurate, and precise representations. Recall that children are able to acquire a general representation of a new word with as little as a single exposure through *fast mapping* (Carey, 1978). After fast mapping occurs, children engage in slow mapping, during which they gradually refine representations with time and multiple exposures to the word in varying contexts. In fact, children may be refining meanings for as many as 1,600 words at any given time (Carey & Bartlett, 1978).

E. Dale (1965) described vocabulary knowledge development as a four-stage process:

STAGE 1	No knowledge of a word	"I never saw it before."
STAGE 2	Emergent knowledge	"I've heard of it but don't know what it means."

Preschoolers might use the principle of novel name–nameless category (N3C) to infer that a novel label refers to a novel object.

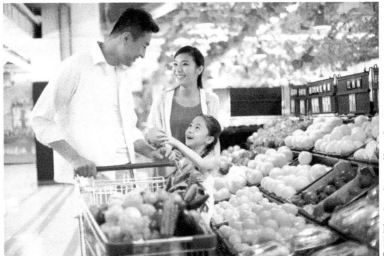

© BJI/Blue Jean Images/Getty Images

| Stage 3 | Contextual knowledge | "I recognize it in context—it has something to do with …" |
| Stage 4 | Full knowledge | "I know it." |

During the preschool period, children's vocabularies include words at each of these levels. Children may require multiple exposures to words in varying contexts to attain what Carey (1978) called extended mapping, or a full and complete understanding of the meaning of a word.

Preschoolers, like toddlers, use the principle of *novel name–nameless category* (N3C) to match novel labels to nameless objects and can then fast map novel words through this process. For example, if you were to show a preschooler three familiar objects (an apple, a chair, and a ball) and one novel object (a corkscrew) and tell him or her, "Find the dax," the child should be able to eliminate the familiar objects from contention and select the novel object as the *dax*. Furthermore, using fast mapping, he or she should have a general understanding of what a dax is and will refine his or her understanding of daxes with time and additional exposures to the word and the object. See Figure 7.2 for an example of a fast-mapping task during which a preschooler selects an unfamiliar object as the referent of a novel label.

Knowledge of Semantics and Syntax

In the preschool years, children know many vocabulary words and have a well-developed syntax, so when they learn new words, they rely on their knowledge of semantics and syntax to incorporate (or assimilate) the new words into their vocabulary. As we discussed in Chapter 6, toddlers learning new words may overgeneralize as many as one-third of word meanings on the basis of categorical, analogical, and relational similarities. The perceptual features of objects weigh heavily in toddlers' overgeneralizations (e.g., calling all round objects "balls"). In the preschool years, children continue to overextend object names on the basis of information they have about other objects, but they weigh the *function* of an object more heavily than its perceptual appearance. For example, if children know the name for a certain tool, they might call other tools that perform similar functions by the same name. In one study, 4-year-old children invented names for new artifacts on the basis of the functions of the objects rather than their perceptual properties. The children used the perceptual features to invent names only when they did not know the objects' functions (Kemler Nelson, Herron, & Holt, 2003).

Preschool-age children also use knowledge about the *animacy* of objects when inferring the meaning of new words. Preschoolers select animate objects as referents for novel proper names and inanimate objects as referents for common nouns

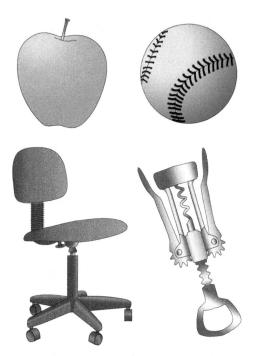

FIGURE 7.2

A fast-mapping task.

ADULT: Find the *dax*.

PRESCHOOLER: **Right here.** (*points to corkscrew, the novel item*)

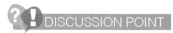 DISCUSSION POINT

What language-development theory (from Chapter 4) could best explain children's ability to use knowledge of the animacy of an object to infer the meaning of a new word?

(Jaswal & Markman, 2001a). For example, if given the choice of a novel inanimate object and a novel animate object, preschoolers will select the inanimate object when you tell them "Find *the dax*" and will select the animate object when you tell them "Find *Dax*."

Another way preschoolers infer the meanings of new words is by recruiting syntactic cues that signal the form class (e.g., noun, verb, adjective) of a novel word to narrow the possibilities for the referent of the word. For example, children who hear "This is *a dax*" interpret *dax* to be a *count noun*, whereas children who hear "This *is* Dax" interpret *Dax* to be a *proper name*. Likewise, children who hear "This is a *dax one*" interpret *dax* to be an *adjective* (Hall et al., 2003). Children are also more likely to assume a novel word is an adjective when it is applied to more than one object (e.g., "This is *round*, and that is *round*, too") because count nouns and proper names rarely take more than a single label (Hall, 1996).

Preschool-age children can also recognize the difference between sentences that refer to objects in a generic way ("Birds lay eggs") and sentences that refer to an object in a specific way ("This bird lays eggs"; Gelman & Raman, 2007), and may use the syntactic cues in these two different types of sentences to learn about the meanings of new words. For example, imagine a preschooler, Jess, is reading a storybook about animals with her mother. As they are reading, they encounter an animal Jess has never seen before and for which she doesn't know the name (a raccoon). If Jess's mother uses a sentence that refers to raccoons in a generic way, by saying "Raccoons like to get into garbage cans," Jess will likely infer that getting into garbage cans is something many raccoons do. If her mother were instead to use a sentence that refers to a specific raccoon, by saying "This raccoon likes to get into garbage cans," Jess might instead infer that getting into garbage cans is a pastime unique to the individual raccoon her mother is describing.

Shared Storybook Reading

In addition to learning words through single and multiple incidental exposures, preschoolers acquire new words as they participate in shared storybook interactions with other people. The language contained within storybook readings is exceptionally rich. In fact, maternal language in storybook-reading activities contains a more diverse array of syntax and vocabulary, and typically has a higher level of abstraction than that in other language contexts, including play (Sorsby & Martlew, 1991).

Although storybook-reading interactions present opportunities for word learning, individual differences in the frequency of these interactions and the quality of the language children hear as they engage in such interactions are related to children's language development. For example, variations in reading interactions with young children are related to children's receptive and expressive vocabulary abilities (Whitehurst et al., 1988). Research results indicate children can learn new words through incidental exposure to words during storybook-reading sessions in which the meanings of target words are not discussed (Robbins & Ehri, 1994). However, storybook readings that include repeated and elaborated exposures to new words, as well as an active (or dialogic) reading style on the adult's part, improve children's learning of new words from storybooks more than shared storybook readings that do not include these components (e.g., Coyne, McCoach, Loftus, Zipoli, & Kapp, 2009; Justice, Meier, & Walpole, 2005). Furthermore, preschoolers better comprehend stories when adults read them with an expressive style (using variation in pitch, tone, volume, pace, and pausing) than with a less expressive style (Mira & Schwanenflugel, 2013).

Relational Terms

Now that we have discussed some processes by which preschoolers acquire new words, we introduce some of the specific kinds of language content preschoolers acquire. One such set of words is relational terms, which are terms that allow speakers to express logical relationships. Preschool-age children become able to understand and use relational terms once they can grasp the concepts underlying the terms. For example, to understand and use temporal terms, children must first have a concept of time. Relational terms include deictic terms, interrogatives (questions), temporal terms, opposites, locational prepositions, and kinship terms.

Deictic Terms.   Deictic terms are words whose use and interpretation depend on the location of a speaker and listener within a particular setting. Examples of English deictic terms include the words *here* and *this*, which indicate proximity to the speaker, and the words *there* and *that*, which indicate distance from the speaker. Young children only slowly develop a mastery of these terms. The second author saw evidence of this when her then 3-year-old daughter Addie, paddling across a swimming pool toward her mother, happily exclaimed, "I'm almost here!" To use deictic terms correctly, children must be able to adopt their conversational partner's perspective. Therefore, using deictic terms signals more advanced cognitive and pragmatic processes than those used in earlier developmental phases. Children master proximal deictic terms such as *this* and *here* more easily than they master distal deictic terms such as *that* and *there*. Generally, children master the contrast between deictic terms by the time they enter school (Clark & Sengul, 1978).

Interrogatives.   Preschoolers become increasingly adept at answering and asking questions. They understand and use question words with more concrete applications, such as *what*, *where*, *who*, *whose*, and *which* before they understand and use other interrogatives with more abstract applications, such as *when*, *how*, and *why*. Preschoolers may respond inappropriately to questions they do not understand, as in the following example of a conversation between a teacher and a preschool-age child:

TEACHER: Why did the girl get so many presents?

CHILD: She got a bike, a doll, and coloring books.

Temporal Terms.   Temporal terms describe the order of events (*before*, *after*), the duration of events (*since*, *until*), and the concurrence of events (*while*, *during*). Preschoolers understand temporal terms describing order before they understand temporal terms describing concurrent events. When preschoolers do not understand the meaning of temporal terms, they often interpret sentences according to word order (e.g., Weist, 2002). For example, preschoolers might interpret the sentence *Before you eat breakfast, take your vitamin* to mean "Eat breakfast, then take your vitamin." Preschool-age children might also interpret temporal terms according to their experience, so a child who takes a vitamin *before* breakfast each day might interpret the preceding example correctly. Preschoolers also often use nouns that describe time-based concepts, such as *yesterday* and *tomorrow*, with some confusion, as shown by Griffin, at age 3, who once questioned: "Is it yesterday?"

Opposites.   Opposites are another aspect of language content that preschoolers learn to understand and use. Some opposite pairs that preschoolers learn include *hard–soft*, *big–little*, *heavy–light*, *tall–short*, *long–short*, and *large–small*. Preschoolers learn opposites that they can perceive physically (such as *big–small*) before they learn more abstract opposites (such as *same–different*).

Locational Prepositions.   Although children begin to use some locational prepositions as toddlers (e.g., *in*, *on*), they do not begin to use many other prepositions until preschool age. Locational prepositions, which describe spatial relations, include *under*, *next to*, *behind*, *in back of*, and *in front of* (Grela, Rashiti, & Soares, 2004). By the end of the preschool period, most children have a solid understanding of these terms.

Kinship Terms.   Children initially interpret kinship terms such as *mommy*, *daddy*, *sister*, and *brother* to refer to specific individuals. Preschoolers eventually fathom the general meaning of these and other kinship terms, including *son*, *daughter*, *grandfather*, *grandmother*, and *parent*. Children tend to learn less complex kinship terms before more complex kinship terms, and they tend to learn kinship terms that refer to the family member with whom they are most familiar earlier than kinship terms that refer to family members with whom they are less familiar (Haviland & Clark, 1974). Thus, children learn the words *mother* and *father* before they learn the words *aunt* and *uncle* because the former concepts are simpler. Children who see their aunts and uncles regularly should also learn these kinship terms before children who are not familiar with their aunts and uncles. Interestingly, preschoolers have difficulty with the reciprocity of some kinship terms (Deák & Maratsos, 1998). For example, children understand when they *have* a brother or a sister, but they have more difficulty understanding that they can *be* a brother or sister to someone else.

Language Use

Use describes how people use language to meet personal and social needs. Preschool-age children implement many new discourse functions, improve their conversational skills, and begin to use narratives.

Discourse Functions

Recall from Chapter 6 that toddlers who are combining words can use language to satisfy seven communicative functions: instrumental, regulatory, interactional, personal, heuristic, imaginative, and informative. Preschoolers begin to use language for even more complex discourse functions, including interpretive, logical, participatory, and organizing functions (Halliday, 1975, 1977, 1978). *Interpretive functions* make clear the whole of a person's experience (e.g., "I was pretty scared after watching that movie."). *Logical functions* express logical relations between ideas (e.g., "Let's put our boots on so our feet don't get wet."). *Participatory functions* express wishes, feelings, attitudes, and judgments (e.g., "I don't like this game. Let's play a different one."), and *organizing functions* manage discourse (e.g., "First we added the flour, and next we added the eggs."). Although preschoolers use these new discourse functions, the informative function continues to be most prevalent at this age (Hage, Resegue, Viveiros, & Pacheco, 2007). Informative functions use language to convey information.

Besides expressing additional pragmatic functions, preschool children continue to detect and use the pragmatic information other people convey. Such information helps preschoolers better understand messages. For example, research results show that children understand an indirect request better when the speaker uses nonverbal pointing in addition to the request. Preschoolers who watched researchers point to an open door (nonverbal cue) while saying "It's going to get loud in here" (indirect request) were more likely to close the door than were preschoolers who heard only the indirect request to close the door (Kelly, 2001). This example demonstrates the importance of pragmatic information to language comprehension, even for preschoolers who can already use an array of pragmatic functions when communicating with other people.

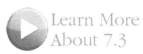

Learn More About 7.3

In the video titled "Preschool-Age Girl Language Sample," the 4-year-old begins by recounting events that occurred over the course of the day in her preschool classroom and then later she spontaneously creates a short song.

Learn More About 7.3 *(Continued)*

She demonstrates that she is becoming quite a proficient conversationalist. For example, near the beginning of the video, she provides corrective feedback to her mother when her mother mistakenly summarizes that she had something to eat three times during the school day. Later, she uses her pragmatic knowledge to prepare her mother for some potentially disappointing news (that she didn't take a nap during nap time like most of the other students) by gently touching her on the hand. Addie uses a variety of complex and compound sentences and connects clauses using coordinating conjunctions (e.g., and, but) and subordinating conjunctions (e.g., then, when, because). Addie also demonstrates an understanding that the kinship terms mommy and daddy refer to other children's parents, and not just her own, when she describes the upcoming field trip at her school, and when she makes up a song spontaneously.

Conversational Skills

Preschoolers begin to improve their conversational skills as they learn how to take turns in a conversation. Most preschoolers can maintain a conversation for two or more turns, particularly when they select the topic for discussion. Although they still have some difficulty realizing when communication breakdowns occur and giving listeners the appropriate amount of feedback to facilitate understanding, preschoolers are becoming increasingly sophisticated conversationalists. They understand they should respond to questions and discover that speaking at the same time as another person results in ineffective communication.

Initiating conversations is another area in which preschoolers make interesting developments. Like adults, preschoolers often find themselves in situations where they must initiate conversations or small talk with their peers. You may wonder how exactly preschoolers initiate conversations with one another and what topics they talk about. One interesting study analyzed the snack-time conversations of a sample of 25 preschoolers for 21 weeks to answer such questions (O'Neill, Main, & Ziemski, 2009). Over the course of their videotaped observations, researchers captured nearly 12 hr of footage that included more than one child at the snack table. Of the total time, children spent 45% in conversation with others at the snack table, 44% in silence, and 11% conversing with others who were not at the table. One of the study's main findings was that 77.5% of children's conversational initiations were person related (e.g., "I drank my juice and spit it back in"; "Where did Julia go?", p. 410), as opposed to object related (14%) (e.g., "There's things in the apple juice."; "Oh! Spill!", p. 410), or about fantasy topics (6.9%) or games, jokes, or tricks (1.6%). Another finding was that children initiated conversation using nonquestions (such as comments or directives) more than 80% of the time and questions less than 20% of the time. Also, the preschoolers' initiations were as often about a topic relevant to the listener (e.g., "We forgot our cups," p. 408) as to themselves (e.g., "My leg is tired of walking," p. 408). Finally, the researchers found that almost one-third of the preschoolers' initiations included mention of a mental state (e.g., "I don't like raisins"; "You know how to get to my house, but the other kids don't, do they?", p. 411). The researchers concluded that preschoolers seem to have a developing understanding of people, their behaviors, characteristics, mental worlds, and interests, and that they use this developing understanding to find common ground with their peers as they initiate conversations and small talk. Finding common ground with others contributes to children's development of social connections with others and allows them to participate in enjoyable forms of communication, such as comparing likes and dislikes, talking about future plans, and joking.

Conversational Pragmatics

One area in which preschoolers begin to develop understanding is conversational pragmatics. Grice (1975, 1989) described a principle of conversational logic that he posited speakers and listeners should be expected to observe, namely: "Make your conversational contribution such as required, at the stage at which it occurs, by the accepted purpose or direction of the talk exchange in which you are engaged" (Grice, 1989, p. 26). He termed the principle the Cooperative Principle. There are four categories pertaining to the Cooperative Principle (quantity, quality, relation, and manner), each with its own adages. People now commonly call the adages Grice's maxims.

The category of quantity concerns the amount of information speakers should provide. The maxims related to quantity include that the speaker should: (1) make the conversational contribution as informative as necessary to facilitate the listener's understanding; and (2) not provide excess information that could lead the listener off track.

The category of quality concerns the truthfulness of the language the speaker should use. The maxims related to quality include that the speaker should: (1) not say something he or she believes to be false; and (2) not to say something for which he or she lacks adequate evidence.

The category of relation concerns the idea that the speaker should "be relevant" (p. 27) in communicative exchanges. Finally, the category of manner concerns not what the speaker says, but how the speaker says it. The maxims related to manner include that the speaker should: (1) avoid being unclear; (2) avoid being ambiguous; (3) be brief; and (4) be orderly.

Some research indicates that preschoolers (3- to 5-year-olds) are sensitive to speakers' violations of the Gricean principles of relation, quantity, and quality (manner was not assessed; Eskritt, Whalen, & Lee, 2008). In the study, children had three chances to follow one of two puppets, one of which adhered to one of Grice's maxims and the other of which did not, to locate a sticker under one of four cups. In the condition examining relation, the puppet violating Grice's maxims said, "I like these cups" or "These are pretty cups." In the condition examining quantity, the puppet violating Grice's maxims said, "It's under a cup" or "It's under one of the cups." In the condition examining quality, the puppet violating Grice's maxims would lie about which cup the sticker was under. Children demonstrated sensitivity to the principle of relation on the first trial about 68% of the time. However, they did not demonstrate significant sensitivity to the quantity principle or the quality principle on the first trial, as they did not listen to the advice of the puppet that adhered to the Gricean maxim significantly more than the puppet that did not follow the Gricean maxim. There was also an effect of age, such that 5-year-olds outperformed 3-year-olds, providing some preliminary evidence of an emerging sensitivity to Grice's maxims in the preschool years.

Other research reveals that preschoolers expect conversational partners to be consistent when using particular referential descriptions for objects. In one study, Graham, Sedivy, and Khu (2014) had an experimenter introduce an object to a preschooler and label it with a specific expression (i.e., the striped ball) before leaving the room. Using an eye tracking device, they found preschoolers could more quickly locate the target object (i.e., the yellow striped ball) when the speaker used the original expression to describe the object (i.e., the striped ball) than when the speaker used a new expression to describe another salient property of the same object (i.e., the yellow ball). In contrast, there was no difference in how quickly preschoolers located the target object when a different speaker used either the original expression (i.e., the striped ball) or a new referential expression (i.e., the yellow ball). The findings demonstrate preschoolers presume that speakers intend to signal a change in meaning if they change the expression they use to refer to a specific object.

Narrative Skills

A narrative is a child's spoken or written description of a real or fictional event from the past, the present, or the future. W. Labov (1972) defined a narrative as minimally containing two sequential independent clauses about the same past event. "Hey, Mom, guess what we did in gym today" is one way a preschooler might begin a narrative, followed by "We got to play with a big parachute."

Preschool children's narratives serve as a showcase for multiple language achievements, including those in syntax, morphology, semantics, phonology, and pragmatics. Children must use syntax to arrange words and ideas, verb morphology to signal the time of events, vocabulary to represent events and persons precisely, phonology to pronounce words clearly and with proper intonation, and pragmatics to share an appropriate amount of information with the listener. Narratives use decontextualized language to describe people or characters not immediately present and events removed from the current context. Narratives differ from conversations in that two or more persons carry on conversations, whereas narratives are largely uninterrupted streams of language from a single person. Children who produce narratives must take responsibility for the effectiveness of the communication.

To produce a narrative, the child introduces a topic and organizes the information pertaining to the topic in such a way that the listener can assume a relatively passive role, providing only minimal support to the speaker. Two important types of narratives are the personal narrative, in which an individual shares a factual event, and the fictional narrative, in which an individual shares an imaginary event. Both types of narratives generally thread a sequence of events together in a causal or temporal manner. A *causal* sequence unfolds following a cause-and-effect chain of events, or provides a reason or rationale for some series of events (e.g., "Kathy locked her keys inside her house, so she had to call a neighbor"). A *temporal* sequence unfolds with time (e.g., "First, we rode our bikes around the lake. Next, we fed the ducks").

Although narrative skills begin to develop as early as age 2 years, most children cannot construct true narratives with a problem and a resolution (or high point) until around age 4 years (Kaderavek & Sulzby, 2000; Peterson, 1990). Children who have not yet mastered narrative discourse might try to describe an event for a listener without providing a clear introduction, middle, or end to their story. Children's early narratives may include only a minimal description of the participants, time, and location relevant to the event and may contain only a series of events, as in the following example:

CHILD: Cody brought a rabbit and left it on the porch and Dad said Cody should go hunting with him.

ADULT: Just one second. Who is Cody?

CHILD: My dog.

ADULT: Where did this happen?

CHILD: At home.

ADULT: So, your dad likes to hunt and he thinks Cody could help him to catch some rabbits because he brought a rabbit home?

CHILD: Yep.

Preschoolers' narratives become clearer as their ability to consider the listener's perspective emerges. Children's repertoire of linguistic devices, including adverbial time phrases (e.g., *yesterday, this morning*) and verb morphology (signaling the time of activities), grows during the preschool period, which helps increase the comprehensibility of their narratives. Some research suggests that a brief intervention can improve preschoolers' narrative comprehension and production skills, with even greater gains for preschoolers who have the opportunity to choose some story elements and manipulate the trajectory of the narrative as part of the intervention, as compared to preschoolers not offered choices (Khan, Nelson, & Whyte, 2014). See Theory to Practice: *Effects of Telephone Conversations on Preschooler's Narrative Skills* to discover another way in which preschoolers might hone their narrative skills in an everyday activity.

Because narratives are a complex multidimensional language activity, narrative skills are a good predictor of concurrent and later school outcomes for preschoolers exhibiting difficulties in developing language skills (Justice, Bowles, Pence, & Gosse, 2010; Paul & Smith, 1993). The decontextualized language inherent in narratives likely plays a crucial role in the acquisition of early literacy skills and in subsequent school achievement (Peterson, Jesso, & McCabe, 1999).

One well-known method for investigating children's narrative abilities is ethnographic research. Ethnographic research is a qualitative research method that involves gathering data about different societies and cultures with the aim of describing the nature of the populations of interest. Miller, Cho, and Bracey (2005) presented an ethnographic review of their own research and the research of others, documenting similarities and differences in the narratives of children from two different socioeconomic backgrounds: working-class families and middle-class families. Before considering the findings, it is important to note that the researchers added appropriate qualifications to their discussion (e.g., the findings may not be representative of the general population; the findings may not adequately characterize the overlap between the groups). In terms of similarities, the researchers found that parents and caregivers from both socioeconomic backgrounds encourage children to tell stories about their past experiences (personal narratives) from an early age, and that these narrative styles persist throughout adolescence and adulthood. In terms of differences, the researchers summarized that children from working-class communities tend to talk about negative

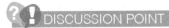

DISCUSSION POINT

Why do you think the telephone intervention described earlier helped develop children's narrative skills?

7.2

Check Your Understanding

Click here to gauge your understanding of the concepts in this section.

experiences and serious physical harm (e.g., animal bites, getting burned) more often than their middle-class counterparts; children from middle-class communities tend to talk more about sustaining minor injuries (e.g., falling down at the park). The researchers also summarized that children from working-class families use more dramatic language than their middle-class counterparts. Specifically, children from working-class families were found to use two times as many verbs of emotion, attributions, and expletives as children from middle-class families. For example, "instead of saying 'I was mad!' which would break up the flow of dramatic action, these young narrators [from working-class families], said, for example, 'I *smashed* him more!'" (p. 128). In addition to summarizing the ethnographic findings, Miller, Cho, and Bracey raise some educational implications for varying narrative styles. For example, the researchers point out that teachers' and children's narrative styles may "clash." It is thus important that educators learn to recognize and value narratives representing a variety of cultural and socioeconomic perspectives.

WHAT FACTORS CONTRIBUTE TO PRESCHOOLERS' INDIVIDUAL ACHIEVEMENTS IN LANGUAGE?

As is true of infancy and toddlerhood, in the preschool period language development varies both individually and among any given group of children. Because language comprises different domains (phonology, morphology, syntax, semantics, and pragmatics), language development is not an all-or-nothing phenomenon. Instead, a child acquires competence in different domains at slightly different times and may be stronger in some areas and weaker in others. In addition, among a group of preschoolers, patterns of language and literacy vary, and factors such as familial socioeconomic status and gender continue to contribute to language development.

Intraindividual Differences

Intraindividual Variation in Language Profiles

An individual preschooler usually grows more rapidly in some areas and more slowly in other areas. As such, a preschooler will exhibit one of many *language profiles* (Fey, 1986; J. Miller, 1981)—simultaneous patterns of language in multiple domains. A language profile encompasses only the language domains (phonology, morphology, syntax, semantics, or pragmatics) and not competencies (such as narrative discourse). Within his or her language profile, an individual child will have strengths and weaknesses in different areas. For instance, in Figure 7.3, Child A exhibits relatively poor language comprehension *and* production skills for his or her age. By comparison, Child B exhibits good language comprehension skills but relatively poor language production skills. Child C exhibits good language comprehension skills and production skills, with the exception of phonology, which is not as strong as the other areas of his or her language production.

Intraindividual Variation in Early Literacy Profiles

An individual preschooler may also differ in terms of his or her early literacy abilities. *Literacy profiles* are simultaneous patterns of literacy, including competencies such as narrative discourse and metasemantics (the ability to think about and explain the meaning of words and sentences). Figure 7.4 illustrates how individual children may exhibit relative strengths and weaknesses in semantics, syntax, phonemic awareness, metasemantics, and narrative discourse, as measured by standardized assessments. For example, Child 2 has strong narrative discourse abilities

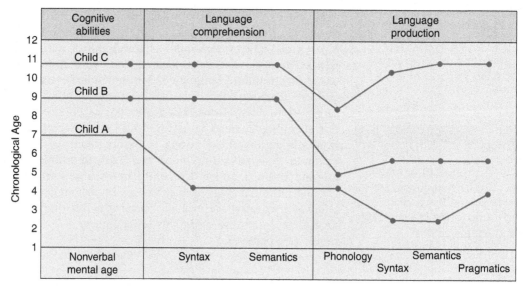

FIGURE 7.3
Three language profiles.

Source: From J. Miller, ASSESSING LANGUAGE PRODUCTION IN CHILDREN, "Language functions required of school-age children," p. 169, © 1981. Reproduced by permission of Pearson Education, Inc.

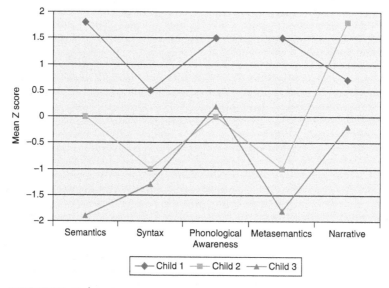

FIGURE 7.4
Three sample literacy profiles.

but relatively weak abilities in semantics, syntax, phonemic awareness, and metasemantics. Knowing a preschooler's strengths and weaknesses with regard to his or her early literacy abilities can help educators tailor early literacy instruction to the child's individual needs.

Interindividual Differences

If you observe a *group* of preschoolers, they also exhibit a variety of language and early literacy profiles. Likewise, they differ in language achievements as a result of their families' socioeconomic status and their gender.

Interindividual Variation in Language Profiles

If you were to compare a group of preschoolers, they would exhibit a variety of language profiles. For example, in Figure 7.3, Child A exhibits poor language comprehension and language production abilities relative to those of his or her peers of the same chronological age. This 7-year-old child's syntax comprehension abilities are similar to what would be expected for a 4-year-old, and his or her syntax production abilities are similar to what would be expected for a 3-year-old. Child B's comprehension of syntax and semantics are consistent with his or her age, but when considering language production skills, this 9-year-old's performance is similar to what would be expected for a child who is 3 to 4 years younger. Child C's performance matches that of his or her on-target peers in all areas except phonology.

Interindividual Variation in Early Literacy Profiles

Groups of preschoolers also differ from one another in terms of their early literacy abilities. Such differences can also be illustrated in terms of profiles. For example, early literacy profiles might be created based on a preschooler's scores on measures of semantics, syntax, phonological awareness, metasemantics, and narrative language; see Figure 7.4. Early literacy profiles are similar to language profiles in that they illustrate how a group of same-age children can exhibit varying performance levels across early literacy domains.

Effects of Socioeconomic Status

As in toddlerhood, familial socioeconomic status (SES) continues to relate to children's language development in the preschool years. Differences may become even more prominent in the preschool years because not all children attend preschool programs, and those who do are subject to varying levels of program quality. Because the United States does not have universal prekindergarten, parents who can afford to send their children to quality preschool programs often do, and parents who cannot afford preschool may take advantage of nationally funded programs such as Head Start. Fortunately, research results suggest that the quality of teacher–child interactions in the classroom and the quality of teacher language relate positively to children's language growth in preschool and that teachers can be trained to incorporate high-quality language interactions throughout the day (e.g., Girolametto & Weitzman, 2002; J. Huttenlocher, Vasilyeva, Cymerman, & Levine, 2002).

Effects of Peers and Siblings

A number of research lines indicate that a preschooler's peers and siblings may contribute to their language development in positive ways. As one example, preschoolers from low-SES backgrounds appear to benefit from attending classes in which children have mixed-SES backgrounds (Bagby, Rudd, & Woods, 2005). Researchers found that children in heterogeneous classes (low SES and high SES) experiences more language interactions, fewer negative interactions, and fewer physical interactions than children in homogeneous classes (low SES only), providing some preliminary evidence on the positive effects of mixed-SES grouping on children's language, cognitive, and socioemotional development.

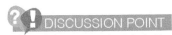

DISCUSSION POINT

How might a researcher study the quality of teachers' language use within the preschool classroom?

In another study, researchers found that preschoolers with disabilities attending classrooms with peers of higher average language skills had language scores (measured in the spring) about 40% higher than preschoolers with disabilities attending classrooms with peers of lower average language skills (Justice, Logan, Lin, & Kaderavek, 2014). The results suggest that peers have an impact on language development. Heterogeneous grouping may have a facilitative effect on language development for preschoolers with disabilities because they have opportunities throughout the day to observe, imitate, and model the language of their classmates who do not have disabilities.

With regard to sibling effects, research indicates that preschoolers with more than three siblings tend to have smaller receptive vocabularies than preschoolers with fewer siblings (presumably because they engage in fewer language interactions with their parents). However, preschoolers with an older sibling who is attuned to the preschooler's language abilities and adjusts his or her own language to match, do not exhibit lower receptive vocabulary abilities (Prime, Pauker, Plamondon, Perlman, & Jenkins, 2014). Findings indicate that older siblings who are sensitive to the cognitive needs of their younger siblings provide a rich environment for language development. This, in turn, moderates the negative impact of having several siblings on one's language development.

Effects of Gender

Recall from Chapter 6 that boys and girls differ in terms of their language development in toddlerhood. The results of longitudinal studies confirm that differences between girls and boys remain stable through the preschool years. Bornstein, Hahn, and Haynes (2004) hypothesized that several issues account for gender differences in language development, including maturation rates, neurological development, interests, opportunities to learn because of gender role stereotypes, and boys' and girls' role models for their language (i.e., girls usually model their language on that of their mothers, who are typically more verbal than fathers).

Gender differences in language can be identified for the areas of form, content, and use, although differences in language use (or the domain of pragmatics) are probably the easiest to spot when observing preschool-age boys and girls together. As one example, Nohara (1996) found that although preschool-age boys and girls use the word *no* with similar overall frequency, they tend to use it in different ways. For example, boys tend to use *no* more often than girls to correct or prohibit the behavior of their playmates ("No! I was playing with that truck"). In another study, researchers found that preschool-age boys and girls differ in the types of stories they narrate. Libby and Aries (2006) found that when given story prompts to complete, 3- to 5-year-old girls included greater numbers of friendly, assistance-providing characters and talked more about responding to the needs of others, whereas boys included more aggressive behavior and more attempts to resolve situations by using such behavior. Girls also tended to tell more stories about girls, whereas boys tended to tell more stories about boys.

The work of Bornstein et al. (2004) suggests that both nature and nurture play a role in the relation between gender and language development. What remains

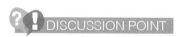

DISCUSSION POINT

In what ways does the contribution of gender to language development support both positions in the nature–nurture debate?

Boys and girls tend to differ from one another in their language development throughout the preschool-age years.

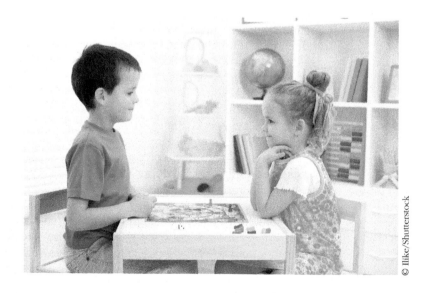

© Ilike/Shutterstock

7.3
Check Your Understanding
Click here to gauge your understanding of the concepts in this section.

unclear is whether gender differences in language (and in other areas) have implications for education, such as whether children benefit from attending single-sex schools or single-sex classes. Organizations such as the National Association for Single Sex Public Education (http://www.singlesexschools.org/) strongly support this idea, whereas other organizations (e.g., U.S. Department of Education, 2005) report limited support for the idea, citing neither benefit nor harm in implementing same-sex schooling.

HOW DO RESEARCHERS AND CLINICIANS MEASURE LANGUAGE DEVELOPMENT IN THE PRESCHOOL PERIOD?

Researchers

Language Sample Analysis

One method researchers continue to use throughout the preschool years to study children's language achievements is language sample analysis. Although the general premise is the same as in toddlerhood, researchers investigating preschoolers' language development have a wider range of analysis tools at their disposal and, more important, a larger amount of language to analyze. Researchers who measure preschoolers' language development can analyze children's language form, content, and use in many ways. Some common measures of semantics include total number of words (TNW), number of different words (NDW), and type–token ratio (TTR, computed by dividing NDW/TNW). Popular measures of syntax include mean length of utterance (MLU) and developmental sentence scoring (see Research Paradigms: *Developmental Sentence Scoring*). Researchers can also assess preschoolers' pragmatic abilities by coding language samples for the communicative functions the child uses—such as requesting, commenting, or responding to questions—and by coding for communication acts—such as repair strategies, interruptions, and false starts. See Table 7.2 for examples of measures applied to spontaneous language samples.

When collecting a language sample from a child, researchers must follow some general rules to obtain the most representative sample possible. Language samples should be representative in terms of both their reliability and their validity. *Reliable* language samples are similar across multiple recording contexts for the same child. *Valid* language samples accurately represent the quantity and quality of language a child can produce.

J. Miller and Chapman (2000) recommend the researcher or examiner collecting a language sample try to establish rapport with the child as soon as the session

RESEARCH **PARADIGMS**

Developmental Sentence Scoring

Developmental sentence scoring (DSS) is a tool researchers can apply to language samples to quantify children's expressive syntax development (Lee, 1974). DSS involves examining structures from eight grammatical categories and assigning points to each category, on a scale from 1 point for the simplest developmental form to 8 points for the most complex developmental form. DSS assesses the following categories: indefinite pronouns, personal pronouns, main verbs, secondary verbs, negatives, conjunctions, interrogative reversals, and *wh-* questions. A sentence may also receive an additional point if it is syntactically and semantically adultlike. For example, if a child said, "He ate the cookie," the child would receive 1 point for personal pronoun use (*he*), 1 point for primary verb use (*ate*), and 1 point for a syntactically and semantically adultlike sentence. To determine the developmental sentence score, the researcher calculates the average number of points for each utterance. Norm references are available for DSS, so some researchers may want to compare children's scores before and after a particular language intervention.

TABLE 7.2

Measures applied to spontaneous language samples

MEASURE	GENERAL GOAL	SPECIFIC GOAL	CALCULATION
Mean length of utterance (MLU) in morphemes	To measure syntactic complexity	To measure the average length of utterances in morphemes	Total number of morphemes/ total number of utterances
Percentage of complex sentences	To measure syntactic complexity in later stages of syntactic development	To determine the percentage of sentences in a sample containing more than one clause	Number of complex sentences/number of complete sentences
Total number of words (TNW)	To measure lexical productivity	To determine the total number of words in a sample	Raw frequency of number of main-body words
Number of different words (NDW)	To measure lexical diversity	To determine the number of different words in a sample	Raw frequency of different main-body word roots (e.g., *girl* and *girls* would be counted only once)
Type–token ratio (TTR)	To measure lexical diversity	To determine the ratio of different words to the total number of words in a sample	NDW/TNW
Conjunction use	To measure syntactic complexity and the ability to organize discourse	To determine the number of coordinating conjunctions (e.g., *and, or, but, so*) and subordinating conjunctions (e.g., *because, still, although*) in a sample	Raw frequency of conjunctions in a sample *or* Percentage of utterances containing conjunctions
Percentage of responses to questions	To measure discourse abilities	To determine the percentage of questions responded to in a sample	Number of responses immediately following a question/ number of questions from another speaker
Percentage of intelligible utterances	To measure intelligibility (i.e., phonological abilities)	To determine the percentage of complete utterances that are intelligible	Number of complete and intelligible utterances/ number of complete utterances
Number of mazes (language disruptions)	To measure fluency	To measure false starts, filled pauses (e.g., *um, uh*), repetitions, and reformulations	Raw frequency of mazes in a sample *or* Percentage of utterances containing mazes

begins by introducing himself or herself and describing his or her job. They also recommend introducing the recording equipment to the child and explaining what they will discuss during the recording session (e.g., "We're going to talk about your family and the kinds of things you like to do"). Once the researcher establishes rapport with the child, introduces the recording equipment, and describes the purpose of the session to the child, the researcher should begin obtaining the language sample, using the following three strategies to establish shared interests with the child (J. Miller & Chapman, 2000):

1. For children who are particularly reticent or who appear to be self-conscious about their speech, try not to say anything beyond the initial greetings for the first 5 min.

2. Engage in parallel play by directing talk to the toys rather than to the child (e.g., "These cookies look delicious!").

3. Engage in interactive play but ensure that the activity does not preclude talking. Encourage discussion once the activity is underway.

Once the interaction begins, the researcher can use the following six strategies to maintain a productive interaction (J. Miller & Chapman, 2000):

1. Be enthusiastic by using eye contact, vocal inflection, and by smiling.

2. Be patient by allowing the child plenty of time to initiate conversation and to respond to your questions and directions.

3. Listen and follow the child's lead by encouraging the child to elaborate on his or her ideas, by adding new information when appropriate, and by maintaining the child's pace.

4. Demonstrate that you value the child's communication efforts by giving the child your undivided attention, maintaining eye contact, and nodding to indicate agreement and interest.

5. Treat the conversation as if it were a genuine adult conversation by refraining from asking questions with obvious answers.

6. Keep the child's perspective in mind and adapt your language to the child's needs—for example, by shortening the length of utterances, simplifying vocabulary, and reducing sentence complexity.

Grammaticality Judgment Tasks

Researchers can use grammaticality judgment tasks to investigate various kinds of syntactic development in the preschool period. Grammaticality judgment tasks are metalinguistic in the sense that they require children to think about language and make judgments about the appropriateness of specific forms or interpret sentences. There are two types of grammaticality judgment tasks: well-formedness judgments and judgments about interpretation (McDaniel & Smith Cairns, 1998). To make a *well-formedness judgment*, the child must decide whether a sentence is syntactically acceptable. For example, Sentence A, which follows, would be syntactically acceptable, but Sentence B would not:

A. "What is your favorite movie?"

B. "What your favorite movie is?"

In the case of Sentences A and B, the researcher would ask the child whether each sentence is appropriate by saying, "Does this sentence sound good or bad?"

Judgments about interpretation are different. To make a judgment about interpretation, the child must interpret one or more parts of a sentence; for example, he or she might have to determine pronoun reference. In Sentence A, which follows, the child would need to indicate that *herself* refers to the baby, and in Sentence B, that *her* refers to someone other than the mother:

A. "The baby is feeding *herself*."

B. "The mother is feeding *her*."

The researcher could introduce props or pictures to facilitate this interpretation task. In Sentence A, the researcher could say, "We have a baby and a mother here, and the baby is eating. Would it be okay to say the baby is feeding *herself*?" In this case, a child who understands the pronoun *herself* refers to the baby would say, "Yes." In Sentence B, the researcher might say, "Now the mother is eating. Would it be okay to say the mother is feeding *her*?" In this case, a child who understands the pronoun *her* refers to someone other than the mother would say, "No."

Because preschoolers may not be accustomed to metalinguistic tasks such as the grammaticality judgment task, the researcher must introduce the task and be certain the child understands it and has had sufficient practice with it before proceeding (McDaniel & Smith Cairns, 1998). For example, the researcher should tell the child they will be thinking about language together, and explain that the child's job is to listen for things that "sound funny." After providing examples, the researcher should introduce some practice items about which a preschooler can reasonably be expected to make grammaticality judgments (e.g., number: "That boy *are* running"). Only after the researcher establishes that the child understands the task, by attending to language form rather than language content, should the researcher proceed to the target items.

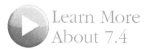

Learn More About 7.4

The video titled "Measuring Preschoolers' Print Awareness" features a 4-year-old child participating in a study using the Eye-gaze Response Interface Computer Aid (ERICA) in Dr. Laura Justice's former research lab, the Preschool Language and Literacy Lab at the University of Virginia.

Learn More About 7.4 *(Continued)*

ERICA is a computer system developed by engineers at the University of Virginia that tracks an individual's eye movement. In this video, the experimenter reads a book to the child as she tracks the print with her finger. As the experimenter reads, she ensures that an image of the child's pupil is visible on the monitor just to the right of the storybook presentation. The purpose of the study is to determine the extent to which 4-year-old children attend to print when engaged in shared storybook reading. The study tests four different conditions of reading to determine if any are associated with greater visual attention to print by the children. In the first condition, the experimenter reads the text without any comments or questions. In the second condition, the experimenter reads the text and additionally asks questions and makes comments about pictures. In the third condition, the experimenter reads the text and additionally asks questions and makes comments about print. In the fourth condition, the experimenter reads the text verbatim but tracks the print when reading.

After the storybook reading session is complete, the computer indicates where the child was looking during the session, and also provides information concerning the order and length of her visual fixations. The computer additionally calculates the amount of time children spent in "print zones" and "non-print zones" on the page. These data will be used to estimate the amount of time children spent looking at regions of print (i.e., print zones) during the different storybook reading conditions.

Researchers and clinicians can use props, such as photo albums, to elicit language samples from preschoolers.

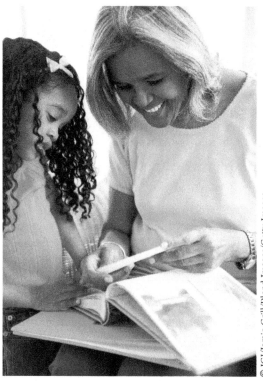

© JGI/Jamie Grill/Blend Images/Getty Images

Clinicians

Preschoolers, who better understand and produce language than their toddler and infant counterparts, can participate in considerably more assessments to directly measure many oral language components and emergent literacy skills. As is true in toddlerhood, screenings, comprehensive evaluations, and progress monitoring tools are popular ways to measure children's language and emergent literacy abilities. Clinicians can use screening measures in educational settings to determine which children might be at risk for difficulties with language and emergent literacy development, for example. Clinicians can also use comprehensive evaluations to gain a deeper understanding of children's language abilities and possibly make a formal diagnosis of a speech or language problem if they suspect a child may be lagging behind his or her peers in particular areas. Finally, clinicians may use progress monitoring tools to chart students' progress across a period of time and may also use these tools to adjust instruction to meet the language and early literacy needs of the children.

Next, we provide descriptions of several language and emergent literacy assessments that clinicians (and sometimes early childhood educators) may use to measure English-speaking preschoolers' language and early literacy achievements. We end with a brief discussion of assessment of children who are bilingual.

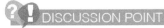

DISCUSSION POINT

In the previous section, we described some strategies for obtaining a representative language sample. What are some repercussions of *not* using these strategies? How might a language sample be affected?

Screening

In Chapter 6, we described screening measures as those a clinician would use to determine whether a child is experiencing difficulty with particular aspects of language, and to determine whether a child might need a more comprehensive language evaluation. For preschool-age children, clinicians are also concerned with screening children's emergent literacy abilities. One example of a screening measure for language abilities is the Expressive Vocabulary Test—Second Edition (EVT-2; Williams, 2007). The EVT-2 can screen for difficulties with expressive language and word retrieval. It is particularly useful for screening preschoolers' knowledge of high-frequency words, such as body parts, common household objects, foods, colors, and numbers. In addition to being appropriate for preschool-age children, the EVT-2 is normed for use with children as young as 2 1/2 years of age and adults through age 90. To administer it, the clinician shows the child a picture and reads a question aloud (e.g., "What do you call this?"). The child must respond with a single word that provides an appropriate label or synonym for the picture or that answers a question about the picture. The EVT takes approximately 10 min to administer and has been reported to be a culturally fair test of expressive vocabulary (e.g., Thomas-Tate, Washington, Craig, & Packard, 2006).

An example of a screening measure for emergent literacy is the Phonological Awareness Literacy Screening—PreK (PALS–PreK; Invernizzi, Sullivan, Meier, & Swank, 2004). Early childhood educators can use the PALS–PreK to identify children's strengths and weaknesses in early literacy to plan instruction for the school year. The PALS–PreK measures children's knowledge of phonological awareness and print knowledge in six subtests: Name Writing, Alphabet Recognition and Letter Sounds, Beginning Sound Awareness, Print and Word Awareness, Rhyme Awareness, and Knowledge of Nursery Rhymes.

Comprehensive Evaluation

As we described in Chapter 6, clinicians may use a comprehensive evaluation to determine whether a child has a language disorder and, if so, to learn more about the nature of the disorder. Clinicians also complete comprehensive evaluations of preschoolers' emergent literacy skills. One popular comprehensive evaluation tool for language development is the Preschool Language Scale—Fifth Edition (PLS–5; Zimmerman, Steiner, & Pond, 2011). The PLS–5 is a norm-referenced, play-based measure of vocabulary, grammar, morphology, and language reasoning that contains two scales. The Auditory Comprehension scale measures children's language comprehension abilities, including receptive vocabulary, comprehension of concepts and grammatical markers, and the ability to make comparisons and inferences. The Expressive Communication scale measures children's language production abilities, including using expressive vocabulary, using grammatical markers, segmenting words, completing analogies, and telling a story in its proper sequence. The PLS-5 is normed for use in children from birth through age 7 years, 11 months. As compared to its predecessor (the PLS-4), the PLS-5 includes items that assess preschoolers' emergent literacy skills, such as letter naming and book handling, as well as items that measure theory of mind.

A popular comprehensive assessment of emergent literacy abilities is the Test of Early Reading Ability—Third Edition (TERA–3; Reid, Hresko, & Hammill, 2002). The TERA–3 is a norm-referenced measure of children's mastery of early developing reading skills. Its three subtests include Alphabet Knowledge (measures children's knowledge of the alphabet and its uses), Conventions (measures knowledge of print conventions), and Meaning (measures children's ability to construct meaning from print). The three subtests combine to form an overall reading quotient.

Progress Monitoring

As we described in Chapter 6, progress monitoring tools measure and monitor a child's progress in a certain area of language development. Again, in preschool, clinicians can also monitor children's progress in emergent literacy abilities. One example of a progress monitoring measure for language abilities is the Oral and Written Language Scales, Second Edition (OWLS-II; Carrow-Woolfolk, 2011). The OWLS-II measures both expressive and receptive language skills of children and young adults between 3 and 21 years of age. Clinicians can use the OWLS-II to provide a record of students' language growth across a school year. Because the OWLS-II is a norm-referenced assessment, clinicians can compare children's performance on this measure to that of their same-age peers. The OWLS-II includes four scales: the Listening Comprehension scale, which measures receptive vocabulary; the Oral Expression scale, which measures expressive vocabulary; the Reading Comprehension scale, which measures reading and comprehending written language; and the Written Expression scale, which measures written language expression. Each of the four scales assesses four linguistic structures: lexical/semantics, syntax, pragmatics, and supralinguistics (such as figurative language, inference, and double meaning).

An example of a progress monitoring assessment of emergent literacy skills is the Test of Preschool Early Literacy (TOPEL; Lonigan, Wagner, Torgesen, & Rashotte, 2007). The TOPEL includes three subtests that combine to form a composite score representing the child's emergent literacy skills. The first subtest is the Print Knowledge subtest. This subtest measures a child's alphabet knowledge and early knowledge about written language conventions and form. To assess these areas, the clinician asks the child to identify or name certain letters, identify letters associated with specific sounds (e.g., /b/ is associated with the letter *B*), and say the sounds that correspond to specific letters (e.g., the letter *T* makes the /t/ sound). The second subtest is the Definitional Vocabulary subtest. This subtest measures a child's vocabulary, including the ability to define words. To administer it, the clinician shows the child a picture and asks him or her to say what the picture is and to describe one of its important features. The third subtest is the Phonological Awareness subtest. This subtest measures preschoolers' elision and blending abilities. To measure elision, the clinician asks the child to say a word (e.g., *boat*) and then to say what remains

DISCUSSION POINT

What types of information about a child's language might be gathered from an interview that could not be obtained from standardized assessments or language samples?

7.4

Check Your Understanding

Click here to gauge your understanding of the concepts in this section.

after removing a specific sound (e.g., "What word do we have if we take the /b/ from *boat*?"; answer = *oat*). To measure blending, the clinician asks the child to listen to separate sounds (e.g., /p/ /ɪ/ /n/) and then to combine them to make a word (answer = *pin*). In addition to monitoring students' progress throughout the year, clinicians can use the TOPEL for identification purposes (to document their abilities in print, oral vocabulary, and phonological awareness) and for research purposes.

Formal Assessment of Bilingual Children

Assessing the language and early literacy skills of children who are bilingual presents a unique challenge, and in most cases, norm-referenced measures developed for English-speaking children may not paint an accurate picture of bilingual children's competencies. See Language Diversity and Differences: *Informal Interviews with Caregivers and Teachers* for an alternative to formal assessment of bilingual children.

LANGUAGE DIVERSITY AND DIFFERENCES

Informal Interviews with Caregivers and Teachers

An alternative way to assess children's language abilities is to use structured interviews with parents, caregivers, or teachers (Gutiérrez-Clellen, Restrepo, Bedore, Peña, & Anderson, 2000). These persons, who know the children well, can provide valuable information on their English proficiency. The person conducting the interview should inquire about the length of time the child has been speaking his or her native language, the length of time the child has been speaking English, the context in which the child acquired English, and the relative proficiency in both languages across situations. Parent interviews are also useful for determining whether language performance is related to patterns of language loss by comparing the child's language development and loss to that of siblings or other family members. The interviewer can then explain the child's performance in each language in terms of the child's prior learning experience and language history.

SUMMARY

This chapter begins with a discussion of the major language milestones preschoolers achieve, including the use of decontextualized language, developments in theory of mind, and important emergent literacy skills such as alphabet knowledge, print knowledge, and phonological awareness. In the next section of this chapter, we discuss preschoolers' achievements in language form, content, and use. Preschoolers' achievements in language form include additions to their speech sound repertoires and suppression of several phonological processes that began in toddlerhood. Preschoolers also acquire new grammatical and derivational morphology and new sentence forms. Preschoolers' achievements in language content include fast mapping and slow mapping as a means

of acquiring new words, using knowledge of semantics and syntax to acquire new words, learning new words through shared storybook reading, and acquiring new and more complex language content, including various types of relational terms, such as deictic terms, interrogatives, temporal terms, opposites, locational prepositions, and kinship terms. Preschoolers' achievements in language use include new discourse functions, improved conversational skills, and narrative skills.

We then describe some of the intraindividual and interindividual differences in preschoolers' language development, including different types of language and early literacy profiles, as well as language differences related to one's SES, peers and siblings, and gender. Finally, we describe some ways researchers and clinicians measure preschoolers' language development. Some methods researchers use include language sample analysis and grammaticality judgment tasks. Clinicians may use screening, comprehensive evaluation, and progress monitoring.

Apply Your Knowledge

Click here to apply your knowledge to practical scenarios.

BEYOND THE BOOK

1. Recall from our discussion in Chapter 5 that although young children tend to comprehend certain language forms before they produce them, understanding language is still a challenging task. What are some of the specific semantic and syntactic abilities preschoolers must use to understand the differences between the following three sentences: (a) "Find Dax," (b) "Find the dax," and (c) "Find the dax one"?

2. Search the Web to find some strategies for promoting preschoolers' alphabet knowledge, print knowledge, and phonological awareness while reading books to them. Report back to the class on what you found and discuss any ways in which you might modify the suggested practices and why.

3. Find a wordless storybook and have a preschool-age child tell you a story using the pictures in the book. Make note of the child's narrative abilities, such as whether he or she includes a clear beginning, middle, and end to the story, whether he or she uses causal or temporal sequences, and any use of decontextualized language.

4. Observe a group of preschool-age children and identify any phonological processes you hear. In addition to noting the phonological processes, note the specific words the preschoolers use as they produce the phonological processes. Do you notice any patterns with regard to the length or phonological complexity of the words?

5. Collect a language sample (approximately 5 min long) from a preschooler or download a sample from the CHILDES Web site (http://childes.psy.cmu.edu/) and use at least three of the measures in Table 7.2 to analyze the sample.

Check Your Understanding

Gauge your understanding of the chapter concepts by taking this self-check quiz.

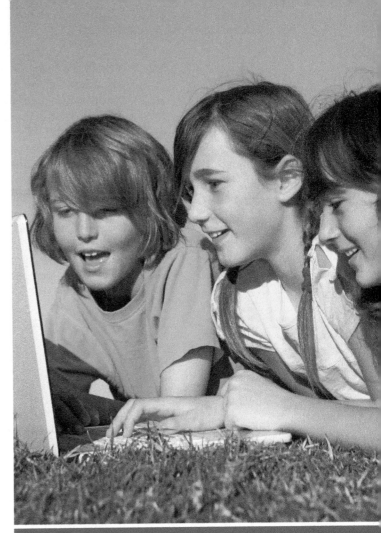

8

School-Age Years and Beyond

Developing Later Language

LEARNING OUTCOMES

After completion of this chapter, the reader will be able to:

1. Identify major language-development milestones that occur in the school-age years and beyond.

2. Describe major achievements in language form, content, and use that characterize the school-age years and beyond.

3. Explain factors that contribute to school-age children's, adolescents', and adults' individual competencies in language.

4. Describe how researchers and clinicians measure language development in the school-age years and beyond.

Now that we have discussed language development in infancy, toddlerhood, and the preschool years, you may wonder what language and communication achievements remain for school-age children and adolescents to master. After all, by the time children leave preschool, they can pronounce almost all the sounds of their native language, they can create sentences that include complex clauses and phrase structures, and they can use language for a number of communicative functions. In actuality, substantial development and refinement of syntax, pragmatics, and semantics occurs throughout the school-age years and adolescence. In this chapter, we begin with an overview of some of the major language-development milestones school-age children and adolescents achieve. Then we discuss accomplishments in language form, content, and use that occur in the school-age years and beyond. We also explore factors that contribute to the language competencies of individual school-age children, adolescents, and adults. In the final section, we describe methods for measuring language development in the school-age years and beyond.

WHAT MAJOR LANGUAGE-DEVELOPMENT MILESTONES OCCUR IN THE SCHOOL-AGE YEARS AND BEYOND?

In infancy and toddlerhood, identifying language milestones is fairly straightforward. Researchers can note when children typically speak their first word or begin to combine words into short sentences. However, pinpointing language milestones in the school-age years and adolescence is not as simple. During these years, language development is more subtle than in early childhood. People do not usually notice the *products* of language development unless they know what to look for. Therefore, this section on major language-development milestones focuses on the *process* of language development in the school-age years and beyond. Two processes that differentiate school-age children from their younger counterparts are shifting sources of language input and the acquisition of metalinguistic competence.

Shifting Sources of Language Input

Before the school-age years, children's sole source of language input is oral. However, once children learn to read, they can acquire language input from text as well. Beginning at around age 8–10 years, children shift to gaining more and more of their language input from text. As a result of increased exposure to language through reading, children develop language in an increasingly individualized manner (Nippold, 1998). For example, a child who is interested in cars and reads books about cars will likely acquire a set of car-related vocabulary words, including *carburetor, transmission,* and *spark plugs.*

Reading not only helps build children's lexical knowledge, but also has a role in developing the phonological, semantic, and pragmatic aspects of oral language. Menyuk (1999) suggested that reading gives children opportunities to reflect on language because, unlike oral language, reading allows children to review and think about the written words that remain in front of them. Because oral language plays a crucial role in developing reading and writing abilities, and vice versa, oral language must develop both independently of reading and writing activities *and* in a symbiotic relationship with reading and writing development (Menyuk, 1999). This symbiotic relationship is evident in the classroom when you consider the reading and writing activities that take place, and the opportunities for oral language exchanges between students and teachers and between peers.

Being able to read requires the child's successful understanding of grapheme-to-phoneme (letter-to-sound) correspondence. Children's success in understanding this correspondence rests on how well they have established print and phonological awareness in the preschool period. (Recall from Chapter 7 that *print awareness* is the child's knowledge of print forms and functions, whereas *phonological awareness* is the child's sensitivity to the sound structure of language.) Children who enter school with skills in these areas are more likely to succeed at beginning reading (Chaney, 1998).

Between the preschool years and adulthood, children learning to read generally progress through a predictable series of qualitatively distinct developmental stages (Chall, 1996). Chall presented these stages in what she termed a "model" or "scheme" instead of a theory of reading development. She organized her scheme for understanding reading development in much the same way Piaget organized his theory of stages and his stages of cognitive development (Inhelder & Piaget, 1958; Piaget, 1970). The prereading stage, which spans the period from birth to the beginning of formal education, is witness to some of children's most critical developments, including oral language, print awareness, and phonological awareness. An abundance of research results demonstrate the importance of prereading achievements to later reading success (e.g., Burgess, Hecht, & Lonigan, 2002; Bus, Van Ijzendoorn, & Pellegrini, 1995; Oliver, Dale, & Plomin, 2005; Whitehurst & Lonigan, 1998). After the prereading stage, children progress through five stages that build on this early foundation (Chall, 1996):

1. *Initial reading, or decoding, stage:* Stage 1 covers the period of kindergarten through first grade, when children are about 5–7 years old. During this stage, children begin to decode (or sound out) words by associating letters with corresponding sounds in spoken words. During Stage 1, children usually move sequentially through three phases (Biemiller, 1970, cited in Chall, 1996). In the first phase, when children read, they make word substitution errors in which the substituted word is semantically and syntactically probable. For example, they might read the sentence, *The dog is growling* as *The dog is barking*, substituting the semantically and syntactically plausible word *barking* for a word they do not know (*growling*). In the second phase, when children read, they make word substitution errors in which the substituted word has a graphic resemblance to the original printed word. They might read the sentence, *The dog is growling* as *The dog is green*, substituting for the word *growling* a word that looks similar but does not make sense semantically. In the third phase, when reading, children make word substitution errors in which the substituted word has a graphic resemblance to the original printed word but is also semantically acceptable. For example, they might read the sentence, *The dog is growling* as *The dog is growing* or *The dog is going*, either of which involves substituting a semantically plausible and perceptually similar word. Children who are more proficient at reading move through these phases more quickly than do children who are less proficient.

2. *Confirmation, fluency, and ungluing from print:* Stage 2 covers the period of second to third grade, when children are about 7–8 years old. During this stage, children hone the decoding skills they learned in Stage 1 and experience confirmation as they become more confident in the reading skills they have gained. As children read familiar texts, they become particularly proficient with high-frequency words, and use the redundancies of language to gain fluency and speed in reading. *Fluency* refers to reading that is efficient, well paced, and free of errors. It improves as children practice reading with texts that are familiar to them and that closely match their reading abilities. *Ungluing from print* refers to the idea that as children become more confident and fluent in their reading abilities, their reading becomes more automatic. They can thus focus less on the print itself and begin to focus more on gaining meaning from the text—they become *unglued* from the print. To illustrate this process, imagine a young boy reading the sentence, *Kit's pants got lost at camp*. Before he experiences confirmation, fluency, and ungluing from print, the boy will likely sound out each individual word in the sentence in a slow and

LANGUAGE DIVERSITY AND DIFFERENCES

Reading to Learn

Students learning English as a second language may struggle not only with oral language but also with aspects of reading comprehension. However, there are a number of strategies educators can implement that draw on students' native language, social skills, and cognitive abilities to help them learn to read in English (Anderson & Roit, 1996). One strategy involves using culturally familiar informational texts in the classroom that provide a balance of familiar information and new information. A *culturally familiar text* contains content about animals, foods, events, activities, and

experiences that would be relevant to a student's culture. There are three main advantages to using culturally familiar informational texts. First, students can read about something that sparks their interest. Second, students can demonstrate their intelligence by sharing knowledge with their peers and by relating their personal experiences to the class. Third, and most important, using culturally familiar informational texts allows students to identify with text, react to text, and connect text to their prior knowledge.

deliberate manner. By the time he reaches the end of the sentence, because he has devoted so many resources to decoding, he might have forgotten some of the words in the sentence, ultimately losing the sentence's meaning. After he experiences confirmation, fluency, and ungluing from print, the same boy will likely read the example sentence quickly and efficiently, allowing him to devote most of his resources to comprehending the sentence. As children become more confident and fluent readers, and as they become unglued from the print in Stage 2, they gradually begin to transition from *learning to read* to *reading to learn.*

3. *Reading to learn the new—a first step:* Stage 3 lasts from grade 4 to grades 8 or 9, when children are about age 9–14 years. During Stage 3, children read to gain new information and are solidly reading to learn by the end of this stage. Chall suggested thinking about Stage 3 in two distinct phases. In the first phase, Stage 3A (grades 4–6, or ages 9–11 years), children develop the ability to read beyond egocentric purposes so that they can read about and learn conventional information about the world. By the end of Stage 3A, children can read works of typical adult length, but not at the adult level of reading difficulty. In Stage 3B (grades 7–8 or 9 and ages 12–14 years), children can read on a general adult level. Reading during Stage 3 helps expand children's vocabularies, build background and world knowledge, and develop strategic reading habits. See Language Diversity and Differences: *Reading to Learn* for an example of how to encourage children learning English as a second language to read to learn.

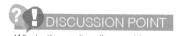

DISCUSSION POINT

What other culturally sensitive strategies could educators use to facilitate reading comprehension for children learning English as a second language?

4. *Multiple viewpoints—high school:* Stage 4 covers the high school period, between ages 14 and 18 years. During Stage 4, students learn to navigate increasingly difficult concepts and the texts that describe them. The most important difference between reading in Stage 3 and reading in Stage 4 is that in Stage 4, children can consider multiple viewpoints on an issue. Stage 4 necessarily builds on the knowledge in Stage 3, when children read to learn, because without the background knowledge from Stage 3, children would not be able to read more difficult texts with multiple sets of facts, theories, and viewpoints.

5. *Construction and reconstruction—a world view: college:* Stage 5 occurs from about age 18 on. During Stage 5, readers read selectively to suit their purposes. Reading selectively involves knowing which portions of a text to read—whether it be the beginning, middle, or end of the text or some combination thereof. Readers also make judgments about what to read, how much to read, and at what level of detail to achieve comprehension. Readers at Stage 5 use advanced cognitive

Between ages 9 and 14 years, children refine their reading abilities, enabling them to read text to learn new information. Most children are no longer learning to read but are reading to learn.

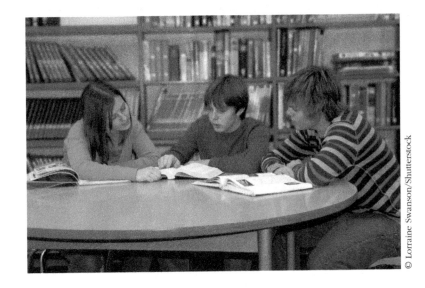

© Lorraine Swanson/Shutterstock

processes, such as analysis, synthesis, and prediction, to construct meaning from text. The following responses to the question, *Is what you just read true?* help illustrate the difference between Stage 5 reading and reading in Stages 3 and 4:

STAGE 3: Yes, I read it in a book. The author said it was true.

STAGE 4: I don't know. One of the authors I read said it was true; the other said it was not. I think there may be no true answers on the subject.

STAGE 5: There are different views on the matter. But one of the views seems to have the best evidence supporting it, and I would tend to go along with that view. (Chall, 1996, p. 58)

Acquisition of Metalinguistic Competence

Although children begin to acquire some metalinguistic competence—or the ability to think about and analyze language as an object of attention—in the preschool years, their competence increases significantly in the school-age years and beyond. One important reason children's metalinguistic abilities undergo dramatic growth in the school-age years is that many of the activities children engage in during these years draw on language analysis. For example, children in first-grade classrooms may have to identify the number of phonemes in a word, and children in seventh-grade classrooms may have to determine the meaning of an unfamiliar word by using their knowledge of the word's root. Some specific types of metalinguistic competence children achieve in the school-age years are phonological awareness and figurative language.

Phonological Awareness

In Chapter 7, we defined *phonological awareness* as children's sensitivity to the sound structure of language. Although children generally master some early-developing phonological awareness abilities in the preschool years (segmenting words from sentences, segmenting multisyllabic words, detecting and producing rhymes), they usually do not master some of the later-developing abilities until kindergarten or first grade. The later-developing abilities in phonological awareness involve awareness of the smallest units of sound (phonemes) and include blending sounds, segmenting sounds from words, and manipulating sounds (see, for example, Schuele & Boudreau, 2008). This level of phonological awareness is termed *phonemic awareness* to indicate the child must attend to the phonemes, or individual speech sounds in syllables and words.

The awareness of the distinct sounds in syllables and words usually develops by kindergarten or first grade (around age 5–6 years). Blending tasks might take the following form: "What word is /b/ /æ/ /t/?" "What word is /p/ /ɪ/ /n/?" The ability to blend sounds to make words supports a child's reading development, particularly his or her decoding skills. However, this relationship between phonemic awareness skills, such as blending, and reading development is bidirectional in that learning to read also improves a child's phonemic awareness.

The ability to segment sounds from words also develops by kindergarten or first grade. Segmentation tasks might involve asking the following questions: "What is the first sound in *car*?", "What is the last sound?", and "What are the three sounds in *cat*?" The ability to segment words into their onset-rime segments (/b/ /ot/ for *boat*; /k/ /ot/ for *coat*) and their individual phonemes (/b/ /o/ /t/; /k/ /o/ /t/) is related to children's awareness of spelling sequences in words and their reading development (Goswami & Mead, 1992). Children can use their knowledge of spelling patterns in words to help them read new words they encounter in texts. For example, if a child knows the spelling pattern of words such as *boat* and *coat*, he or she should be able to recruit this knowledge to infer how to pronounce the word *moat*.

Sound manipulation is the most complex phonological awareness ability and usually develops by second grade (at around age 7 years). A sound manipulation task might resemble the following: "Say *rate* without the /r/." "What word do you have if you switch the /p/ and /t/ sounds in *pat*?" Such tasks require children to intensively analyze and manipulate the sound structures of individual words. Phillips, Clancy-Menchetti, and Lonigan (2008) explain that nearly all of the phonological awareness intervention studies with evidence of efficacy have two key elements in common: (a) They have all been conducted with individual children or with small groups of children (rather than with large groups of children or with entire classrooms), and (b) many of the successful interventions have emphasized that teachers provide clear, explicit models of phonological awareness skills and support children's practice with the tasks. Conversely, Phillips and colleagues find no published studies indicating a positive effect of large-group, implicit phonological awareness activities, such as having a whole class clap the syllables in words together or simply sing rhyming songs. These researchers thus suggest that practitioners who would like to implement phonological awareness activities supported by scientific research consider the evidence base from research pertaining to small-group or individual, systematic, and explicit instruction in phonological awareness skills. For example, Carson, Gillon, and Boustead (2013) detected gains for 5-year-olds with and without specific language impairment in the areas of phonological awareness, spelling, and reading abilities, following an intensive intervention provided for 30 minutes per day for 10 weeks.

Figurative Language

Language that people use in nonliteral and often abstract ways is called **figurative language**. Using figurative language is a metalinguistic ability because children must recognize language as an arbitrary code (Westby, 1998). People use figurative language to evoke mental images in the minds of their listeners, or to provide emphasis or highlight something in an interesting way. Figurative language includes metaphors, similes, hyperboles, idioms, irony, and proverbs.

Metaphors. A metaphor conveys similarity between two ideas or objects by stating that those two ideas or objects are the same (see Figure 8.1 for an example). Metaphors consist of a term called the *topic* or the *target*, which is compared to another term called the *vehicle* or the *base*. The topic (target) and the vehicle (base) share features, and form the basis of comparison called the *ground*. Metaphors can be of at least two types: predictive and proportional (Table 8.1). We use metaphors often in our everyday conversations and using metaphors seems to help us communicate about and reason with abstract concepts, such as time and emotion (Bowdle &

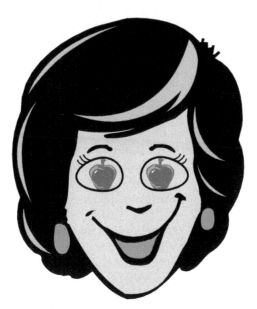

FIGURE 8.1

Literal interpretation of the metaphor *the apple of my eye.*

Gentner, 2005). Children begin to understand metaphors in the preschool years, and their comprehension improves throughout the school-age years and into adulthood as their ability to use figurative language increases. Recall that in Chapter 5, we introduced the terms *basic-level category*, *superordinate-level category*, and *subordinate-level category*. Some research indicates that similar to children's first words, children understand basic-level metaphors (e.g., *the girl in the pool is a fish*) before they understand subordinate-level metaphors (e.g., *the girl in the pool is a dolphin*; Purser, Thomas, Snoxall, & Mareschal, 2009). This research suggests that in order for children to understand more complex subordinate-level metaphors, they must first have a strong grasp of the very specific concepts subordinate-level words express. So, to understand the metaphor, *the girl in the pool is a dolphin*, the child would need to recognize the specific attributes of dolphins that make them different from other fishlike creatures (e.g., they swim gracefully, can do flips and other tricks in the water, and need to surface periodically for air).

TABLE 8.1

Types of metaphors

TYPE	DEFINITION	EXAMPLE	EXPLANATION
Predictive	Contains one topic and one vehicle	*All the world's a stage.*	*World* is the topic and *stage* is the vehicle.
Proportional	Contains two topics and two vehicles and expresses an analogical relationship	*The artist was an apple tree with no fruit* (Nippold, 1998, p. 89).	The analogy is "apple tree is to fruit as artist is to artwork." The topics are artist and artwork (implied from the analogy) and the vehicles are apple tree and fruit.

Source: Information from *Later Language Development: School-Age Children, Adolescents, and Young Adults,* 3rd ed. (p. 159), by M. A. Nippold, 2007, Austin, TX: PRO-ED. Copyright 2007 by PRO-ED, Inc.

Similes.   Similes are similar to predictive metaphors in that they contain a topic, a vehicle, and the ground. They are different in that they make the comparison between the topic and vehicle explicit by using the word *like* or *as*. Common similes using *like* include *like water off a duck's back* and *sitting like a bump on a log.* Common similes using *as* include *quiet as a mouse* and *flat as a pancake.* Nippold (1998) summarized research results indicating that the extent to which children use similes (and metaphors) relates to situational factors, including whether the children are engaging in a formal writing task or comparing dissimilar objects. Children's ability to understand and produce similes and metaphors is related to their performance on measures of general cognition, language, and academic achievement. However, whether these abilities are prerequisites to understanding and producing metaphors and similes is unclear.

Hyperboles.   Hyperbole is a form of figurative language that uses exaggeration for emphasis or effect. Examples of hyperbole include *I'm so hungry, I could eat a horse,* and *I nearly died laughing.* Research examining children's understanding of hyperbole (and other forms of figurative language) is somewhat inconclusive. For example, Creusere (1999) summarized research results showing that salient intonation patterns may help 8- and 10-year-olds' comprehension of hyperbole, or children may make use of the discrepancy between the literal and intended meanings of an utterance to determine the speaker's intent. In the first case, to understand the hyperbole, children would exploit paralinguistic cues (intonation patterns), whereas in the second case they would exploit pragmatic cues.

Idioms.   Idioms are expressions containing both a literal and a figurative meaning. *I've put that on the back burner,* and *We're in the same boat* are examples of idioms. Illustrations of two common idioms appear in Figure 8.2. People use two major types of idioms: opaque and transparent (Gibbs, 1987, cited in Nippold, 1998). *Opaque idioms* demonstrate little relationship between the literal interpretation and the figurative interpretation (e.g., *drive someone up the wall*), whereas the figurative meaning of a transparent idiom is an extension of the literal meaning (e.g., *hold one's tongue*). Gibbs's study showed that children ages 5, 6, 8, and 9 years could

DISCUSSION POINT

Do you think school-age children use hyperbole more than other types of figurative language? Why or why not?

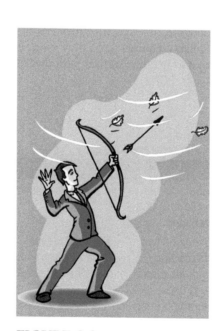
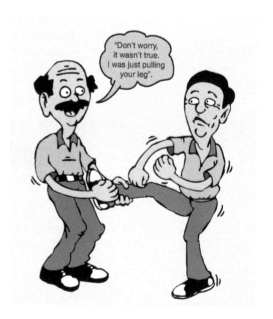

FIGURE 8.2

Literal interpretations of the idioms (A) *shoot the breeze* and (B) *pull someone's leg.*

TABLE 8.2

Mean idiom familiarity and transparency ratings for adolescents and adults

	FAMILIARITY		TRANSPARENCY	
IDIOM	ADOLESCENTS	ADULTS	ADOLESCENTS	ADULTS
Go through the motions	2.35	1.70	1.90	1.65
Skating on thin ice	1.30	1.30	1.35	1.55
Take down a peg	4.30	3.30	2.60	2.70
Vote with one's feet	4.55	4.35	2.65	2.80

Familiarity measures how often a person reported hearing or reading the idiom before: 1 = many times, 2 = several times, 3 = a few times, 4 = once, 5 = never. *Transparency* measures reports of how closely the literal and nonliteral meanings of the idiom compare: 1 = closely related, 2 = somewhat related, 3 = not related.

Source: Information from *Later Language Development: School-Age Children, Adolescents, and Young Adults,* 3rd ed. (pp. 204–207), by M. A. Nippold, 2007, Austin, TX: PRO-ED. Copyright 2007 by PRO-ED, Inc.

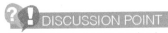

DISCUSSION POINT

How might you assess a school-age child's understanding of idioms?

explain transparent idioms more easily than opaque idioms. Furthermore, children could interpret the meanings of idioms more correctly in multiple-choice tasks than in explanation tasks, and had more success interpreting idioms when they received contextually supportive information than when they did not. Children's ability to comprehend the text they read predicts their understanding of idioms presented in context (Levorato, Nesi, & Cacciari, 2004). In general, understanding of idioms improves throughout the school-age years and adolescence and into adulthood. Opaque and less frequently used idioms are the most difficult to understand. In Nippold's (1998) study, adolescents and adults rated how familiar they were with certain idioms and how transparent the idioms were. Table 8.2 provides a sample of their mean ratings.

Irony and Sarcasm. *Irony* and *sarcasm* are types of figurative language for which a speaker's intentions differ from the literal meaning of the words he or she uses. Although the terms *irony* and *sarcasm* both refer to unmet expectations, they differ according to whether the statement relates to an expectation about a specific individual or a general expectation (Glenwright & Pexman, 2010). More specifically, irony refers to unmet general expectations that are not the fault of an individual, whereas sarcasm refers to a specific individual's failure to meet an expectation. Consider the following two sentences (Glenwright & Pexman, 2010, p. 432):

1. On the way to the park, Tim comments to Jan that the weather is perfect for a picnic. As they unpack their food, it begins to rain. Jan comments, "What perfect weather for a picnic."

2. Tim and Jan walk to the park to have a picnic. As they unpack their food, it begins to rain. Jan comments, "What perfect weather for a picnic."

The first sentence is an example of sarcasm, because Jan is criticizing Tim's inaccurate weather forecast. By contrast, the second sentence is an example of verbal irony, because Jan is not criticizing Tim, or any individual in particular, when she speaks about how the bad weather does not meet the generally agreed-upon expectations for a picnic. In their study, Glenwright and Pexman found that although 5- to 6-year-olds are not yet able to distinguish between speakers' intentions when they use sarcasm versus irony, 9- to 10-year-olds are able to distinguish speakers' intentions, and they consider sarcastic comments to be more negative or "mean"

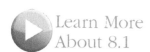

Learn More About 8.1

In the video titled "Adolescent Interpreting Proverbs", an examiner asks an adolescent to interpret a number of proverbs. Although she expresses uncertainty about the meaning of the proverbs, she provides reasonable interpretations for all of them. Proverbs are one of the most difficult types of figurative language to master.

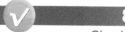

8.1

Check Your Understanding

Click here to gauge your understanding of the concepts in this section.

than ironic comments. Even though 5- to 6-year-olds cannot distinguish between sarcasm and irony, they are able to use specific cues to distinguish between a literal statement and a sarcastic statement. More specifically, 5- to 6-year-olds better understand the nonliteral meaning of sarcastic statements when there is a large reduction in the pitch of the speaker's voice as compared to the preceding sentence (Glenwright, Parackel, Cheung, & Nilsen, 2014).

In addition to verbal irony, which occurs when a speaker says one thing but means another, writers can also use dramatic irony. With *dramatic irony*, an audience is aware of facts of which characters are unaware. Shakespeare used both forms of irony in his plays. Some research results suggest people use both acoustic cues and contextual information to infer ironic intent in other persons' spontaneous speech (Bryant & Tree, 2002).

Research also suggests that school-age children's understanding of sarcasm and irony is related to their theory of mind (e.g., Peterson, Wellman, & Slaughter, 2012), which continues to develop well into adolescence (e.g., Bosco, Gabbatore, & Tirassa, 2014; Dumontheil, Apperly, & Blakemore, 2010).

Proverbs.   Proverbs are statements expressing the conventional values, beliefs, and wisdom of a society (Nippold, 1998). Nippold reported that of the types of figurative language, proverbs are one of the most difficult to master. Proverbs serve a variety of communicative functions, such as the following:

Commenting: *Blood is thicker than water.*

Interpreting: *His bark is worse than his bite.*

Advising: *Don't count your chickens before they hatch.*

Warning: *It's better to be safe than sorry.*

Encouraging: *Every cloud has a silver lining.*

Proverb understanding improves gradually during the adolescent years, and the presence of a supportive linguistic environment can facilitate adolescents' understanding of proverbs. The degree to which adolescents understand proverbs has been correlated with measures of academic success in literature and mathematics (Nippold, 2000), likely because proverb understanding requires that students be able to contend with abstract and metalinguistic aspects of language.

WHAT MAJOR ACHIEVEMENTS IN LANGUAGE FORM, CONTENT, AND USE CHARACTERIZE THE SCHOOL-AGE YEARS AND BEYOND?

As children mature to school age and into adolescence, they continue to make significant gains in language form, content, and use. In doing so, they increase—among other things—their receptive and expressive vocabularies, their ability to clarify language ambiguities, their use of decontextualized language, the number of functions for which they use language, their conversational skills, and their narrative abilities. We discuss such gains next. (See Developmental Timeline: School-Age Years for a summary of specific achievements.)

Language Form

As students move through the elementary grades into high school, their achievements in language form progress in a slow and subtle manner. Three notable areas of school-age development in language form are (a) phonological development, (b) morphological development, and (c) complex syntax development.

Phonological Development

A few developments in phonology remain to be achieved during the school-age years. Previously in this chapter, we described school-age children's accomplishments in phonological awareness, including their ability to segment syllables from multisyllabic words and their ability to blend and manipulate the sounds in words. In addition, children make progress in their morphophonemic development.

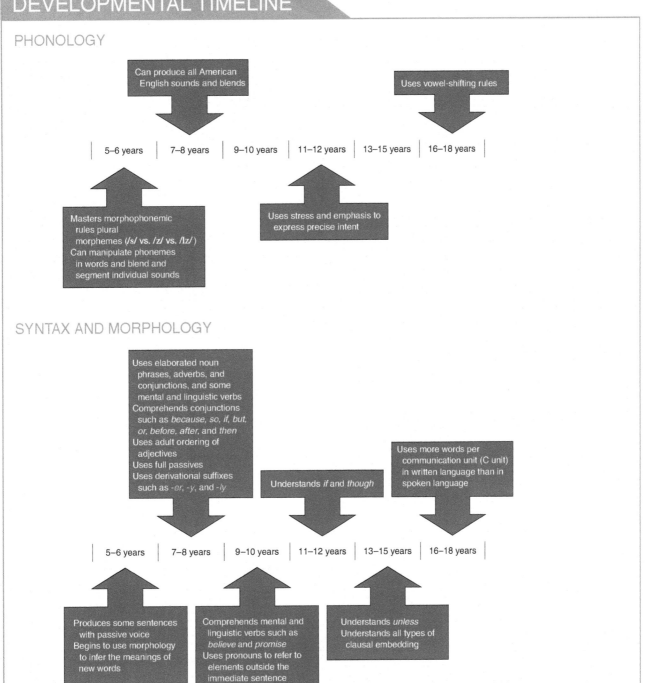

DEVELOPMENTAL TIMELINE

PHONOLOGY

Can produce all American English sounds and blends

Uses vowel-shifting rules

| 5–6 years | 7–8 years | 9–10 years | 11–12 years | 13–15 years | 16–18 years |

Masters morphophonemic rules plural morphemes (/s/ vs. /z/ vs. /ɪz/) Can manipulate phonemes in words and blend and segment individual sounds

Uses stress and emphasis to express precise intent

SYNTAX AND MORPHOLOGY

Uses elaborated noun phrases, adverbs, and conjunctions, and some mental and linguistic verbs
Comprehends conjunctions such as *because, so, if, but, or, before, after,* and *then*
Uses adult ordering of adjectives
Uses full passives
Uses derivational suffixes such as *-er, -y,* and *-ly*

Understands *if* and *though*

Uses more words per communication unit (C unit) in written language than in spoken language

| 5–6 years | 7–8 years | 9–10 years | 11–12 years | 13–15 years | 16–18 years |

Produces some sentences with passive voice
Begins to use morphology to infer the meanings of new words

Comprehends mental and linguistic verbs such as *believe* and *promise*
Uses pronouns to refer to elements outside the immediate sentence

Understands *unless*
Understands all types of clausal embedding

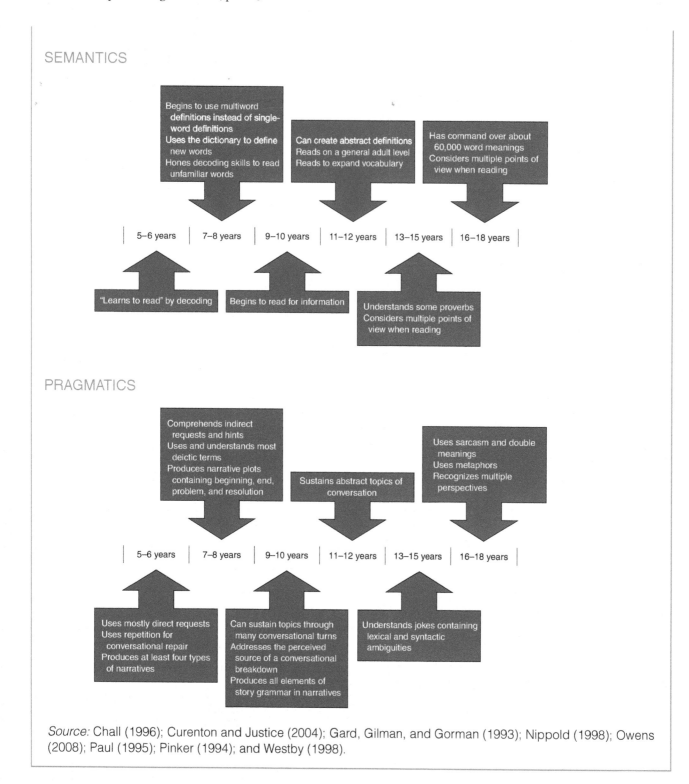

SEMANTICS

Begins to use multiword definitions instead of single-word definitions
Uses the dictionary to define new words
Hones decoding skills to read unfamiliar words

Can create abstract definitions
Reads on a general adult level
Reads to expand vocabulary

Has command over about 60,000 word meanings
Considers multiple points of view when reading

| 5–6 years | 7–8 years | 9–10 years | 11–12 years | 13–15 years | 16–18 years |

"Learns to read" by decoding

Begins to read for information

Understands some proverbs
Considers multiple points of view when reading

PRAGMATICS

Comprehends indirect requests and hints
Uses and understands most deictic terms
Produces narrative plots containing beginning, end, problem, and resolution

Sustains abstract topics of conversation

Uses sarcasm and double meanings
Uses metaphors
Recognizes multiple perspectives

| 5–6 years | 7–8 years | 9–10 years | 11–12 years | 13–15 years | 16–18 years |

Uses mostly direct requests
Uses repetition for conversational repair
Produces at least four types of narratives

Can sustain topics through many conversational turns
Addresses the perceived source of a conversational breakdown
Produces all elements of story grammar in narratives

Understands jokes containing lexical and syntactic ambiguities

Source: Chall (1996); Curenton and Justice (2004); Gard, Gilman, and Gorman (1993); Nippold (1998); Owens (2008); Paul (1995); Pinker (1994); and Westby (1998).

Morphophonemic development relates to development in the interaction between morphological and phonological processes. One type of morphophonemic development concerns the use of sound modifications we make when joining certain morphemes. For example, at around age 5 or 6 years, children correctly use the plural ending /ɪz/, as in *matches* and *watches*, which differs phonologically from sound modifications in other pluralized words (e.g., *hats, dogs*).

A second type of morphophonemic development involves vowel shifting, which occurs when the form class of a word (e.g., noun, verb, adjective) changes when adding a derivational suffix. Examples of vowel shifting include /aɪ/ to /ɪ/ (*decide–decision*), /eɪ/ to /æ/ (*sane–sanity*), and /i/ to /ɛ/ (*serene–serenity*). Most children do not master vowel shifting until about age 17 years (Owens, 2008). Finally, a third type of morphophonemic rule school-age children learn is how to use stress and emphasis to distinguish phrases from compound words (*hot dog* vs. *hotdog*, *green house* vs. *greenhouse*) and to distinguish nouns from verbs (*record* vs. *record*, *present* vs. *present*). Children usually master stress and emphasis by 12 years of age (Ingram, 1986, as cited in Owens, 2008).

Morphological Development

Children's morphological development is closely related to their syntactic development. Major morphological developments in the school-age years include use of derivational prefixes and derivational suffixes. When we add a *derivational prefix* to the beginning of a word, it changes the word's meaning. For example, when we add the derivational prefix *un-* to the word *healthy*, to make *unhealthy*, the meaning of the word changes to its negative counterpart. Other derivational prefixes include *dis-* (as in *disengage*), *non-* (as in *nonconformist*), and *ir-* (as in *irregular*).

Derivational suffixes include *-hood* (as in *childhood*), *-ment* (as in *excitement*), *-er* (as in *protester*), *-y* (as in *jealousy*), and *-ly* (as in *weekly*), among others. When we add a derivational suffix to the end of a word, it can change the word's form class, meaning, or both. For example, we can change the verb *encroach* to a noun by adding the derivational suffix *-ment* (*encroachment*). Some of the more difficult derivational suffixes include *-y* (to form adjectives such as *squishy* and *tasty*), which children acquire at around age 11 years, and *-ly* (to form adverbs such as *correctly* and *aptly*), which children learn in adolescence. Children's morphological awareness abilities are associated with other language and literacy skills, such as receptive vocabulary, word-level reading, and spelling (Apel & Masterson, 2001b; Apel &

THEORY TO PRACTICE

Morphological Awareness Interventions

Like phonological awareness, morphological awareness is associated with important areas of literacy development and is amenable to instruction. However, unlike phonological awareness, morphological knowledge continues to develop throughout the upper elementary years and beyond (Nagy, Carlisle, & Goodwin, 2013). For these reasons, morphological awareness has been the focus of a number of literacy interventions for students in the school-age years.

As one example, Wolter and Dilworth (2013) randomly assigned second-grade students with spelling difficulties to receive either an intervention featuring phonological and orthographic awareness (spelling) activities, or an intervention featuring phonological, orthographic, and morphological awareness activities. Results revealed that students receiving the combination with morphological awareness activities performed better on measures of spelling, reading

comprehension, and morphological patterns than their peers whose intervention addressed only phonological awareness and spelling.

As another example, McCutchen, Stull, Herrera, Lotas, and Evans (2013) found that fifth-grade students participating in a morphological awareness intervention using words drawn from their science curriculum and targeting writing outcomes, outperformed students in a control group. Specifically, students in the intervention condition included more morphologically complex words in a sentence combining task, and used more morphologically complex words from the intervention in their writing responses than students in the control group. Also, notably, students in the intervention with lower pretest scores had even greater gains in using morphologically complex words at posttest than students with higher pretest scores.

Thomas-Tate, 2009) and at least one feasibility study has demonstrated that it is both appropriate and beneficial to provide explicit instruction in inflectional and derivational morphology as early as kindergarten (Apel, Brimo, Diehm, & Apel, 2013).

See Theory to Practice: *Morphological Awareness Interventions* to learn more about how morphological awareness interventions can facilitate students' language and literacy abilities.

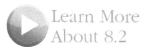

Learn More About 8.2

In the video titled "Complex Syntax Use in Narrative", a 7-year-old provides an account of how his parents adopted him from China.

Learn More About 8.2 *(Continued)*

He provides a clear beginning and end to the story, and even lets the listener know ahead of time that his story is about China. He demonstrates that he is beginning to use the passive voice construction ("when I was a baby, I had to be tooken to another person"), even though he overextends the past tense form of the word *take* to the passive form (i.e., *took-tooken*). Throughout the narrative account, this boy uses several adverbs of time, including *next*, *now*, and *then*. Just as is common with adults who are telling stories, this boy deviates during his narrative to talk about the size of girls' and boys' eyes in China. He then returns to his story to finish explaining how his parents had to complete paperwork in the United States and some additional paperwork in China in order to complete the adoption.

Complex Syntax Development

The most important achievements in form for school-age children involve complex syntax. *Complex syntax* refers to developmentally advanced grammatical structures that mark a "literate," or decontextualized, language style (Paul, 1995). These structures occur relatively infrequently in spoken language, but when students use them in written language, it indicates they have achieved more advanced levels of grammar. Examples of complex syntax include noun-phrase postmodification with past participles (*a dance called the waltz*), complex verb phrases using the perfective aspect (*Stephanie has arrived from Vancouver*), adverbial conjunctions (*only, consequently*), and passive voice construction (*The fish were caught by an experienced fisherman*). Children's development of complex syntax seems to be related to the complexity of their caregivers' syntax (Vasilyeva, Waterfall, & Huttenlocher, 2008).

Children rarely use complex syntactic forms, such as the passive voice, in conversation, so it can be difficult to witness their accomplishments with these forms. However, children do use complex syntax in their writing. Persuasive writing in particular is a vehicle for the expression of more complex syntax. The goal of *persuasive writing*, as the name suggests, is to adopt a particular point of view and convince the reader to adopt the same stance or to take action consistent with that point of view. Some examples of persuasive writing include letters to support the reelection of a political official, and e-mail messages to persuade colleagues to help with an important project. According to Nippold (2000), persuasive writing is a challenging communicative skill that students develop during the school-age period. It requires that children have an awareness of what other people believe and value, as well as the ability to present personal ideas in a logical sequence. Between childhood and adulthood, students incorporate an increasing amount and variety of complex language forms in their persuasive writing. With regard to complex syntax, in particular, increases are evident in students' use of relative clauses and their mean length of utterance in words (MLU-W; Nippold, Ward-Lonergan, & Fanning, 2005).

Another vehicle for measuring complex syntax development is narrative tasks, particularly those involving fables. Research indicates that adolescents participating in a narrative task that involves listening to fables and then retelling them exhibit greater syntactic complexity than when participating in a more traditional conversational task (Nippold, Frantz-Kaspar, Cramond, Kirk, Hayward-Mayhew, & MacKinnon, 2014). The researchers hypothesize that adolescents exhibit greater syntactic complexity during the narrative task because the fables themselves provide a model of highly sophisticated language, which might prime the adolescents to use complex language as well. Additionally, fables include complex story content, which might prompt adolescents to draw on their cognitive and linguistic resources more fully than when engaging in a conversation.

Language Content

The typical school-age child makes considerable gains in several language content areas. Most of these gains occur as a result of reading text, which provides students with access to words and concepts not typically the topic of everyday conversations. Gains in content during the school-age years also occur as a result of the classroom environment, where the topic of conversation is generally decontextualized. Four areas of notable content development for school-age students are (a) lexical development, (b) understanding of multiple meanings, (c) understanding of lexical and sentential ambiguity, and (d) development of literate language.

Lexical Development

School-age students' receptive and expressive vocabularies expand so much that upon graduation from high school, they have command over about 60,000 words (Pinker, 1994). According to Nippold (1998), school-age children learn new words in at least three ways: through direct instruction, contextual abstraction, and morphological analysis.

Direct Instruction.   *Direct instruction* involves learning the meaning of a word directly from a more knowledgeable source. This source may be another person or a reference such as a dictionary. A person learns new words throughout his or her life, either because the person asks for the definitions of words or because another person presupposes he or she should learn the definitions. For example, the first author (K.P.T.) learned the definition of the term *scut work* after requesting that her colleague, who had used it in a sentence, define the term. The colleague explained that his mother (who was in her mid-90s at the time) had always used the word to describe a tedious, monotonous, unrewarding task, so he assumed that others used it as well. Regarding learning words from other sources, children do not begin to use dictionaries to learn the meanings of words until about second grade (age 7 or 8 years). The first author remembers that during second-grade independent reading activities, whenever a student raised his or her hand to ask for the definition of a word, the teacher would always reply, "Use the dictionary to look it up." Students continue to use this method throughout middle school and high school.

Contextual Abstraction.   *Contextual abstraction* involves using context clues in both spoken and written forms of language to determine the meanings of unfamiliar words. In Chapter 7, we discussed the process by which children learn new words in context: Children form an initial representation of a word through *fast mapping*. After repeated exposure, children refine a word's representation through the process of *slow mapping*. School-age children, adolescents, and adults learn the meanings of words in the same way when they encounter unfamiliar words in context. When encountering new words in text, we make either pragmatic inferences or logical inferences about the meanings of the words (Westby, 1998). *Pragmatic inferences* about the meaning of a word bring an individual's personal world knowledge or background knowledge to the text. *Logical inferences* use only the information the text provides and are more difficult to make than pragmatic inferences. Westby explained

During the elementary grades, children begin to use dictionaries to learn the meanings of new words directly.

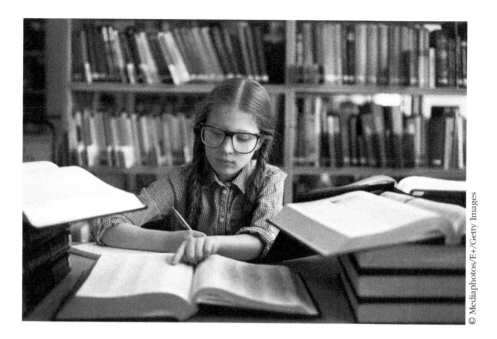

© Mediaphotos/E+/Getty Images

that people make pragmatic inferences more often when they are reading narrative texts (such as storybooks), and logical inferences when they are reading expository texts (such as textbooks). See Table 8.3 for examples of context clues readers can draw on to abstract the meanings of new words from a text.

Morphological Analysis. *Morphological analysis* involves analyzing the lexical, inflectional, and derivational morphemes of unfamiliar words to infer their meanings. For instance, a child who encounters the word *homophone* in a language arts textbook can use knowledge of the morphemes *homo-* (meaning "same") and *-phone* (meaning "sound") to make an educated guess about the meaning of the word. Although younger children (ages 6–10 years) become proficient at using morphemes to infer the meanings of new words, their older counterparts (ages 9–13 years) are proficient at using both morphological information and context clues to arrive at the meanings of unfamiliar words. Examples of morphemes with clear lexical meaning that older children (age 9 years and older) might use to decipher the meanings of unfamiliar words include the common prefixes *un-, re-, dis-, en-, em-, non-, over-, mis-, sub-, fore-, de-, trans-, super-, semi-, anti-, mid-,* and *under-,* as well as the "not" prefixes (*in-, im-, ir-, il-*; White, Sowell, & Yanagihara, 1989).

Understanding of Multiple Meanings

As the lexicons of school-age children grow and they encounter more and more words, they realize many words have multiple meanings. As students develop, they become able to provide multiple definitions for words with several similar meanings, but they have particular difficulty understanding the secondary meanings of words that bear little or no relation to the primary meaning. Being able to supply multiple meanings for words requires not only lexical knowledge but also metalinguistic knowledge, both of which are necessary to achieve full competence at the literate end of the oral–literate language continuum, which we discuss in the subsequent section entitled, "Development of Literate Language."

Understanding of Lexical and Sentential Ambiguity

Another notable area of achievement in language content for school-age children is the understanding of lexical and sentential ambiguity. Lexical ambiguity occurs for words and phrases with multiple meanings, such as *That was a real bear*, in which

TABLE 8.3

Examples of context clues for abstracting the meanings of words from text

SYNTACTIC CUES	EXAMPLE
Appositives	*Quinoa,* the seed of a leafy plant native to the Andes, is often mistaken for a grain because of its taste and appearance.
Relative clauses	The *Incas,* who were people indigenous to the Andean region, fed quinoa to their armies.
The conjunction *or*	The Incas were *indigenous,* or native, to the country of Ecuador.
Direct explanation	If you visit Ecuador, you can visit Incan ruins known as *Ingapirca.*
Linked synonyms	While driving through Ecuador, you will experience scenic views of the rolling, meandering, *undulating* countryside.
Participial phrases	The travelers, exhausted from a long day at the Otavalo market, vowed to practice their *bargaining* strategies.
Categorical sequence	Some of Ecuador's popular produce items include mangoes, pineapples, papayas, and *plantains.*
Restatement	Persons in some regions of Ecuador must be careful of *landslides.* They must guard against the downward sliding of earth and rock.
Illustrations or examples	The flag of Ecuador is *multicolored.* For example, it contains the colors yellow, blue, and red, among others.
Similes	The *thermal baths* in Ecuador are like outdoor hot tubs.
Metaphors	The Andes mountains are a colorful *tapestry.*
Personification	Clouds *scatter* rain over the region on some afternoons.
Summary	When traveling, be especially cautious in or avoid areas where you are likely to be *victimized.* These areas include crowded subways, train stations, elevators, tourist sites, marketplaces, festivals, and marginal areas of cities.
Cause and effect	Because the Galapagos Islands are so *isolated,* they are home to species of animals and plants not found anywhere else in the world.

Source: Information from *Later Language Development: School-Age Children, Adolescents, and Young Adults,* 3rd ed. (p. 31), by M. A. Nippold, 2007, Austin, TX: PRO-ED. Copyright 2007 by PRO-ED, Inc. Adapted with permission.

bear has several meanings. Lexical ambiguity at the level of the individual word may take one of three forms:

1. *Homophones:* Homophones are words that sound alike but have different meanings. Homophones may be spelled alike (*brown bear* vs. *bear weight*) or may be spelled differently (*brown bear* vs. *bare hands*), in which case they are called heterographs.

2. *Homographs:* Homographs are words that are spelled the same way but have different meanings. Homographs may sound alike (*row a boat* vs. *row of homes*)

or may sound different from each other (*record player* vs. *record a movie*), in which case they are called heteronyms or heterophones.

3. *Homonyms:* Homonyms are words that are alike in spelling and pronunciation but differ in meaning (*brown bear* vs. *bear weight*). They are both homophones and homographs.

Lexical ambiguity regularly fuels the humor in jokes, riddles, comic strips, newspaper headlines, bumper stickers, and advertisements, such as the joke, *Is your refrigerator running? ... You'd better go catch it!* (Nippold, 1998). When students encounter ambiguous words, they must first notice the ambiguity and then scrutinize the words to arrive at the appropriate meaning. Students with weak oral language skills are often not adept at noticing when lexical ambiguities are present and are less likely than other students to seek clarification of the ambiguity, both of which can result in a communication breakdown (Paul, 1995).

Sentential ambiguity involves ambiguity within different components of sentences. It includes not only lexical ambiguity but also phonological ambiguity, surface-structure ambiguity, and deep-structure ambiguity. Phonological ambiguity occurs with a sound sequence that carries more than one interpretation; it often occurs when a listener confuses the boundaries between words (*I can't wait for the weekend* vs. *I can't wait for the weak end*). Surface-structure ambiguity results when words within a sentence can be grouped in two different ways, with each grouping conveying a different interpretation (*I fed her bird seed* vs. *I fed her bird seed*), or as in the joke, "Can you tell me how long cows should be milked? They should be milked the same as short ones, of course" (Chapman & Foot, 1996, p. 13). With deep-structure ambiguity, a noun serves as the subject of a sentence in one interpretation and as an object in another (e.g., *The duck is ready to eat* can mean "The duck is hungry" or "The duck is ready to be eaten"; Nippold, 1998, p. 140), or the joke, "Did you know that natives like potatoes even more than missionaries? Yes, but the missionaries are more nutritious" (Chapman & Foot, 1996, p. 13).

Development of Literate Language

Recall that in Chapter 7, we described the difference between contextualized and decontextualized language. When children enter school, the language they hear and use becomes increasingly decontextualized, or removed from the here and now. *Literate language* is the term used to describe language that is highly decontextualized. The literate language style characterizes language used to "monitor and reflect on experience, and reason about, plan, and predict experiences" (Westby, 1985, p. 181). To understand literate language, a child must be able to use language without the aid of context cues to support meaning; he or she must rely on language itself to make meaning. Developing a literate language style, or progressing from contextualized to decontextualized language, is crucial for children's participation in the type of discourse used in school settings. Imagine the following conversation taking place between 4-year-old Addie and her 8-year-old sister, Lily:

ADDIE: That's my toy!

LILY: No, remember we have to share this toy? Mom and Dad bought it for both of us to play with. Let's take turns playing with it.

Children's discourse development moves along a continuum reflecting oral language at one end and literate language at the other (Westby, 1991). In the preceding example, Addie's and Lily's utterances represent opposite ends of this continuum. At the lower level of the discourse continuum is *oral language,* or the linguistic aspects of communicative competence necessary for communicating basic desires and needs (phonology, syntax, morphology, and semantics). Westby described children at this end of the continuum as "learning to talk." Children learning to talk can achieve some basic language functions, including requesting and greeting. They can also produce simple syntactic structures. For example, English speakers can form yes-or-no questions by inserting *do* before the subject of the sentence (*You like ice cream* becomes *Do you like ice cream?*) and can mark the past tense by adding *-ed* or by retrieving the appropriate irregular past tense verb. The most salient characteristic of oral language is its highly contextualized style. Highly contextualized language depends heavily on the immediate context and environment. Markers of highly contextualized language include *referential pronouns*, or pronouns that refer to something physically available to the speaker ("I want *that*"), as well as gestures and facial expressions. Only when children have mastered oral language can they begin to "talk to learn" or to use language to reflect on past experiences and reason about, predict, and plan for future experiences using decontextualized language (Westby, 1991).

Children who talk to learn are at the literate language end of the discourse continuum. At this end, children use language to communicate, but also to engage in higher-order cognitive functions, such as reflecting, reasoning, planning, and hypothesizing. Highly specific vocabulary and complex syntax that expresses ideas, events, and objects beyond those of the present typify literate language. Four specific features of literate language that children learn to use are as follows (Curenton & Justice, 2004):

1. *Elaborated noun phrases:* An elaborated noun phrase is a group of words consisting of a noun and one or more modifiers providing additional information about the noun, including articles (*a, an, the*), possessives (*my, his, their*), demonstratives (*this, that, those*), quantifiers (*every, each, some*), *wh-* words (*what, which, whichever*), and adjectives (*tall, long, ugly*). Children's elaborated noun phrases become increasingly complex as they age. More specifically, by age 5, children can produce simple designating noun phrases. Simple designating noun phrases include a determiner followed by a noun (e.g., *the boy, some candy*). By age 8, children can produce simple descriptive noun phrases, which consist of a determiner and a descriptive element followed by a noun (e.g., *the garage door, a small toy*). By 11 years of age, children can produce elaborated noun phrases with postmodification, which consist of a determiner and a noun followed by a prepositional phrase or a clause (e.g., *a boy named Dillon, a girl with red hair*; Eisenberg et al., 2008).

2. *Adverbs:* An adverb is a syntactic form that modifies verbs and enhances the explicitness of action and event descriptions. Adverbs provide additional information about time (*suddenly, again, now*), manner (*somehow, well, slowly*), degree (*almost, barely, much*), place (*here, outside, above*), reason (*therefore, since, so*), and affirmation or negation (*definitely, really, never*).

3. *Conjunctions:* Conjunctions are words that organize information and clarify relationships among elements. *Coordinating conjunctions* include *and, for, or, yet, but, nor,* and *so. Subordinating conjunctions* are more numerous and include *after, although, as, because,* and *therefore,* as well as others.

4. *Mental and linguistic verbs:* Mental and linguistic verbs refer to various acts of thinking and speaking, respectively. *Mental verbs* include *think, know, believe, imagine, feel, consider, suppose, decide, forget,* and *remember*. Linguistic verbs include *say, tell, speak, shout, answer, call, reply,* and *yell*.

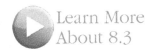

Learn More About 8.3

In the video titled "Literate Language Use in Narrative", a 9-year-old tells a fictional narrative about wearing pajamas to school in response to an examiner's prompt.

Learn More About 8.3 *(Continued)*

In telling the story, he uses literate language in a number of ways. For example, he uses elaborated noun phrases to provide additional detail ("all of this crazy hair"). He also uses adverbs of time ("I *suddenly* thought that there was somebody that was making fun of me outside") and affirmation ("He remembered that he should *always* ask if there was holidays"). The boy also uses conjunctions, such as the coordinating conjunction *because* ("I can't *because* I made a mistake and it was just embarrassing"), and he uses mental verbs to refer to acts of thinking ("I just *felt* strange"), and linguistic verbs to refer to acts of speaking ("I was *yelling* and I *said* what?").

Consider the extent to which these four literate language features are present in the following example of decontextualized language:

Yesterday, after I arrived at work, I was about to sit down at my desk when I decided I would make a cup of coffee first. You see, I was desperate for some caffeine, given that I had not had a cup of coffee at home. I started to grab some coffee from the machine, at which point I heard a familiar voice in the hallway. Now, before I tell you who it was …

This speaker paints a picture for the listener using a variety of techniques that go well beyond using correct vocabulary and syntax. The speaker provides lexical specificity by using elaborated noun phrases (*my desk, a cup of coffee*), adverbs (*yesterday, now*), and mental and linguistic verbs (*decided, tell*). The speaker also spreads conjunctions liberally throughout the story to weave together events in a causal (*given*) and temporal (*at which point*) manner. These devices provide the listener with context that would not otherwise be available. As children move through the elementary grades into adolescence and high school, they should be able to use literate language structures—both when they speak and when they write—to create context for other individuals.

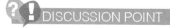
DISCUSSION POINT

Describe in writing something you did yesterday. Document the use of literate language features in this written sample. Which features occur most frequently? Least frequently?

Language Use

During the school-age years and beyond, individuals develop the ability to use language for many reasons. People also further refine their conversational and narrative abilities during this period. Three important achievements in language use during this time period are (a) functional flexibility, (b) conversational abilities, and (c) narrative development.

Functional Flexibility

Functional flexibility refers to the ability to use language for a variety of communicative purposes or functions. This flexibility is increasingly important for school-age children, who must be able to compare and contrast, persuade, hypothesize, explain, classify, and predict in the context of their classroom activities. Figure 8.3 provides a more complete list of language functions school-age children must use in the classroom. Each function requires a distinct set of linguistic, social, and cognitive competencies, all of which develop during the school-age years. Next, we elaborate on two specific language functions that exhibit notable development during the school-age years—expository discourse and persuasive discourse.

Expository Discourse.   Expository discourse is language used to convey information. Developments in this area are particularly relevant to the school-age years and beyond because students must regularly use their listening and speaking skills, their reading and writing skills, and analyze new concepts in academic domains and with respect to new and challenging concepts (Nippold & Scott, 2010). A number of factors facilitate the comprehension and production of expository discourse and text in the school-age years and beyond.

Three important factors related to the comprehension of expository text include domain-specific topic knowledge, text coherence, and text cohesion (Snyder & Caccamise, 2010). Research indicates that domain-specific topic knowledge (also called world knowledge) is more highly associated with comprehending expository text than general background knowledge because expository text communicates very specific information about a domain. For example, someone highly familiar with scuba diving would be more likely than someone who has only general knowledge about diving to comprehend an expository text about the topic

1. *To instruct:* To provide specific sequential directions

2. *To inquire:* To seek understanding by asking questions

3. *To test:* To investigate the logic of a statement

4. *To describe:* To tell about, giving necessary information to identify

5. *To compare and contrast:* To show how things are similar and different

6. *To explain:* To define terms by providing specific examples

7. *To analyze:* To break down a statement into its components, telling what each means and how they are related

8. *To hypothesize:* To make an assumption to test the logical or empirical consequences of a statement

9. *To deduce:* To arrive at a conclusion by reasoning; to infer

10. *To evaluate:* To weigh and judge the relative importance of an idea

FIGURE 8.3

Ten higher-level functions of language required of school-age children.

Source: Based on *Teaching Disadvantaged Children in the Preschool*, by C. Bereiter and S. Engelmann, 1966, Upper Saddle River, NJ: Prentice Hall.

because they would understand domain-specific vocabulary such as *regulator* and *buoyancy compensator*. With regard to coherence, expository text that is highly coherent (e.g., relationships between pieces of information are clear) is generally easier to comprehend than text that is not as coherent, especially for students with lower domain knowledge about a topic (Caccamise & Snyder, 2005). Additionally, expository text that is highly cohesive (e.g., the text is explicit with regard to relations within and across sentences) is generally easier to comprehend than text that is less cohesive.

Three key factors contributing to the quantity and quality of one's productive expository discourse include domain-specific topic knowledge, an interest in the topic, and a genuine need to express that knowledge (Nippold, 2010). Age also appears to play a role in the quantity and quality of productive discourse. In one study, Nippold, Hesketh, Duthie, and Mansfield (2005) found that in a study asking children, adolescents, and adults to explain the rules of their favorite game or sport, the mean length of T-units (a measure of syntactic complexity we discuss later in the chapter) increased with age. Researchers attributed the lengthier explanations to the older speakers' greater knowledge base; however, they also acknowledged that additional research that objectively measures a speaker's degree of knowledge would be helpful. Furthermore, despite the statistically significant effect of age on the syntactic complexity of expository discourse, Nippold and colleagues (2005) also cited wide individual differences. They reported, for example, that some of the younger children used elaborate syntax, and that some adults used more simple sentence constructions, providing evidence for variability along the age continuum.

Persuasive Discourse.   Like expository discourse, persuasive discourse is an important development in the school-age years and beyond, and it requires the coordination of a number of language areas, including syntax, semantics, and pragmatics. Persuasive discourse is language used to convince another listener or an audience to adopt a certain stance or to take action consistent with a particular point of view. As school-age children and adolescents mature, they exhibit gradual improvements in at least seven skills required for successful persuasion (Nippold, 2007):

1. Adjust to listener characteristics (e.g., age, authority, familiarity).
2. State advantages as a reason to comply.
3. Anticipate and reply to counterarguments.
4. Use positive techniques such as politeness and bargaining as strategies to increase compliance.
5. Avoid negative strategies such as whining and begging.
6. Generate a large number and variety of arguments.
7. Control the discourse assertively.

To use persuasive discourse successfully, a speaker must be flexible so as to adjust to relevant interpersonal and situational factors (Nippold, 2007). For example, a preschooler might persuade a friend to share his toy by using a polite request ("Can I have a turn with the truck?"). As another example, a high school–age student might persuade his father to let him borrow the car by adjusting to listener characteristics (e.g., authority) and by generating a number of arguments for his position ("Dad, you know I am always careful when I borrow something from you. You can trust me to return it as soon as I am finished at the store. Also, if you let me borrow the car rather than drive me to the store yourself, you'll have extra time to do something you'd rather be doing."). As yet another example, an adult campaigning for a politician's reelection might additionally control the discourse assertively, and be prepared to use a number of arguments (and counterarguments) when talking with a voter ("I understand you are concerned that Mr. Smith might vote to raise property taxes, but let me assure you his record demonstrates that he has not voted for an increase throughout his tenure. Instead, he has a number of creative solutions for generating much-needed revenue for improvements that will benefit all of our community members.").

Like it or not, children's ability to lie also improves during the school-age years. To be successful at lying, the speaker must not only produce a false statement, but must also ensure any subsequent statements are consistent with the lie. In a study involving children ages 6 to 11 years, Talwar, Gordon, and Lee (2007) found that children's ability to lie and to maintain the consistency of statements following lies increase with age. The researchers also found that children with better theory of mind abilities were more effective at lying than children with poorer theory of mind abilities, which suggests theory of mind, or the ability to recognize that others have intentions, beliefs, and desires that are different from one's own, plays an important role in being able to lie consistently.

Conversational Abilities

During the school-age years and into adolescence, children gradually improve their conversational abilities—for example, by doing the following (Nippold, 1998):

1. Staying on topic longer
2. Having extended dialogues with other people that last for several conversational turns
3. Making a larger number of relevant and factual comments
4. Shifting smoothly from one topic to another
5. Adjusting the content and style of their speech to the listener's thoughts and feelings

Children also become more proficient at understanding and using indirect requests as they develop. By about age 7 years, they begin to use indirect language, including hints, and they recognize other people's indirect requests for action (e.g., "Do you know what time it is?"). Likewise, children become more adept at detecting conversational breakdowns and repairing them. Whereas younger children favor using repetition to provide additional information during breakdowns, at around age 9 years, school-age children begin to use more sophisticated strategies, such as providing additional background information and defining terms to repair breakdowns when they occur.

Narrative Development

School-age children and adolescents use narration in both classroom and social settings. Narration is more complex than conversation because the speaker carries the linguistic load and the listener or audience takes a relatively passive role; by contrast, in conversation, multiple participants share responsibility for the give-and-take of information.

Types of Narratives. Younger children (about 5–6 years old) can produce at least four types of narratives (Owens, 2008):

1. *Recounts* involve telling a story about personal experiences, or retelling a story the person has heard or read. An adult who has shared an experience with a child usually prompts a recount. For example, a teacher might ask, "Can someone remind the class what happened in the story we read yesterday?" Because the experience is shared, the adult can provide additional detail when the child does not provide enough. Recounts are also called *personal narratives*.

2. *Accounts*, like recounts, are also a type of personal narrative. However, they are spontaneous. Unlike a recount, an account does not describe a shared the experience. Accounts are thus highly individualized because adults cannot prompt the child or supply missing information.

3. *Event casts* are similar to how sportscasters narrate during a sporting event. Event casts describe a current situation or event as it is happening (speaking on the phone: "Wow, you should see this new trick the dog has learned. He's doing it right now. Do you hear that? He's ringing a bell by the back door to let us know he wants to go outside"). Children often use event casts while they play to direct other people's actions ("Alright, I'm bringing my clothes to the counter so I can pay at your register").

4. *Fictionalized stories* are invented narratives and usually have a main character who must overcome a challenge or solve a problem. These stories are also called *fictional narratives*.

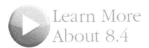 Learn More About 8.4

In the video titled "Advanced Elements of Mature Narratives", a 13-year-old tells a fictional narrative about a monkey village that has run out of bananas.

Learn More About 8.4 *(Continued)*
There is a clear beginning and end to the story, as well as a resolution to the problem. The boy uses a great deal of specific and advanced vocabulary throughout the story, including such words as *sprinted, burst, phenomenon, catastrophe, alerted, snatched, bruised, bestowed,* and *valor*. As the boy tells his story, he uses several instances of embedding. For example, he clarifies the meaning of *sprinted* in the following sentence: "As soon as he realized this, he sprinted up, or climbed very fast, up to the hall of the monkey king." He also emphasizes key words, such as *burst* and he uses a different voice to aid the listener in understanding when he is speaking in the role of the monkey king.

Elements of Mature Narratives.   Early in the school-age years, children begin to manipulate the content, plot, and causal structure of their narratives. With respect to causality, school-age children learn how to move both forward and backward in time as they narrate, whereas younger children can only move forward in time. School-age children's narratives also begin to describe other individuals' physical and mental states and motivations for actions. As children mature, their narratives grow to include multiple episodes. An *episode* includes a problem or challenge and all the elements that relate to solving the problem or challenge. Whereas children ages 5–6 years may include only one episode in their narratives, older children may include two or more.

   Story grammar refers to the components of a narrative (e.g., characters, setting, episodes), as well as the rules that govern how these components are organized. Usually, story grammar in English consists of the setting and an episode structure. See Table 8.4 for a description of the components of story grammar. By the end of the elementary grades, children often include many or all of these features in their narratives.

TABLE 8.4
Components of story grammar

COMPONENT	DESCRIPTION	EXAMPLE
Introduction	Child introduces the characters and describes the setting in which the story takes place	*There was this little boy who woke up on his own one morning. Normally, his parents would wake him up, but on this day, they were still sleeping.*
Initial event	Child introduces an event that begins the story	*The boy saw it was 8:00, and he remembered he had to be ready for the school bus at 8:15.*
Character development	Child mentions the main character and all supporting characters, and discriminates clearly between the main and supporting characters	*The boy decided to get ready for school on his own because his parents were still sleeping.*
Mental states	Child describes the mental states of the characters using various mental state words	*The boy was so worried that he might miss the school bus.*
Referencing	Child uses pronouns so others understand what the pronouns refer to consistently throughout the story	*After the boy ate breakfast, he decided to brush his teeth quickly.*
Cohesion*	Child describes the story's events in a logical order, places greater emphasis on important events and less importance on minor events, and transitions smoothly between events	*After he brushed his teeth, the boy grabbed his books and ran out the front door. He then saw the Saturday morning newspaper on the front porch.*
Resolution	Child clearly states all resolutions to conflicts that are important in moving the story along	*It turns out he wasn't late for school at all. It was Saturday.*
Conclusion	Child finishes the story by using general conclusion statements	*The boy and his parents had a good laugh about what happened.*

Sources: Based on Miller, J. F., & Heilmann, J. (2009). New tool assesses narrative structure. Advance Magazine for Speech–Language Pathologists and Audiologists, 19, 10.; Boudreau, D. M., & Hedberg, N. L. (1999). A comparison of early literacy skills in children with specific language impairment and their typically developing peers. American Journal of Speech–Language Pathology, 8, 249–260.

*Note. Cohesion is often considered a microstructural measure rather than a macrostructural measure (or a measure of story grammar). However, because aspects of cohesion are necessary for producing coherent narratives, Miller and Heilmann (2009) examine cohesion in conjunction with story grammar.

Expressive Elaboration. Ukrainetz and colleagues (2005) described the combination of narrative elements in an expressive or artful manner of storytelling as expressive elaboration. Expressive elaboration adds to a narrative's story grammar and enhances its overall expressive quality. Researchers examined the narratives of 293 children ages 5–12 years to study the development of children's expressive elaboration in three main categories:

1. *Appendages:* Cues that a narrator is telling or ending a story (e.g., a formal introduction to a story, such as "Once upon a time ..."; a summary prior to beginning a story; a formal ending to a story, such as "The end")

2. *Orientations:* Elements that provide more detail to the setting and characters (e.g., characters' names, relations between characters, personal attributes of characters)

3. *Evaluations:* Ways to convey narrator or character perspectives (e.g., using interesting modifiers, repetition for emphasis, internal-state words, or dialogue)

Results revealed that the presence of all three major categories of expressive elaboration increased with age. When the children were divided into three age clusters, 5- to 6-year-olds consistently differed from 7- to 9-year-olds and 10- to 12-year-olds in their use of all three categories of expressive elaboration. However, 7- to 9-year-olds and 10- to 12-year-olds differed statistically only in their use of orientations.

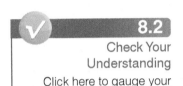

8.2
Check Your
Understanding
Click here to gauge your
understanding of the
concepts in this section.

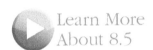

Learn More
About 8.5

In the video titled "Expressive Elaboration in Narrative", a 6-year-old tells a fictional narrative about an alien invasion in response to an examiner's prompt.

Learn More About 8.5 *(Continued)*

In telling the story, he uses expressive elaboration in a number of ways. For example, the boy uses an appendage to begin the story ("One sunny day ..."), as a cue to the listener that the story has begun. The boy also uses orientations, such as when he provides detail about the main character ("There was a boy that thought that aliens were true but all of his friends said it was a myth."). He also uses dialogue as a form of evaluation to convey characters' perspectives ("A real alien!"; "I thought it was a myth!").

WHAT FACTORS CONTRIBUTE TO SCHOOL-AGE CHILDREN'S, ADOLESCENTS', AND ADULTS' INDIVIDUAL ACHIEVEMENTS IN LANGUAGE?

Like infants, toddlers, and preschoolers, school-age children, adolescents, and adults differ from one another in certain ways in language development. In this section, we focus on language differences with respect to gender and aging in these groups.

Language and Gender

In the school-age years and adolescence, gender differences between males and females become apparent in terms of the vocabulary and conversational styles they use. Many people are aware of just how significant these differences are, in large part as a result of popular books such as Deborah Tannen's (1991), *You Just Don't Understand: Women and Men in Conversation* and John Gray's (1993), *Men Are from Mars, Women Are from Venus: A Practical Guide for Improving Communication and Getting What You Want in Your Relationships*. These books illustrate how important gender differences in language are to relationships and day-to-day interactions with other people.

As we have discussed in previous chapters, differences in language development between males and females begin to emerge at an early age, perhaps from birth. Research results demonstrate that language socialization, whereby children learn how to use language in ways consistent with their gender, plays a large role in these differences. For example, parents refer more frequently to emotion with daughters than with sons, describing negative emotions such as sadness and dislike more often with daughters (Adams, Kuebli, Boyle, & Fivush, 1995). Differences in the emotional content of parent–child conversations are related to children's own references to emotion by age 6 years as well; girls use more unique emotion terms than boys (Adams et al., 1995). Next, we discuss two main areas of language in which gender differences may play a role: (a) vocabulary use and conversational style and (b) conversational pragmatics.

Gender Differences in Vocabulary Use and Conversational Style

Research results from the 1960s through the early 1980s revealed larger differences in vocabulary use and conversational styles between the genders than more recent research. For example, earlier research showed that women use more polite words, such as *please* and *thank you*, whereas men use coarser words and swear more often (Grief & Berko Gleason, 1980). Other previous research results demonstrated that men's language is more assertive than women's language and that certain features of women's language reflect this less assertive style, including the following three (Lakoff, 1975):

1. Use of more tag questions ("You like lasagna, don't you?")
2. Use of rising intonation in declarative sentences, whereby declarative sentences sound more like questions
3. Use of polite requests more often than commands

In a more recent review of language and gender, Talbot (2010) summarizes research suggesting that men and women have different ways of being friendly in conversations. For example, women tend to use more politeness strategies than men, including hedges, boosting devices, compliments, and apologies. Hedges modify the intensity of a statement by weakening it. Speakers use hedges to avoid sounding too sure of themselves ("I *sort of* wanted to take a bike ride today rather than hike"; "I *kind of* like turkey better when it's roasted"). Boosters add friendly enthusiasm to a conversation and express intense interest ("I'm *really* surprised to hear that"; "It's *so* great to see you"). Speakers use compliments to create or maintain rapport in conversations ("I love your dress. Is that new?"), and use apologies to express concern or to avoid offending the other person ("I'm sorry to hear about your situation"; "I'm sorry to ask, but would you mind turning the TV down a bit?").

By contrast, other research findings suggest context and social status effects on language use may be stronger than gender effects (e.g., Dixon & Foster, 1997; Hannah & Murachver, 1999; Koike, 1986; Robertson & Murachver, 2003). One example concerns *hedges*, or linguistic devices that soften utterances by signaling imprecision and noncommitment, such as *about, sort of, you know, possibly,* and *perhaps.* Dixon and Foster (1997) found no effect of gender on speakers' use of hedges in conversation, but they did find effects of speaking contexts on hedging. Specifically, their research results revealed that both men and women use fewer hedges in competitive contexts than in noncompetitive contexts and more hedges when addressing males than when addressing females.

School-age children can also adjust their speech style regardless of their conversational partner's gender (Robertson & Murachver, 2003). For example, children use more instances of tag questions and compliments when their conversational partner uses this style, and more negative comments, disagreements, and directives when their conversational partner uses this speech style.

Some research also explores what we can learn by observing men and women converse with one another. For example, one such study found that the way in which married men and women talk with one another may provide clues about their marital satisfaction (Seider, Hirschberger, Nelson, & Levenson, 2009). Specifically, these researchers found that greater use of *we-words* among married couples is related to interactions characterized by relatively higher levels of positive emotional behavior, lower levels of negative emotional behavior, and lower levels of cardiovascular arousal than use of *separateness words* such as *you* and *I*. By contrast, separateness words were found to be associated with relatively higher levels of negative emotional behavior and greater marital dissatisfaction. These researchers concluded that although pronouns may seem to be small and unimportant words, they appear to provide an important window into the emotional connections married couples share and the ways these couples express and regulate their emotions when conflicts arise.

Gender Differences in Conversational Pragmatics

It appears that gender relates not only to the *kinds* of language speakers use, but also to *how* they use language. For example, body posture and eye contact tend to differ for men and women in the United States. Women usually face their conversational partners and make eye contact, whereas men are more likely to take a more distant stance and make less eye contact (Tannen, 1994). Men also change conversational topics more frequently than women, whereas women tend to exhaust conversational topics more thoroughly (Tannen, 1994). Also, women indicate their attention by using fillers such as *uh-huh* and *yeah* more often than men, and women usually interrupt a speaker only to clarify the message and support the speaker. As with vocabulary use, men's and women's conversational pragmatics may be more a function of context than of gender. See K. J. Anderson and Leaper (1998) for a meta-analysis of 43 studies comparing men's and women's conversational interruptions across a variety of situational contexts as an excellent summary of these between-gender differences.

Some research suggests men and women differ in the kinds of language they use, as well as how they use language.

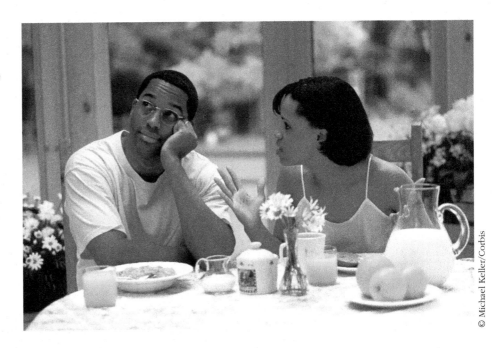

© Michael Keller/Corbis

Language and Aging

Research in the field of developmental psychology and cognitive aging, in particular, has illuminated a number of language differences between younger and aging adults. Such research reminds us that one's language abilities continue to develop and change not only throughout the school-age years but throughout life.

Have you ever had a conversation with someone and experienced difficulty thinking of a specific word you had wanted to use? Maybe you have even announced, "Wow, the word is right on the tip of my tongue." This is called the *tip-of-the-tongue phenomenon* and describes the inability to produce the spoken form of the word one intends to use. Older adults report, and experimental research confirms, that they have more difficulty producing the spoken forms of familiar words than younger adults. Older adults also have more difficulties retrieving the spelling of familiar words than younger adults. Research suggests that the tip-of-the-tongue phenomenon and other word-finding problems seem to result from difficulties in retrieving the sounds of words (Burke & Shafto, 2004). Another noticeable difference between older and younger adults is that older adults tend to speak more slowly; speech rate tends to decrease as adults age (e.g., Benjamin, 1997).

You have probably experienced another issue that increases with age—forgetting someone's name. Maybe you have attended a social function where you recognized someone you had met a month or so earlier, but you could not remember her name. Or maybe at that same social function you were introduced to someone, and before a few seconds had passed, you had already forgotten his name. Although this situation is common among people of all ages, the ability to remember proper names (e.g., Fred Smith) seems to decline with age (James, 2004).

Naming ability (naming the word a picture represents) is another area in which adults exhibit decline. In a study that examined adults ages 25–35 years, 50–59 years, 60–69 years, and above 70 years, Verhagen and Poncelet (2013) demonstrated naming accuracy is worse for adults in their 60s (with an average of 90.3% pictures named correctly in the study) and 70s (with an average of 76.4% pictures named correctly) as compared to adults ages 25–35 years (with an average of 98.5% pictures named correctly) and adults in their 50s (with an average of 96.0% pictures named correctly in the study). Furthermore, adults in their 50s, 60s, and 70s (with picture-naming latencies of about 1,500 ms, 1,700 ms, and 3,500 ms respectively, in the study) are slower to name pictures than adults ages 25–35 years (about 1,250 ms in the study).

Older adults also have more difficulty than younger adults in understanding others' affective prosody, or the phonological characteristics of one's speech that convey emotion, such as happiness or sadness. The ability to understand others' affective prosody is particularly important when a speaker's words do not match the emotions they intend to convey, such as when a speaker uses sarcasm or irony. Orbelo, Grim, Talbott, and Ross (2005) found that older adults' ability to interpret affective prosody seems to be independent of their hearing and cognitive abilities. This means older adults who have very good hearing and strong cognitive abilities experience more difficulties interpreting affective prosody than younger adults. Researchers hypothesize that the loss of affective prosodic comprehension might result from an age-related processing deficit in the right hemisphere of the brain. Other research suggests older adults may be able to overcome this challenge simply by repeating the other person's sentence before responding; this way, the emotional context of the speaker's utterance becomes clearer, and the listener can better able make a judgment about the speaker's intent (Dupis & Pichora-Fuller, 2010).

Some neuroimaging research suggests that in general, older adults have more difficulties with higher-order language processes, such as constructing sentence-level

8.3

Check Your
Understanding

Click here to gauge your
understanding of the
concepts in this section.

or message-level meaning, than with lower-order language processes, such as understanding individual words and their meanings (Federmeier, Van Petten, Schwartz, & Kutas, 2003). Despite the many differences between language in older and younger adults, Tyler and colleagues (2010) emphasize that many complex cognitive processes, including language comprehension, remain stable as adults age.

HOW DO RESEARCHERS AND CLINICIANS MEASURE LANGUAGE DEVELOPMENT IN THE SCHOOL-AGE YEARS AND BEYOND?

Researchers and clinicians measure language development in the school-age years and beyond in various ways, such as by using formative and summative evaluations, naturalistic language situations for collecting language samples, and elicitation procedures. In this section, we describe different assessment types and explore ways to measure the development of language form, content, and use during the school-age years and beyond.

Assessment Types

There are a number of assessment types a clinician, researcher, or teacher could use to measure language in the school-age years and beyond. In general, the method for assessing a person's language abilities should reflect the reason for doing so. Practitioners may use formative evaluations to inform potential language-learning activities, or to measure the language-development *process*. For example, before beginning a new curricular unit, a teacher might informally administer a formative assessment of a child's vocabulary knowledge by having the child define specific words he or she will encounter in the unit. The teacher might then devote additional attention to the words the child does not know as they progress through the unit.

Conversely, practitioners use summative evaluations to measure the *products* and final outcomes of language learning and development. For example, a clinician might administer a summative assessment of vocabulary knowledge—such as the Peabody Picture Vocabulary Test—Fourth Edition (PPVT–4; Dunn & Dunn, 2007)— to evaluate a child who has participated in a year-long vocabulary intervention designed to raise his or her vocabulary level to that of same-age peers.

Besides focusing on process versus product, practitioners may have more specific goals in mind for assessing school-age children's language development. To accomplish such goals, they use three types of assessments, as we have described in Chapters 6 and 7:

1. Screenings are brief assessments usually performed at the beginning of the school year (or at another key developmental juncture) to help identify students who need extra assistance in certain areas.

2. Comprehensive evaluations can be conducted any time during the school year to obtain an in-depth probe of a specific child's instructional needs. These assessments are typically used to identify the presence of a language disability.

3. Progress monitoring assessments are conducted routinely (at least three times a year) to document a child's rate of improvement in an area and to monitor the efficacy of curricula and interventions.

Assessment of Language Form

Assessment of language form involves measuring phonological and syntactic development. We describe some measurement procedures for these two areas of language development next.

Measurement of Phonological Development

To measure a school-age child's phonological development, clinicians can use a standardized assessment such as the Goldman–Fristoe Test of Articulation–2 (GFTA–2; Goldman & Fristoe, 2000) (The GFTA–3 was in preparation as the current text went to press). This assessment is appropriate for children and adolescents through age 21 years. To conduct it, the examiner uses pictures and verbal cues to sample the child's or adolescent's spontaneous and imitative sound production of consonants. The examiner can then determine whether he or she correctly produces specific speech sounds or sound sequences in different contexts (e.g., medial vs. final position of a word).

Measurement of Syntactic Development

To measure syntactic development in the school-age years and beyond, examiners can use language samples, elicitation procedures, judgment tasks, and standardized measures. Language samples are useful for measuring advanced syntax. To do so, the researcher or clinician segments the transcript of spoken or written language into communication units (C units) or terminable units (T units). C units and T units both consist of an independent clause and any of its modifiers, such as a dependent clause. The difference between C units and T units is that C units apply to oral language analysis; they can include incomplete sentences and sentence fragments. T units, by comparison, apply to written language transcripts (e.g., a written essay) and include only complete sentences. After segmenting a transcript into T or C units, the researcher or clinician analyzes the units in various ways, such as calculating the mean length of the units in words or the percentage of units containing dependent clauses. Simply counting the number of units a sample contains also provides an informative measure of *language productivity*, or the amount of language a child produces. The researcher or clinician who has collected a language sample might also be interested in examining the number and types of noun phrases, verb phrases, questions, and negation strategies a student uses in spoken or written language samples.

Elicitation procedures are also useful for examining advanced syntax, including complements, verb clauses, multiclause utterances, question forms, and negation. For example, presenting a student with improbable pictures is a good method for eliciting verb clauses because the student can describe what is wrong with the picture (e.g., "The baby is holding an elephant!"). To elicit negative forms, the examiner can create the need for objects that are not present. For example, to elicit a negative form ("The pen doesn't work"), the examiner can present the student with a nonfunctioning pen and a piece of paper and ask him or her to draw something. Other broken or nonfunctioning materials should also elicit negative forms.

We introduced judgment tasks in Chapter 7 as metalinguistic tasks that require children to think about language and make judgments about the appropriateness of specific forms or interpret sentences. In addition to the grammaticality judgment tasks we described in Chapter 7, there are also judgment tasks appropriate for use with school-age children and adults. One such task is the graded grammaticality judgment paradigm (e.g., Ambridge, Pine, Rowland, & Young, 2008; Theakston, 2004). Ambridge (2012) describes the graded grammaticality judgment paradigm as a measure in which participants judge the extent to which a language form is acceptable using a scale (e.g., Likert scale; smiley face scale) rather than a binary judgment, such as indicating whether a particular form is acceptable or unacceptable. The graded grammaticality judgment paradigm is appropriate for use with children no younger than age 4 years, 6 months and researchers may use it with older school-age children and adults as well. Using the paradigm, researchers can obtain ratings of past tense forms of novel verbs, prefix forms, and verb argument structures (e.g., transitive; intransitive).

One standardized test that measures syntactic development is the Test of Language Development—Intermediate, Fourth Edition (TOLD–I:4; Hammill & Newcomer, 2008). The TOLD–I:4 is appropriate for children ages 8 years through

17 years, 11 months. It assesses a student's understanding and meaningful use of spoken words, as well as different aspects of grammar. The subtests of the TOLD–I:4 that measure syntax include Sentence Combining, Word Ordering, and Morphological Comprehension. The TOLD–I:4, like other standardized tests of language, is also used to identify students whose language skills are significantly depressed, which possibly indicates the presence of a language disorder.

Assessment of Language Content

Researchers and clinicians can assess children's language content by analyzing spontaneously generated language samples and structured elicitation procedures. Standardized tests are also available for measuring school-age children's language content, including achievements in lexical meaning, abstract relational meaning, and figurative language.

Measurement of Lexical Meaning

Using language samples and elicitation procedures, researchers and clinicians can examine children's understanding of lexical meaning (Lund & Duchan, 1993). Lund and Duchan suggested the following procedure for analyzing language samples:

1. Examine transcripts for instances in which the child used a word differently than an adult would use it (e.g., overextensions, underextensions, and incorrect referents).

2. Examine transcripts for gestures, pronouns, and indefinite and idiosyncratic terms that replace specific words, which may indicate the child has a deficit in a particular class of meaning (e.g., verbs of motion, superordinate terms). Determine whether the deficit is in one class or multiple classes.

3. Examine transcripts for the absence of particular word classes, including noun modifiers and conjunctions.

Elicitation procedures for examining a child's lexical meaning include having the child define words (if he or she might potentially be using them incorrectly), and playing games in which the child would need to use the word class of interest. For example, a Simon Says game might prompt children to use motion verbs, such as "Simon says leap forward; now kneel. ..."

Standardized assessments that measure lexical meaning include the aforementioned PPVT–4 and the Test of Word Knowledge (TOWK; Wiig & Secord, 1992). The PPVT–4 is a norm-referenced measure of receptive vocabulary. The examiner presents sets of four pictures on a page and directs the person being assessed to point to one of the pictures. The PPVT–4 is a popular tool because it provides normative references of receptive vocabulary for children and adults of all ages; thus, clinicians and researchers can continue to use it throughout adulthood. Although delays in developing receptive vocabulary can signal a language difficulty or impairment, receptive vocabulary is only one component of language, so clinicians generally use the PPVT–4 in conjunction with other measures of language ability to evaluate a person's language competencies.

The TOWK is appropriate for children ages 5–17 years and evaluates students' semantic and lexical knowledge through their ability to understand and use vocabulary. Compared to the PPVT, it provides a more comprehensive analysis of children's lexical abilities. Researchers and clinicians can use the TOWK as part of a comprehensive evaluation battery. Level 1 of the assessment (for children ages 5–8 years) includes subtests that measure expressive vocabulary, word definitions, receptive vocabulary, and word opposites. An optional subtest for 5- to 8-year-olds measures synonyms. Level 2 of the assessment (for children ages 8–17 years) includes subtests that measure word definitions, multiple contexts, synonyms, and figurative language usage. Supplementary subtests address word opposites, receptive vocabulary, expressive vocabulary, conjunctions, and transition words. Test developers also suggest that clinicians can use the TOWK as a resource for gifted and talented assessment to identify students who excel in semantic knowledge.

Measurement of Abstract Relational Meaning

Researchers and clinicians can also analyze children's understanding of abstract relational meaning by using language samples and elicitation procedures. With language samples, a researcher or clinician examines language transcripts, with particular attention to how children use relational terms such as prepositions. When children use relational terms, such as spatial prepositions (e.g., *among, between, through*), they understand not only something about the *properties* of an object but also something about the *state* of the object. Cognitive psychologists might be particularly interested in children's use of such abstract relational terms.

Elicitation procedures might involve having a child follow directions, retell stories, or complete metalinguistic exercises. When having a child follow directions, the researcher or clinician can assess the child's comprehension of spatial prepositions (*Put the ball under the cup*) and dative relations (*Give the monkey the cat* vs. *Give the cat the monkey*).

To elicit language by having a child retell stories, an examiner tells a story that includes specific linguistic devices (e.g., time markers such as *first, second,* and *third*) as a model for the child . The examiner then prompts the child to retell the story while the examiner listens for inclusion of the modeled features.

To elicit language using metalinguistic exercises, an examiner presents statements for a child to reflect on, analyze, and interpret, such as the following (Lund & Duchan, 1993):

"John will go and Henry will go. Who will go?"

"John will go or Henry will go. Who will go?"

"John will go so Henry will go. Who will go?" (p. 262)

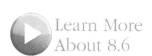

Learn More About 8.6

The video titled "Study of Metaphor Understanding" illustrates a research method that might be used with a school-aged child. In this case, the girl is 6 years of age, and the study takes place at Dr. Roberta Golinkoff's research lab at the University of Delaware.

Learn More About 8.6 *(Continued)*

The purpose of this study is to investigate children's understanding of metaphors involving verbs. The experimenter asks the child to explain a series of stories to her, in three study condititions. In the first condition, the stories include verb metaphors (e.g., "the toaster ate his bread"). In the second study condition, the stories include instrument verbs used in a nontraditional way. For example, the verb *mop* is usually associated with the instrument mop. In one of the example stories, the experimenter asks the girl to explain what it means to say, "the baby mopped the floor with his diaper." In the third condition, stories describe a simple action (e.g., "the girl licked the ice cream cone"). Stories containing simple action descriptions serve as a control to the stories involving instrument verbs used in a nontraditional way and stories involving verb metaphors. The hypothesis is that all children should be able to explain the simple actions and that older children should have an easier time explaining the verb metaphors than younger children.

Measurement of Figurative Language

Because children may use figurative language infrequently in spontaneous speech, elicitation procedures are probably the best choice for assessing children's understanding of figurative language such as metaphors, idioms, and proverbs. To assess children's understanding of metaphors, researchers and clinicians can use an interview-style procedure in which they ask a child to first provide a literal meaning for a word or phrase, and then explain sentences in which words are used metaphorically.

An appropriate way to measure understanding of idioms is to use a picture selection task. In such a task, a researcher or clinician asks a child to find a picture corresponding to an idiomatic expression (e.g., "Which one of these pictures best matches the saying *a dime a dozen*?"). To measure older children's understanding of proverbs, a researcher or clinician can simply ask a child to explain the meaning of one or more proverbs (e.g., "Explain to me the meaning behind 'A stitch in time saves nine.'").

Assessment of Language Use

Measuring conversational skills is one way to assess language use in the school-age years and beyond. We describe three sample assessments, here, to provide an idea of the variety of formats the measures may take and the constructs they might address.

One such measure is the Children's Communication Checklist, Version 2 (CCC-2; Bishop, 2003). The CCC-2 is a parent-report instrument measuring communicative strengths and weaknesses for children and adolescents between ages 4 and 16 years. It includes 70 items divided into 10 scales. The first four scales include the following: (1) speech, which assesses articulation and phonology; (2) syntax, which assesses language structure; (3) semantics, which assesses vocabulary; and (4) coherence, which assesses discourse. The next four scales measure areas of communication for which children with pragmatic difficulties exhibit impairment, including the following: (5) inappropriate initiation, which assesses failing to initiate topics about shared interests, repetitive initiations, and excessive talking; (6) stereotyped language, which assesses overuse of scripted units of language, unusual prosody, and overly precise language; (7) use of context, which assesses politeness and understanding of sarcasm and humor; and (8) nonverbal communication, which assesses understanding of gestures and facial expressions. The final two scales measure behavioral factors relevant to autism: (9) social relations and (10) interests.

The Test of Pragmatic Language—Second Edition (TOPL-2; Phelps-Terasaki & Phelps-Gunn, 2007) is a clinician-administered (e.g., SLP) assessment of pragmatic language skills in children and adolescents ages 6 to 18 years, 11 months. To complete the assessment, an assessor asks a student to respond to a set of hypothetical situations and provide a rationale for each response. The measure takes about 45 to 60 minutes to administer and assesses the ability to use pragmatic language effectively with respect to six areas: (1) physical context; (2) audience; (3) topic; (4) purpose (speech acts); (5) visual and gestural cues; and (6) abstraction.

Another measure, which is available for free download online, is the Conversational Skills Rating Scale (CSRS; Spitzberg & Adams, 2015). The CSRS assesses conversational competence in interpersonal settings. Although the manual does not indicate a target age range, it appears to be an appropriate measure of language use for the school-age years and beyond. The CSRS contains 25 skill items grouped into four skill clusters: (1) attentiveness (attention to, interest in, and concern for one's conversational partner); (2) composure (confidence, assertiveness, and relaxation); (3) expressiveness (animation and variation in verbal and nonverbal expression, topical verbosity); and (4) coordination (conversational initiations and exits, nondisruptive flow in turns, and topical innovation). In addition to the 25 skill items, the instrument includes five general items that serve to validate the behavioral items. The CSRS can be completed as a self-report measure or by another individual (e.g., teacher, peer) and takes about 5–7 minutes to complete.

The three sample measures of language use exhibit some degree of overlap with regard to the skills and competencies they address. For example, all three address nonverbal communication (e.g., gestures, facial expressions) and turn taking within conversations, in some way. The three measures also differ in a number of ways, including whether they are completed by parent, self-report or peer report, or administered by a clinician. As with any measure of language development, it is important to consider the purpose for administration and to select an assessment that best serves that goal.

RESEARCH **PARADIGMS**

Assessment of Later Language Development

To assess later language development of syntax, semantics, and pragmatics, researchers can use written language measures in addition to spoken language measures. In one such study, researchers examined children's, adolescents', and adults' development in these areas using a persuasive writing task (Nippold, Ward-Lonergan, & Fanning, 2005). Participants handwrote a persuasive essay on the controversial topic of animals being trained to perform in circuses; then researchers coded the essays for specific indicators of syntactic, semantic, and pragmatic development. Findings revealed several age-related changes in students' language form, content, and use. With respect to language form, older students' essays were longer, had a longer mean length of utterance (MLU), and used more relative clauses (e.g., "People *who enjoy the outdoors* want to protect the forests.") than younger students' essays. With regard to language content, older students' essays included a greater use of literate language features, including adverbial conjuncts (e.g., *however, meanwhile*), greater use of abstract nouns (e.g., *longevity, diversion*), and greater use of mental verbs (e.g., *hypothesize, doubt*) and linguistic verbs (e.g., *argue, reflect*). Concerning language use, older students included a greater number of reasons to support their point of view than younger students, and they were also more likely than younger students to acknowledge multiple viewpoints in their essays.

Nippold and colleagues suggested the developmental information provided by the 11- to 24-year-old participants could serve as a starting point for establishing expected achievement levels in these areas of later language development. The researchers also suggested the results may have implications for persons who experience difficulties with these areas of language, which are important for persuasive writing.

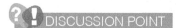
DISCUSSION POINT
What are some other topics that could serve as prompts for a persuasive writing task?

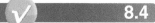
8.4
Check Your
Understanding
Click here to gauge your understanding of the concepts in this section.

One standardized assessment that measures school-age children's language use abilities is the Test of Language Competence—Expanded Edition (TLC–Expanded; Wiig & Secord, 1989). The following subtests of the TLC–Expanded measure students' higher-level language functions: Ambiguous Sentences, Listening Comprehension: Making Inferences, Oral Expression: Recreating Speech Acts, and Figurative Language. The TLC–Expanded also includes a supplemental memory subtest and a screening composite to determine whether students would benefit from more in-depth assessment. Level 1 of the test is appropriate for students between 5 and 9 years old, and Level 2 is appropriate for students between 10 and 18 years old. See Research Paradigms: *Assessment of Later Language Development* to learn about a specific paradigm researchers might use to assess development of later language acquisition, including language use.

Later language development can also be assessed in the written modality.

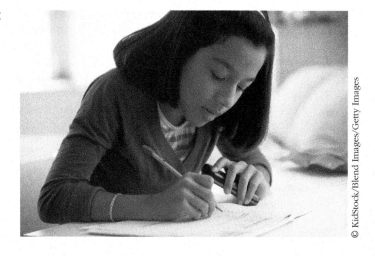

© KidStock/Blend Images/Getty Images

SUMMARY

We open this chapter with a discussion of the major language processes that differentiate school-age language development from earlier language development. These processes include shifting sources of language input and the acquisition of metalinguistic competence. School-age children begin to gain increased language input from text, and their metalinguistic competence improves as they engage in analyzing language as an object of attention, such as when they encounter figurative language.

In the second section, we describe important achievements in language form, content, and use in the school-age years and beyond. Specific achievements in language form include phonological forms, such as morphophonemic changes and the use of stress and emphasis. Other developments in language forms include morphological forms, such as derivational prefixes and suffixes, and complex syntax, some of which occurs mainly in the written modality. Specific achievements in language content include lexical development through direct instruction,

contextual abstraction, and morphological analysis; understanding of multiple meanings; understanding of lexical and sentential ambiguity; and acquisition of a literate language style through the use of elaborated noun phrases, adverbs, conjunctions, and mental and linguistic verbs. Specific achievements in language use include functional flexibility; conversational abilities, such as detecting and repairing conversational breakdowns; and narrative development, including the use of expressive elaboration.

In the third section, we discuss how school-age children, adolescents, and adults differ in their individual language competencies, focusing on gender differences and contextual influences on language forms and use, as well as language in aging adults. Finally, we explore ways researchers and clinicians measure the development of language form, content, and use in the school-age years and beyond. In particular, we discuss the use of naturalistic language samples, elicitation procedures, and standardized assessments to measure language development and competencies.

Apply Your Knowledge

Click here to apply your knowledge to practical scenarios.

BEYOND THE BOOK

1. Create a list of five idioms. Trade lists with a classmate and try to interpret the idioms on his or her list. Rate the extent to which you are familiar with your partner's idioms using the following scale: 1 = heard the idiom many times, 2 = heard it several times, 3 = heard it a few times, 4 = heard it once, 5 = never heard the idiom. *Next, rate the transparency of the idiom using the following scale:* 1 = literal and nonliteral meanings are closely related, 2 = literal and nonliteral meanings are somewhat related, 3 = literal and nonliteral meanings are not related. Discuss your ratings.

2. Think about a new word you learned recently. Did someone tell you its meaning? If so, how did this

happen? If you used another strategy to learn the new word, describe it.

3. Record a school-age child telling a short story about himself or herself (about 2–3 min). List all of the literate language features you hear.

4. Think about the most recent conversation you had. Which language functions did you use to communicate (see Figure 8.3) and why?

5. Thinking about gender and language, what other differences in form, content, and use (not covered in this chapter) are you familiar with from your own experiences?

Check Your Understanding

Gauge your understanding of the chapter concepts by taking this self-check quiz.

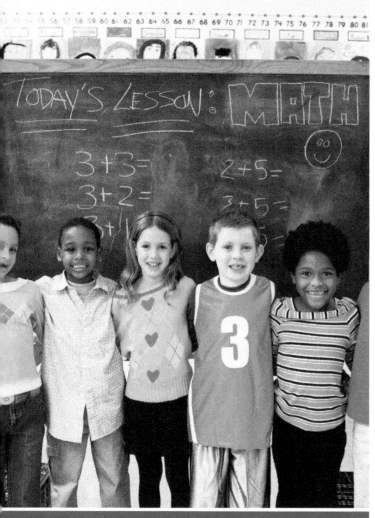

© Digital Vision/Getty Images

9

Language Diversity

LEARNING OUTCOMES

After completion of this chapter, the reader will be able to:

1. Describe the connection between language and culture.

2. Explain how languages evolve and change.

3. Compare and contrast bilingualism and second language acquisition.

4. Describe some theories of second language acquisition and their implications for practice.

In many of the preceding chapters, we introduce major milestones that characterize how most children develop language from infancy to adolescence. However, we have also addressed issues related to individual differences in language acquisition, such as how girls may develop differently than boys, and how children's experiences can affect their rate of language growth. In Chapter 1, we introduced the concepts of *language difference* and *language disorders*; the former is a general term used to describe the normal variability among children in their language development, whereas the latter refers to instances in which children experience significant difficulties in the development of language. In this chapter, we explore the concept of language diversity in greater detail, and emphasize that variability in language acquisition seems to be the rule rather than the exception. For instance, consider Mrs. Riggert's second-grade classroom of twenty-two 7-year-olds at Compass Elementary School, located in a large midwestern American city. If we study the language abilities of each child in this classroom, we notice there are indeed many similarities among the children regarding aspects of form, content, and use. However, we also quickly note that a great deal of variability distinguishes each child from his or her classmates. Haj, for instance, raised in India until age 3 years, speaks an English dialect that differs strikingly from that of Kisha, who just moved from Mississippi to live with her grandparents while her mother serves overseas in the armed services. Kimberly, Jesus, and Dayana are all learning English as a second language and speak primarily Spanish at home. Josephine, Arianna, and Damian all read well beyond the second-grade reading level and have strikingly sophisticated vocabularies. Katinka speaks Dutch and English fluently, and Adelaide knows a number of Italian words and phrases from spending time in Italy last summer. Clearly, there is great benefit to not only understanding the universality of many language accomplishments, as emphasized in much of this book, but also recognizing the ways in which each of us follows a unique pathway.

In this chapter, we address four primary topics related to language diversity. First, we discuss the connection between language and culture. Second, we explore how languages evolve and change. Third, we compare and contrast bilingualism and second language acquisition. Finally, we describe some prevailing theories of second language acquisition and their implications for practice.

Most people in the world acquire or learn more than one language during their lifetime (Grabe, 2002); in fact, an estimated 60%–75% of the global population speaks more than one language (C. Baker, 2000). Multilingualism is even more prevalent in areas of the world where people in neighboring states speak different languages. For example, the European Union encourages multilingualism among its member states, specifically advocating that citizens learn two languages in addition to their native language. When people share a language, they have an important bond in common because language conveys more than the meanings behind individual words. With language comes history, tradition, and identity—in short, the culture of a group of people. In this chapter, we first discuss the connection between language and culture. Second, we examine the process of language change and evolution through dialectical variation, pidgins, and creoles. In the third section, we explore bilingualism and second language acquisition, and, finally, we examine some prevailing theories of second language acquisition and discuss their implications for practice.

WHAT IS THE CONNECTION BETWEEN LANGUAGE AND CULTURE?

The Interrelatedness of Language and Culture

Anthropologist, Franz Boas viewed language as reflecting the conceptual ideas and forms of thinking characteristic of a culture (Lucy, 1992). Linguist and anthropologist, Edward Sapir (1921) further stated that language does not exist apart from culture. These views expressing the interconnectedness between language and culture make sense on many levels. People learn about language through their culture (e.g., pragmatics such as interaction styles and speech registers) and about their culture through language (e.g., vocabulary to describe culturally specific phenomena).

The connection between language and culture is often evident in television shows and in interactions with other individuals, even those who speak the same language. Because the United States is home to persons with numerous backgrounds, Americans have borrowed words and phrases from many world cultures. Yiddish is one such example. Novelist and lecturer, Michael Wex remarked on the National Public Radio program *Fresh Air* that despite the few fluent Yiddish speakers, many Yiddish words and expressions are commonly used in American English. Describing Yiddish words, Wex said,

> They convey something that the basic English translation doesn't have in it. . . . There's an emotional coloring that you just don't get. . . . Because so much of Yiddish life was devoted to dealing with frustration in a way that anticipated a lot of modern North American life, there's this open space for it to enter in and fill up those gaps that English, which was once a very polite language, just doesn't seem to have the words to fill. (Gross, 2005)

Accepting that language and culture are tied to each other seems natural, yet such acceptance raises the question, "Which comes first?" One prominent view on the interrelatedness between language and culture is that from the time humans are born we are socialized both *through* the use of language and *to* the use of language (Schieffelin & Ochs, 1986). The ways in which we interact with infants and young children who are acquiring language provide a window into how we socialize other persons "through and to" language use.

Infant-Directed Speech

All cultures have specific ways of interacting with young language learners. In Western cultures, such as that in the United States, adults speak directly to infants from birth using a unique speech register called *infant-directed (ID) speech*. Noticeable characteristics of ID speech include a high overall pitch, exaggerated pitch contours, and slower tempos than those used in *adult-directed (AD) speech*. ID speech effectively attracts and maintains infants' attention, and infants seem to prefer it to AD speech (Cooper & Aslin, 1990; Fernald & Kuhl, 1987). In addition to eliciting attention, ID speech may facilitate language acquisition in several ways, such as clarifying vowels (Bernstein Ratner, 1986; Kuhl et al., 1997), and aiding acquisition of words (Fernald, 2000; Fernald & Mazzie, 1991; Golinkoff & Alioto, 1995). See Chapter 5 for more information on the role of ID speech in language acquisition.

Although incontrovertible evidence exists for a special speech register in many Western societies, Western ID speech is not universal. Evidence from southern working-class African Americans, Athapaskan Indians, Samoans, and Kaluli indicates that the simplifying characteristics of ID speech are not present in all cultures (Schieffelin & Ochs, 1986). Instead, Schieffelin and Ochs summarized that differences in the communicative interactions between adults and young children "socialize children into different cultural orientations toward communication, meaning, and the social status of children" (p. 174). For example, Athapaskan adults expect their children to repeat the adults' language without understanding the meaning behind it. Furthermore, rather than attempting to reformulate the underlying intentions of children's unintelligible utterances, Athapaskan adults provide a situational and culturally appropriate translation to familiarize children with conventional context-specific responses. In contrast, adults from African American, Samoan, and Kaluli cultures usually ignore unintelligible child speech rather than reformulate it or pursue the child's intentions. The speech adults direct to children thus ranges in its communicative accommodation from highly child-centered to highly situation-centered.

In communicative accommodation that is highly child centered, the adult regularly takes the perspective of the child to foster the child's understanding and production of speech in communicative exchanges. For example, to foster a child's understanding of speech, an adult might use a slower pace and a generous amount of repetition when speaking. To foster a child's production of speech, an adult might extend a child's utterances, or rephrase the child's utterances using correct syntax and pronunciation, while maintaining the child's intended meaning. In communicative accommodation that is highly child-centered, the adult also tends to use child-centered topics and engages with the child, frequently, as a conversational partner. By contrast, in communicative accommodation that is highly situation-centered, the adult expects the child to accommodate to activities and persons within specific communicative situations. The adult also tends to use registers appropriate for each situation, rather than infant-directed speech, in communicative accommodation that is highly situation-centered (Schieffelin & Ochs, 1986).

The extent to which communicative accommodation leans toward the child-centered or situation-centered end of the continuum can vary not only according to one's culture, but also according to the child's age. For instance, Kaluli and Samoan parents emphasize highly situation-centered communication throughout infancy and early childhood, whereas Mayan parents use situation-centered communication with young infants and child-centered communication with toddlers who are beginning to produce intelligible utterances.

HOW DO LANGUAGES EVOLVE AND CHANGE?

Dialects

Everyone has a dialect. *Dialects* are regional or social varieties of language that differ from one another in terms of their pronunciation, vocabulary, and grammar. In comparison, accents are varieties of language that differ solely in pronunciation. The second author of this text (L.J.), born and raised in Ohio, speaks the dialect of English associated with the geographic Midwest, called the Midland dialect. However, her father was born and raised in the Cumberland Gap region of Tennessee, and still has traces of an Appalachian English dialect. By contrast, the first author of this text (K.T.) was born and raised in the Baltimore area and speaks

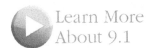

Learn More About 9.1

As you watch the video titled "Infant-Directed Speech", notice how the adult uses a high pitch, rising intonation, and repetition when speaking to the infant. https://www.youtube.com/watch?v=DbW5xHcBpOs

9.1
Check Your Understanding
Click here to gauge your understanding of the concepts in this section.

Dialects are regional or social varieties of language that differ from one another in their pronunciation, vocabulary, and grammar.

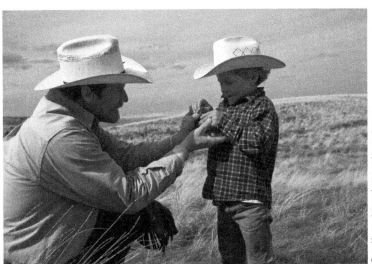

© Ralf Nau/Digital Vision/Getty Images

the Mid-Atlantic dialect, although features of the dialect are more prominent in the speech of her parents and even more so in the speech of her grandparents.

Dialects develop during a prolonged period in which people are separated by geographic barriers, such as mountains and rivers, or by social barriers, such as social-class differences. Almost all languages have a variety of dialects; therefore, everyone speaks some dialect, or variety, of a language. As a general rule, people who speak different dialects of a language can understand one another. However, one's brain might need a period of "calibration" in which it adjusts to variations in how certain sounds are produced in a given dialect. The second author (L.J.) spent some time in New Zealand a few years ago and recalls that it took a short while (and a few instances of confusion!) to become accustomed to how certain vowels were represented in the New Zealand dialect of English as compared to her Midland U.S. dialect.

Because of social-class differences, some dialects are held in higher esteem than others. Unfortunately, this can lead to stereotyping of those persons who speak dialects held in lower esteem within a society. Consider a brief conversation on a Chicago street between two persons—one a male tourist and the other a native Chicagoan—in which the tourist asks for directions to Michigan Avenue. Even in such a brief interaction, each person forms opinions about the other in terms of their intelligence, wealth, success, ambition, and educational attainment—all of which are attributes of status. Importantly, one's dialect strongly influences the opinions of others. Consider it this way: If the tourist speaks a standard dialect of English, he is viewed as smarter, wealthier, more successful, more ambitious, and more educated than if he speaks an Appalachian dialect (Luhman, 1990). Media depictions tend to promulgate such negative stereotyping, as in the long-running *Beverly Hillbillies* television show, which featured pejorative depictions of Appalachian-dialect speakers.

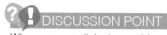

DISCUSSION POINT

Why are some dialects considered more or less prestigious than others?

Generally speaking, Standard American English (SAE; also called *General American English*, GAE) has the highest status in the United States, as does Received Pronunciation (RP) in England. Children develop an awareness of the higher status of these dialects at very early ages, as shown in a great number of studies, such as a now-classic work by Rosenthal (1974). Rosenthal worked with one hundred thirty-six 3- to 5-year-old children, including both Whites and African Americans. Each child had the opportunity to play with two talking Magic Boxes (Kenneth and Steve) that each wanted to give the child a present; however, the child could only pick one box from which to receive the present. The child listened to each box describe the present it wanted to give and then was able to choose (the boxes didn't really talk; inside each was a prerecorded cassette). The critical feature of this study's design was that one Magic Box spoke using an African American vernacular dialect (Kenneth), whereas the other spoke using GAE (Steve). A striking three-fourths of all children, when surveyed, reported that Steve had nicer presents and nearly four-fifths (79%) perceived that Steve "talks better." These language stereotypes are perpetuated over time and transcend a variety of dialectical comparisons. Studies of adolescents and college students, for instance, show that they rate lecturers as smarter and more competent when they use higher- versus lower-status dialects (e.g., Giles & Powesland, 1975). Teachers and other professionals must take these biases extremely seriously, as it is certainly possible that they might hold lower expectations for students who speak dialects they perceive as lower in status (Cross, DeVaney, & Jones, 2001), including both regional and sociocultural varieties.

American English Regional Dialects

American English regional dialects date to colonial America, when people from different parts of the British Isles began to settle in different areas along the East Coast and then moved inland (Wolfram & Schilling-Estes, 2006). These early settlers brought geographically and regionally unique vocabulary and ways of speaking to the New World, and began to incorporate and use vocabulary words from the Native American tribes in the areas where they settled. Several factors contributed to the creation and maintenance of American English regional dialects, including language contact, population movement, expanding transportation and communication networks, and shifting cultural centers (Wolfram & Schilling-Estes, 2006).

Language contact is the process whereby speakers of a language other than English shape the pronunciation, grammar, and vocabulary of English in the surrounding area. Examples include the Hispanic influences on English in areas bordering Mexico, the influences on English of immigrant populations from Asia, and the Native American influences on English in early American settlements (especially with respect to vocabulary, including words such as *raccoon* and *moccasin*).

Population movement, or the migration of persons from one dialect region to another, can affect the maintenance of a dialect in one of two ways. On the one hand, the dialect may begin to vanish in a region that receives an influx of persons from other areas. Such is the case currently for some southern cities: for example, Atlanta, Georgia; Raleigh–Durham, North Carolina; and Charlotte, North Carolina. On the other hand, the dialect may become more pronounced in an area where the cultural and regional identity is strong. For example, the term *fixin'*, which indicates an immediate future action, and the use of double modals, such as *might could* and *useta (used to) could*, remain acceptable grammatical constructions in southern U.S. dialects.

Expanding transportation and communication networks can also affect a regional dialect in the same two ways: It may vanish or it may become more pronounced. Such networks have an impact on once-isolated regions, such as small islands along the eastern seaboard of the United States, which now host tourists from many dialect regions of the country.

Shifting cultural centers also influence dialect change in the United States. Suburban areas are now becoming influential in the development of dialects, just as large urban areas once were. One example of how a large nonurban cultural center can give life to a new regional variety is California English, whose speakers introduced such words as *dude* and *awesome*, as well as the discourse marker *like* to introduce quoted speech rather than using the word *said* (I called my dad and he was *like* "Hey, what have you been up to?" I was *like* "Well, I've been working and studying."). As you study the next section of the chapter, you may be interested to check out an expansive collection of North American English dialects (including many audio samples), maintained by Rick Aschmann, a self-proclaimed collector of dialects, at http://aschmann.net/AmEng/.

Southern Dialects.   Southern dialects are among the more recognizable varieties of American English. Specific southern dialects include Appalachian English, Smoky Mountain dialect, South Carolina dialect, Texas English, New Orleans dialect, and Memphis dialect, although the general dialect of the region is southern American dialect. Southern American dialect differs in its phonology, grammar, and lexicon from other dialects in several ways (Bailey & Tillery, 2006). For example, speakers of southern American dialect pronounce the vowels /ɛ/ and /ɪ/ the same way, which means *pin* and *pen* sound identical (like *pin*). Speakers also use a *monophthong*, or pure vowel sound, in place of a diphthong at the ends of words and prior to voiced consonants such as /d/ and /z/, pronouncing /raɪd/ ("ride") as /raːd/ ("raaad") and /raɪz/ ("rise") as /raːz/ ("raaaz"). Characters in the movie, *Steel Magnolias* speak with a southern American dialect, especially actor, Dolly Parton, who is from Tennessee.

Southern dialects have unique grammatical constructions as well. Some speakers use the contraction *y'all* as a second-person plural pronoun and further use the phrase *all y'all* specifically to acknowledge each individual in a group, as in the sentences *I encourage y'all to visit next summer. I can't wait to see all y'all again.* As mentioned previously, some speakers of southern dialects also use multiple modals

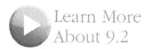

Learn More About 9.2

As you watch the video titled "Example of Southern Dialect", notice the features of the speaker's pronunciation, grammar, and vocabulary.
https://www.youtube.com/watch?v=QUEx1CHZktA

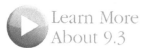

Learn More About 9.3

As you watch the video titled "Example of Appalachian English", notice the features of the speaker's pronunciation, grammar, and vocabulary.
https://www.youtube.com/watch?v=03iwAY4KllU

(*might could, might should, might should oughta*) and the construction *fixin' to*, which indicates an immediate future action, as in *I'm fixin' to call your mother*.

Vocabulary in southern dialects is also distinct. To illustrate, consider the results of Campbell and Plumb's (n.d.) surveys: They showed that speakers of southern dialects often use the word *Coke* to refer to a sweetened carbonated beverage (see Figure 9.1), and the word *sub* to refer to a type of sandwich served on a roll with meats, cheese, lettuce, tomato, and other ingredients (see Figure 9.2).

Northern Dialects. Dialects of the North include New England dialect, Boston dialect, Maine dialect, Pittsburgh dialect, New York City dialect, Philadelphia dialect, and Canadian English. You are likely familiar with the Boston dialect if you have heard reruns of the long-running National Public Radio show, *Car Talk* featuring brothers, Tom and Ray. The late "Mister" Fred Rogers used phonological features common in the Pittsburgh dialect, and Al Pacino is a famous user of the New York City dialect. Distinctive phonological features of northern dialects include dropping postvocalic *r* sounds, as in "cah" for *car* and "yahd" for *yard* (Roberts, Nagy, & Boberg, 2006). Although grammar in northern dialects is not significantly different from that of other regions, some dialects use combinations such as *you all, you guys, youse,* or *y'uns* for the second-person plural pronoun, and Philadelphians specifically eliminate the object of the preposition *with* ("Are you coming with?"; Newman, 2006; Salvucci, 2006). Vocabulary in northern dialects includes such words as *tonic* (Fitzpatrick, 2006) and *soda* (Campbell & Plumb, n.d.) for sweetened carbonated beverages. People of northern dialect regions are also as likely to use the words *grinder, hoagie,* and *hero* as *sub* (see Figure 9.2).

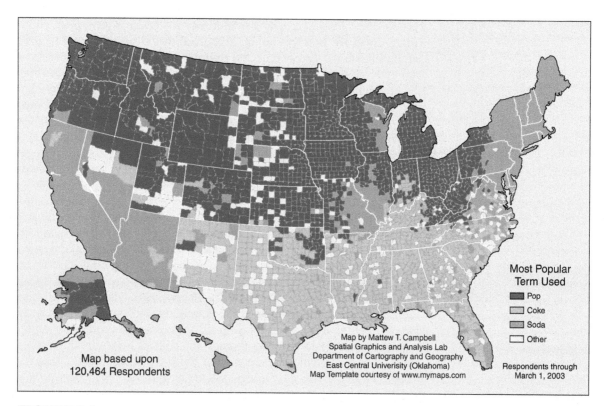

FIGURE 9.1

Names for carbonated beverages by U.S. county.

Source: From "Generic Names for Soft Drinks by County" [Map], by M. T. Campbell and G. Plumb, in *The Great Pop vs. Soda Controversy,* edited by A. McConchie, n.d. Copyright by Matthew T. Campbell and Greg Plumb. Reprinted with permission. Retrieved September 26, 2006, from http://www.popvssoda.com/countystats/total-county.html.

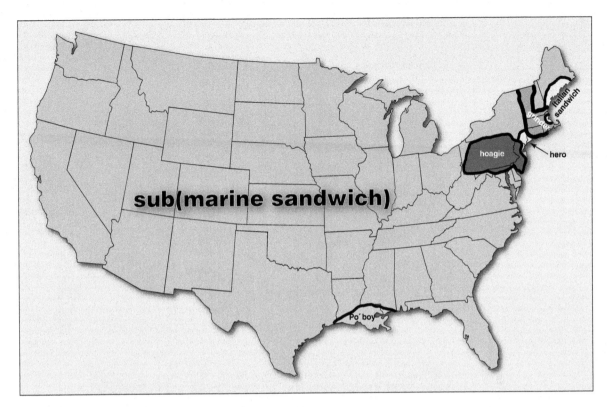

FIGURE 9.2

Sub, grinder, hoagie, or hero?

Source: From "American Dialects," by B. Vaux, in *Let's Go USA 2004*, edited by J. Todd, 2004, New York: St. Martin's Press. Copyright 2004 by Bert Vaux. Reprinted with permission.

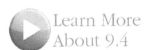

Learn More About 9.4

As you watch the video titled "Example of Boston Dialect", notice the features of the speaker's pronunciation, grammar, and vocabulary. https://www.youtube.com/ watch?v=FiNNsd5Fp80

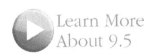

Learn More About 9.5

As you watch the video titled "Example of Pittsburgh Dialect", notice the features of the speaker's pronunciation, grammar, and vocabulary. https://www.youtube.com/ watch?v=BYtTPLit4t4

Midwestern Dialects.   Persons from areas such as Chicago, Illinois, Ohio, St. Louis, Missouri, and Michigan speak midwestern dialects. These dialects, which some people erroneously claim to be accent free or most typical of a "standard" American dialect, actually have phonological, grammatical, and lexical features that differentiate them from other regional dialects. With respect to phonology, midwestern dialects tend to merge the vowel sounds in the words *Don–Dawn, hot–caught, dollar–taller, sock–talk* into a single vowel sound, rendering the words "Don" and "Dawn" virtually indistinguishable. Because of the merging of the vowel sounds in words such as *caught* and *cot*, some people refer to this phenomenon as the caught-cot merger. Figure 9.3 illustrates the caught-cot merger with data from more than 11,000 participants who answered the following question: *Do you pronounce "cot" and "caught" the same?* Another interesting set of mergers is currently occurring within the midwestern dialect, making it more distinctive from other North American dialects. It largely involves the production of six vowels, represented in the words *caught, cot, cat, bit, bet,* and *but* (Gordon, 2006). In such words, the vowels used to distinguish these words are shifting, meaning speakers are pronouncing these sounds with the tongue positioned in a slightly different place in the mouth as compared with speakers in the past. For example, the vowel sound in the word *cat* is shifting to sound more like the vowel sound in the word *bet* or *bit*. As another example, the vowel sound in the word *bet* is shifting to sound more like the vowel sound in the word *but*. This phenomenon is called the *Northern Cities Shift* (NCS) because it is predominant in large cities in the Midwest, such as Buffalo, Cleveland, Chicago, and Detroit (Gordon, 2006). See Figure 9.4 for additional examples of this shift.

Do you pronounce "cot" and "caught" the same?

a. different (60.93%)
b. same (39.07%)
(11050 respondents)

All Results

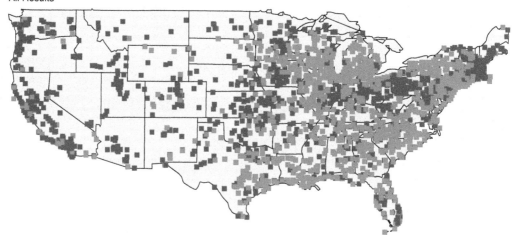

Choice a: different

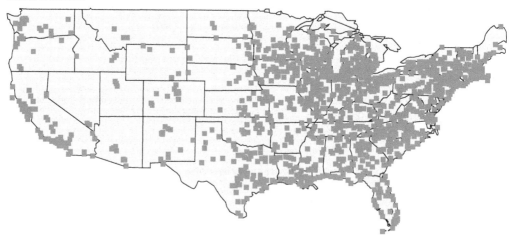

Choice b: same

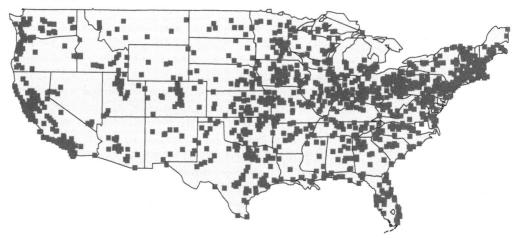

FIGURE 9.3
Maps illustrating the caught-cot merger.

Source: Reprinted by permission from Dr. Bert Vaux.

The Northern Cities Shift

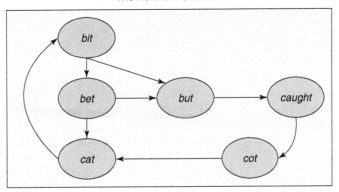

FIGURE 9.4
Vowel changes in the Northern Cities Shift.

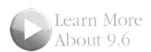

Learn More About 9.6

As you watch the video titled "Example of Midwestern Dialect", notice the features of the speaker's pronunciation, grammar, and vocabulary.
https://www.youtube.com/watch?v=TM72ONyqg9Y

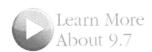

Learn More About 9.7

As you watch the video titled "Example of Michigan Dialect", notice the features of the speaker's pronunciation, grammar, and vocabulary.
https://www.youtube.com/watch?v=Pqhy2ejuGLU

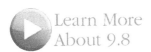

Learn More About 9.8

As you watch the video titled "Example of California English", notice the features of the speaker's pronunciation, grammar, and vocabulary.
https://www.youtube.com/watch?v=duEfACfS-bs

Midwestern dialect grammatical features include the *need/want/like + past participle* construction. For example, a mother leaving her young son with a babysitter for the evening might say, "I'm so sorry that I have to run. Jeremy's diaper needs changed. Buster wants fed, and if he jumps up on your lap, he likes scratched behind the ears."

Western Dialects.   Because the western United States was settled more recently than other regions of the country were, the western dialect area remains largely undefined (Conn, 2006; W. Labov, Ash, & Boberg, 2005). In some respects, western dialects share features with their northern and southern counterparts. Phonologically, many western dialects have a single vowel for the words *caught* and *cot*, as do midwestern dialects. Some western dialects, particularly in California, exhibit *fronted back vowels*, so that *totally* sounds like "tewtally" and *dude* sounds like "diwd" (Conn, 2006). Other western dialects include Utah dialect; Portland, Oregon dialect; and Arizona English.

American English Sociocultural Dialects

Sociocultural dialects differ from geographical dialects of the West, Midwest, North, and South in that they transcend region. Instead, persons from certain socioeconomic classes and cultural orientations speak these dialects. Three examples of sociocultural dialects are African American Vernacular English, Chicano English, and Jewish English.

African American Vernacular English (AAVE) comprises the English dialects that many descendants of enslaved persons speak. AAVE dialects emerged during the period when persons from Africa arrived in the United States. Persons speaking the same African languages were often separated to prevent uprisings. In addition, once the enslaved persons arrived in the United States, they were not permitted to attend schools. As a consequence of these practices, African Americans began to form *pidgins* (discussed later in the chapter), which were combinations of their African languages and the European languages they were exposed to, so they could communicate with their owners and with other enslaved individuals.

AAVE contains many distinct phonological and grammatical regularities (e.g., Baugh, 2006; T. G. Labov, 1998). Speakers may reduce consonant clusters, so that *old* becomes *ol'*, *west* becomes *wes'*, and *kind* becomes *kin'*. Speakers of AAVE may also delete the suffix *-s*—whereby *50 cents* becomes *50 cent*, and *She drives* becomes *She drive*—and the possessive suffix *'s*—so that *my sister's car* becomes *my sister car*. Another common feature of AAVE dialects is phonological

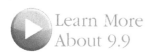

Learn More About 9.9

As you watch the video titled "Example of African American Vernacular English", notice the features of the speaker's pronunciation, grammar, and vocabulary.
https://www.youtube.com/watch?v=Zqohw8nR6qE

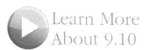

Learn More About 9.10

As you watch the video titled "Example of Chicano English", notice the features of the speaker's pronunciation, grammar, and vocabulary.
https://www.youtube.com/watch?v=p7D0BImQur0

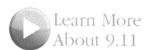

Learn More About 9.11

As you watch the video titled "Example of Miami Dialect", notice the features of the speaker's pronunciation, grammar, and vocabulary.
https://www.youtube.com/watch?v=Y9e84EADpLc

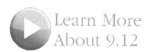

Learn More About 9.12

As you watch the video titled "Example of Jewish English", notice the features of the speaker's pronunciation, grammar, and vocabulary.
https://www.youtube.com/watch?v=hZxcFtBik_U

DISCUSSION POINT

Can you think of some additional phonological, grammatical, and lexical features that characterize the dialect or dialects you speak?

inversion, whereby *ask* becomes *aks*. The AAVE dialect is featured in the speech of the animated characters from *Fat Albert and the Cosby Kids*, which aired from 1978 to 1985. Tracy Jordan, on the television program *30 Rock*, which aired from 2006 to 2013, also exhibits a number of features of AAVE in his character's dialect.

Special grammatical constructions in AAVE include the distinction between habitual and temporary forms of the present progressive and copula *be*. For example, the sentence *Anita be working* is habitual, meaning that Anita works on a regular basis. In comparison, the sentence *Anita working* is temporary, meaning that Anita is working at the time. Another grammatical construction AAVE speakers sometimes use is syntactic alternation, such as "How much it is?"

Chicano English (ChE) is a dialect people of Mexican ethnic origin (generally in California and the Southwest) speak. Although ChE has indicators of contact with Spanish, many ChE speakers are not bilingual and they may not know Spanish at all (Fought, 2003, 2006). In addition to being used in communities such as the Los Angeles area and areas close to the U.S.–Mexican border, ChE has been documented in non-Spanish-speaking midwestern communities (Frazer, 1996). Some features of ChE include final /z/ devoicing in words such as *lies* and *toys*, using a tense-vowel /i/ in place of its lax counterpart in words ending in *-ing* (i.e., pronouncing it as "eeeng"), and using intonation patterns characteristic of Spanish. Another feature of ChE is the use of some Spanish words and phrases, even by speakers who know little Spanish.

There are also a number of dialects that characterize Latino communities in other areas. Some of the more prominent dialects include Puerto Rican English in New York City and Miami dialect (which has influences from Cuba and Nicaragua). A few characteristics of Puerto Rican English include final consonant deletion (e.g., pronouncing the word *boat* as *boa*), cluster reduction (e.g., pronouncing the word *rest* as *res*), and weak syllable deletion (e.g., pronouncing the word *above* as *bove*) (e.g., Goldstein, 2001). Some features of Miami dialect include a heavier /l/ sound than in SAE due to the tongue remaining on the roof of the mouth for a longer duration and fewer vowel sounds than in SAE, which mirror the five vowel sounds of Spanish (e.g., speakers pronounce the word *hand* with a nasal vowel so it sounds like *hahnd*).

The Jewish English dialect is another type of sociocultural dialect. This dialect has characteristics of both the Yiddish and Hebrew languages. Jewish English pronunciation includes a hard *g* sound in words like *singer* (sounds like *finger*), overaspiration of /t/ sounds, and a loud, exaggerated intonation and a fast rate of speech (Bernstein, 2006). Many Jewish English vocabulary words have become a part of mainstream American culture as well, including *schlep, bagel, schmooze, klutz,* and *kosher*. Some celebrities with speech patterns consistent with Jewish English include Jerry Seinfeld, Howard Stern, and the late Joan Rivers.

It is important to recognize that although the use of nonmainstream American English (NMAE) dialects does not indicate a language disorder, children using NMAE dialects may experience greater challenges in learning to read as compared to children who speak mainstream American English (MAE). Some research indicates that when children who speak a nonstandard dialect increase their use of MAE across first and second grade, they experience greater gains in their reading than children whose use of MAE does not increase over these early grades (Terry, Connor, Petscher, & Conlin, 2012). It may be the case that an increasing use of MAE indicates a linguistic awareness or flexibility that is beneficial to learning to read during these early grades when children learn to decode, or translate combinations of written letters into sounds that form words. As we discussed in Chapter 7, children with greater metalinguistic awareness (the ability to think about language as an object of focus) tend to experience an easier time learning to read than children with lesser metalinguistic awareness.

LANGUAGE DIVERSITY AND DIFFERENCES

Nicaraguan Sign Language

The emergence of Nicaraguan Sign Language since the 1970s has presented a unique opportunity to observe the process of language creation and evolution. Before the 1970s, individuals in Nicaragua who were deaf had little contact with one another because of the lack of a unifying national educational system. When individuals who were deaf were finally exposed to one another in the context of schools, they began to form a true deaf community. Because children and adolescents had no common language, to communicate with one another they began to use gestures coupled with any home signs they had. These simple language systems, or *pidgins*, evolved into more complex creoles after new cohorts of children began signing with their older peers.

Evidence that Nicaraguan Sign Language is evolving into an increasingly complex language comes in many forms. One way researchers can study this evolution is by examining the spatial modulations speakers make. *Spatial modulations* are grammatical elements that appear in all sign and spoken languages and perform functions such as indicating number, location, time, and the subject or object of a verb (Senghas & Coppola, 2001). Senghas and Coppola found that newer cohorts of Nicaraguan Sign Language speakers use and understand spatial modulations in ways that earlier users of the language do not. For example, newer cohorts of speakers use spatial modulations to indicate shared reference, whereas their older counterparts do not. Thus, as more generations of children learn Nicaraguan Sign Language, the grammatical specificity and precision of the language improve. Such research provides evidence for the creative and transformational nature of human language and demonstrates the notable role that children can play in language creation.

Pidgins

A *pidgin* is a simplified type of language that develops when speakers who do not share a common language come into prolonged contact. Pidgins have no native speakers; instead, people use them as a second language, particularly when they are conducting business with one another (Southerland, 1997). Pidgins typically use the lexicon of the more dominant of the two languages, and the phonology and syntactic structure of the less dominant language, as is the case for the Hawaiian Pigdin English that Philippine laborers in Hawaii spoke prior to the 1930s (Southerland, 1997). Hawaiian Pidgin English included lexical items of the more dominant language (English), and syntactic structure of the less dominant language (Philippine languages)—for example, by omitting the copula *to be* verb when describing a permanent attribute of a person or an object (e.g., "Da man tall"; "Da lady short").

9.2
Check Your Understanding
Click here to gauge your understanding of the concepts in this section.

Creoles

Pidgins become *creoles* when speakers pass them down through generations as a first language. Creoles continue to evolve and become more elaborate and stable with each new generation of native speakers. Some creoles remain nondominant in their community, whereas others gain status as official languages. See Language Diversity and Differences: *Nicaraguan Sign Language* for a discussion of how Nicaraguan Sign Language evolved among a group of people who did not share a common language.

WHAT ARE BILINGUALISM AND SECOND LANGUAGE ACQUISITION?

According to the 2011 American Community Survey conducted by the U.S. Census Bureau, 21% of people ages 5 years and older reported speaking a language other than English at home. Fifty-eight percent of these people reported speaking English "very well" and another 19% reported speaking English "well" (Ryan, 2013), perhaps because they learned the two (or more) languages simultaneously, or began to learn an additional language within a few years of being born. Other people may have learned English as a second language in school in the United States or as a foreign language in school in another country. Whatever the case, many people living in the United States acquire two or more languages during their lifetime. The generic term for this diverse group of persons is dual language learners (Genesee, Paradis, & Crago, 2004). In this section, we discuss bilingualism, multilingualism, and second language acquisition as important concepts related to language diversity.

Bilingualism and Multilingualism

Bilingualism

Bilingualism is a term that describes the process whereby children essentially acquire *two* first languages. Many young children around the world acquire *more than two* first languages. The term used to describe this process is *multilingualism*. However, for the sake of simplicity, in this text we use the more common term *bilingualism* to describe children who acquire two or more first languages. Some children acquire two or more first languages from birth, whereas others acquire them sequentially.

Simultaneous Bilingualism

With *simultaneous bilingualism*, a child acquires two or more languages from birth, or simultaneously. Simultaneous bilingual children usually receive language input in two or more forms from their parents, grandparents, other close relatives, or child care providers. Simultaneous bilingualism occurs in one of two contexts: A child is part of a majority ethnolinguistic community, or he or she is part of a minority ethnolinguistic community (Genesee et al., 2004). Bilingual children from these two types of communities may experience different degrees of success in acquiring and maintaining proficiency in their two first languages.

A majority ethnolinguistic community is a group that speaks a language the majority of people in an area (e.g., country, state, province) value and assign high social status. The language the majority ethnolinguistic community speaks may be an official language in the community, or it may be the unofficial standard in the community. In general, persons from a majority ethnolinguistic community share cultural and ethnic backgrounds. Examples of majority ethnolinguistic communities include Standard American English (SAE) speakers in the United States, French speakers in France, and German speakers in Germany.

Many children learn more than one language from birth.

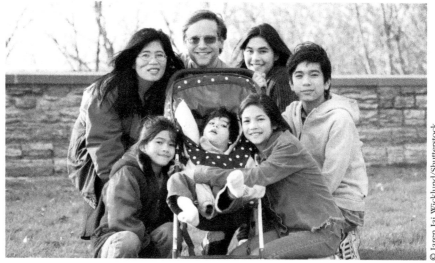

© Jaren Jai Wicklund/Shutterstock

One example of simultaneous bilingualism in a majority ethnolinguistic community would be a young child acquiring both English and French in Montreal, Canada. In Montreal, both English-speaking and French-speaking cultural groups are valued by people in the community. In fact, both languages are the official languages of the province. Children learning both French and English simultaneously in Montreal would likely acquire and maintain equal proficiency in both languages because these children would have the opportunity to use both languages in school, at home, and in the community at such places as the grocery store and the doctor's office.

In contrast to a majority ethnolinguistic community, a minority ethnolinguistic community is a group that speaks a language few people in the community speak or value. Languages that people in minority ethnolinguistic communities speak may have lower social status, and may receive little or no institutional support. Historically, Spanish was considered a minority ethnolinguistic community in the United States, although in many communities that is certainly not the case. For instance, in the Laredo, Texas, metropolitan area, 92% of people speak a language other than English at home—which, in 99% of the cases, is Spanish (Ryan, 2013).

Some children who are simultaneous bilingual individuals in a minority ethnolinguistic community may experience setbacks in acquiring or maintaining the minority language of the community. For instance, in the case of a German–English bilingual family in the United States, the child may hear and speak German only in the home and not in the community, in child care, or in other situations. Without German language input from multiple sources in multiple contexts, the child will most likely begin to use the majority language, English, at the expense of the minority language, German. Shifting to the majority language is common among bilingual children in minority ethnolinguistic communities, especially when they enter formal schooling.

Other children who are simultaneous bilingual individuals in minority ethnolinguistic communities may have more success at maintaining the minority language. For example, although Spanish–English bilingual children in southern California use English in school, they likely use Spanish at home and in their community, where other Spanish speakers live. Support from other people in the minority ethnolinguistic community should increase the chances that children will maintain their bilingualism throughout adulthood.

Sequential Bilingualism

Sequential bilingualism is similar to simultaneous bilingualism in that a child acquires two first languages. The difference is that the child learns the two first languages in succession, usually within the first 3 years of life, before developing proficiency with only one of the languages. Children may acquire two or more languages sequentially rather than simultaneously for two reasons. First, some parents prefer to use a single language from birth and wait to introduce an additional language. Second, input from one language may not be available immediately after birth. For example, a child may start to attend child care with a provider who speaks a different language, or a child's grandparents, who speak a different language, may move to the area after the child has begun to acquire one language. Children who acquire two or more languages sequentially experience the same advantages and setbacks children who acquire multiple languages simultaneously experience, depending on their status in a majority or minority ethnolinguistic community.

Two Systems or One?

Researchers disagree as to whether bilingual children have two separate language systems from the start or begin with a single language system that eventually splits into two. Some time ago, Volterra and Taeschner (1978) proposed that bilingual

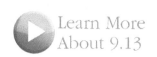

disadvantages

advantages

children begin with a single language system that combines lexical items from both languages they are acquiring. Next, children begin to differentiate between lexical items in the two languages but use a single grammatical system. Finally, between ages 3 and 3.5 years, bilingual children begin to separate both the lexical and the grammatical systems of the two languages. According to the unitary language system hypothesis, then, children are not bilingual until they successfully differentiate between the two languages.

More recently, an opposing viewpoint has emerged countering that bilingual children establish two separate language systems from the outset of language acquisition (Genesee, 1989; Genesee, Nicoladis, & Paradis, 1995). Unlike the unitary language system hypothesis, the dual language system hypothesis does not presuppose that children move through stages whereby they eventually differentiate between two languages. Each hypothesis offers different predictions about how bilingual children's phonology, grammar, and vocabulary should develop. As a result, research into this controversy continues. Genesee and colleagues (2004) suggested that if the unitary language system hypothesis were correct, children would frequently mix words and phrases from both languages without considering the language context or their conversational partners. They would also mix grammatical rules from their two languages, and, most important, their language development would slow to a detrimental pace while they worked to differentiate their two languages.

Research results thus far favor the dual language system hypothesis. For example, a study of 24-month-old German–English bilingual toddlers revealed that their vocabulary size was not inferior to the vocabulary sizes of their monolingual English and monolingual German counterparts (Junker & Stockman, 2002). Furthermore, nearly half of the bilingual toddlers' vocabulary was present in both German and English, which demonstrated that early language separation is possible.

In a separate study in which researchers examined bilingual acquisition across two modalities, three children acquiring Langues des Signes Québécoise (a sign language) and French, and three children acquiring French and English, achieved their early linguistic milestones in each of their languages at the same time and similarly to monolingual children. From the time these bilingual children uttered their first words or used their first signs, they also produced a substantial number of semantically corresponding words in each of their two languages, which demonstrated language separation from an early age. Another way the bilingual children demonstrated language separation was by modifying their language choices, depending on the listener (Petitto, Katerelos, et al., 2001).

Code Switching

A common phenomenon among bilingual individuals is code switching, or *code mixing*. In this process, speakers who have more than one language alternate between the languages. The character, Gloria on the TV show, *Modern Family* uses code switching when she incorporates words and phrases from her native language, Spanish. When the alternation occurs within a single utterance, it is called intrautterance mixing (or, within one sentence, *intrasentential mixing*). These two examples were produced by Isabella, a 3-year-old Spanish–English bilingual speaker (Arias & Lakshmanan, 2005):

1. bueno porque le gusta decir hi sweety good morning

2. We playing mommies, daddies, babies, hermanas.

When the alternation occurs between utterances, it is called interutterance mixing (or, between sentences, *intersentential mixing*). When engaging in code switching, bilingual persons may mix smaller units of language, such as phonemes, inflectional morphemes, and lexical items, or they may mix larger items such as

Learn More About 9.13

As you watch the video titled "Code Switching", notice how the adults switch back and forth effortlessly between English and Japanese and how they tend to use Japanese for direct quotes from a Japanese speaker and for Japanese vocabulary (e.g., gyoza).

https://www.youtube.com/watch?v=qLbQrVvGqw0

phrases and clauses. Children tend to use interutterance mixing more often than intrautterance mixing, especially in the one-word and two-word stages of development (Genesee et al., 2004). This pattern shifts as children develop because as utterances increase in length and grammatical complexity, children have more opportunities to engage in intrautterance mixing. See Table 9.1 for examples of code switching involving different elements of language.

Bilingual children may engage in code switching for three main reasons. One is that children code switch to fill in lexical or grammatical gaps. Evidence for such code switching comes in at least two forms (Genesee et al., 2004). First, children tend to code switch more often while using their less proficient language. Thus, they may code switch to draw on the strengths in their more proficient language when they lack a grammatical construction or lexical item in their less proficient language. Second, children tend to code switch more often when they do not know a translation equivalent for a word, regardless of whether they are using their more proficient or less proficient language.

Another reason bilingual children may code switch is for pragmatic effect (Genesee et al., 2004). For example, they may code switch to emphasize the importance of what they are saying, to convey emotion, or to quote what someone else said in another language.

Third, and finally, bilingual children may engage in code switching according to the social norms of their community. For instance, certain communities may engage in code switching to demonstrate that they belong to two cultures. Children learn to follow the code-switching patterns of the adults who surround them—for example, by engaging in code switching more often in casual and informal situations than in public and formal contexts.

> **DISCUSSION POINT**
>
> Try to produce a few examples of code switching from languages that you know. For instance, if you know a few phrases in Spanish or German, embed these in English to see what you come up with.

[handwritten margin note: reasons for code switching w/ bilingual children]

TABLE 9.1

Zentella's (1997) examples of bilingual code switching in Spanish and English

MIXED ELEMENT OF LANGUAGE	EXAMPLE	TRANSLATION[a]	PAGE NO. IN ZENTELLA (1997)
Phoneme	"*he*"	/xi/, like the *ch* sound in Bach	291
Lexical item	"It's already full, *mira.*"	"look"	119
Object noun phrase	"*Tú estás metiendo your big mouth.*"	"You're butting in"	118
Subject noun phrase	"*Tiene dos strings, una chiringa.*"	"It has two"	118
Independent clause with coordinating conjunction	"My father took him to the ASPCA *y lo mataron.*"	"and they killed him"	118
Subordinate clause without subordinate conjunction	"Because *yo lo dije.*"	"I said it"	118

[a]Translation is of the italicized element in the Example column.

Second Language Acquisition
Second language acquisition

Second language acquisition (SLA), or L2 acquisition, is the process by which children who have already established a solid foundation in their first language (L1) learn an additional language. Second language acquisition usually takes place in the context of a school, either as the majority language for a particular community or as a foreign language. Some researchers use the term instructed second language acquisition (ISLA) to differentiate L2 acquisition that occurs as a result of instruction as opposed to acquisition that occurs implicitly from exposure to authentic L2 input (e.g., Loewen, 2015). As with bilingualism, success at acquiring a second language and maintaining an L1 or L2 depends on a number of factors, including whether an individual is part of a majority or a minority ethnolinguistic community.

A number of developmental processes and influences characterize L2 acquisition (see Hummel, 2014, for a thorough synthesis of common processes and influences), including transfer, interlanguage, overgeneralization, formulaic language, and avoidance.

Transfer is the influence of one's L1 on his or her L2 development. For example, with respect to phonology, Spanish speakers learning English may exhibit spirantization, whereby the stop sound in the English word *caddy* sounds more like the fricative sound in the word *Cathy*. With respect to syntax, Spanish speakers learning English may reverse the order of adjectives and nouns, consistent with Spanish word order (e.g., *the store new* instead of *the new store*). In some cases, greater similarity between an L1 and L2 can lead to greater transfer of L1 features to the L2 (including syntax, semantics, phonology, morphology, and pragmatics). In other cases, greater similarity between an L1 and L2 may lead to less transfer of L1 features to the L2 (possibly because the learner does not believe certain structures work similarly in the L1 and L2), so research has not been fully conclusive as to the predictability of language transfer.

During the process of L2 acquisition, speakers create a language system called an interlanguage that represents the learner's evolving second language knowledge, patterns, and rules. Other terms that characterize an L2 learner's developing language system include learner language, approximative system, and idiosyncratic dialect (Hummel, 2014). The interlanguage includes elements of the L1 and the L2, as well as elements found in neither of the two languages (Gass & Selinker, 2001). For example, evidence of L1 phonology and syntax in the L2 is often evident in the interlanguage (see Table 9.2). In addition to phonology and syntax, one's interlanguage is also evident in morphological, semantic, and pragmatic aspects of language. Depending on a person's exposure to and education in the L2, linguistic forms of the interlanguage may stabilize with time. Language stabilization occurs once the interlanguage stops evolving and L2 learners reach a plateau in their language development. Gass and Selinker (2001) cautioned that because of a lack of research on the extent to which L2 learners experience temporary or permanent plateaus in their development, practitioners should avoid using the term *language fossilization*. To say a student's language has become fossilized conveys that the student is no longer making progress in his or her L2 acquisition, or that that student is permanently trapped in the interlanguage. Regardless of whether an L2 learner stabilizes in his or her development, considering the notion of interlanguage is still important in order to understand the process by which L2 learners transition to a new system, including their potential struggles and errors. See Research Paradigms: *Methods for Studying Second Language Learning* for an overview of several methods for investigating L2 learning.

Overgeneralization is a developmental process we discussed in Chapter 5, with regard to word learning. Overgeneralization also occurs in second language acquisition and refers to situations when a learner incorrectly overextends or applies rules in the L2, such as using the past tense ending -ed with irregular verbs as in, "We *drinked* it."

TABLE 9.2

Examples of L1 influences on the L2

L1	L2	EXAMPLE	EXPLANATION
French	English	"I have ([aev]) no money."	French does not have the phoneme /h/, so the interlanguage of many speakers does not include it.
German	English	"I have ([haef]) no money."	German changes the /v/ in a syllable-final position to /f/, so the interlanguage of many speakers includes this feature.
English	Spanish	"Caro" ([karo]) "Carro" ([karo])	English has neither the tapped /r/ sound nor the trilled /r/ sound that Spanish has, so speakers usually substitute /r/.
German	English	"I bring not the children."	German places negative markers after the verb in the main clause of the sentence.
Italian	English	"How many years you have?"	Some languages (such as Spanish and Italian) describe age in terms of "how many years one has" instead of "how old one is."

L1 = first language; L2 = second language.

Using formulaic language is another developmental process that occurs in second language acquisition, and describes a learner's use of certain language routines or phrases that exist as a unit rather than as individual pieces the learner compiles for meaning. For example, an L2 learner might memorize phrases such as, "How do you say . . . ?" or "I don't know" to ask for assistance or respond to others, rather than constructing the phrases using his or her knowledge of the L2 grammar and vocabulary.

Avoidance is another common developmental process in L2 acquisition and describes when a learner avoids using sounds, words, or grammatical constructions he or she finds to be difficult or does not know. For example, although the first author (K.T.) studied Spanish in classroom settings for more than 10 years, she still avoids using the subjunctive mood (which expresses doubt, uncertainty, and conveys subjectivity) in conversations because she does not have as strong of a grasp on the subjunctive as the indicative mood (which expresses factual information, certainty, and conveys objectivity).

Attitudes and Policies Regarding Dual Language Instruction

Dual language instruction has been an important consideration throughout history. In ancient times, when written materials were scarce, students who wanted to read widely had to learn more than a single language (Lessow-Hurley, 1990). Ancient societies thus valued and endorsed dual language instruction. In later times, dual language instruction became important for religious purposes. For example, Latin remained the language of worship for Catholics, and Hebrew persisted as the language of worship for Jews, well after people ceased to use these languages in their homes and communities. In more modern times, dual language instruction has endured in most areas of the world, especially in countries with official bilingualism, such as Canada, Israel, and Belgium.

The United States, too, has a history of changing attitudes and policies regarding dual language instruction (Lessow-Hurley, 1990). For example, in the 19th century, Native American tribes often provided dual language instruction to their

RESEARCH **PARADIGMS**

Methods for Studying Second Language Learning

As with measuring L1 acquisition, researchers who study L2 acquisition can measure productive language competence in qualitative ways, such as with naturalistic observations, and in quantitative ways, such as with normative tests and measures. Performance data can be elicited from L2 learners in at least a dozen ways, as summarized by Larsen-Freeman and Long (1991, pp. 27–30):

1. Reading aloud: Participants read aloud word lists, sentences, or passages containing sounds under investigation.

2. Structured exercises: Participants perform grammatical manipulations by completing fill-in-the-blank, sentence-rewrite, sentence-combining, or multiple-choice activities that contain the morphemes or syntactic patterns under investigation.

3. Completion task: Participants hear or read the beginning of a sentence and then complete the sentence in their own words.

4. Elicited imitation: Participants hear sentences containing the structure under investigation and then repeat or reconstruct the sentence.

5. Elicited translation: Participants translate sentences from their L1 into their L2.

6. Guided composition: Participants tell a story, or write a composition on the basis of a set of stimuli, such as pictures.

7. Question and answer (with stimulus): Participants view pictures and then answer questions that elicit particular target forms.

8. Reconstruction: Participants read, listen to, or watch a story and then retell the story in their own words.

9. Communication games: Participants play a game, sometimes with a native speaker. They may use materials designed to elicit particular language forms.

10. Role-play: Participants engage in a role-play with a researcher that focuses on target speech acts.

11. Oral interview: Researchers orally interview a participant. They may constrain the interview topic to elicit a particular structure or may allow the participant to choose the topic of conversation.

12. Free composition: Participants write a composition on a given topic.

students. German communities in the Midwest also instituted dual language programs with success and support until the onset of World War I, when such programs began to collapse around the country as a result of intense feelings of nationalism. Consequently, dual language programs were virtually nonexistent between World War I and World War II. Not until the advent of the Cold War and the civil rights movement, did dual language instruction regain importance in the United States, although it remains controversial in many communities and school systems.

English as a Second Language

Learning *English as a second language* (ESL) occurs when a person who speaks *a first language* other than English then learns English in the context of an English-speaking country, such as England or the United States. Sometimes people refer to learning *English as an additional language* (EAL) when a person who speaks *two or more languages* subsequently learns English. Within U.S. schooling, the term English language learner (ELL) or English learner (EL) is often used to describe children identified as having limited English proficiency.

According to the *Local Education Agency Universe Survey, 2011–12*, the number of public school students in the United States who are ELLs was roughly 4.4 million, or 9.1% of students in the 2011–12 school year. In that same school year, states where 10% or more of public school students were English language learners included Alaska, California, Colorado, Hawaii, Nevada, New Mexico, Oregon, and Texas. ELL students constituted 23.2% of public school enrollment in California (U.S. Department of Education, National Center for Education Statistics, 2015).

The U.S. Department of Education, and the U.S. Department of Justice (2015) have provided joint guidance to state education agencies, public school districts, and public schools concerning their legal obligation to ensure English learner (EL) students can participate meaningfully and equally in educational programs. For example, school districts must have procedures for identifying potential EL students and assessing the English language proficiency of those students who are English learners using valid and reliable measures. School districts may choose from among programs for instructing EL students as long as the program is theoretically sound and effective in practice and must make appropriate language assistance services available to all EL students.

There is a good deal of controversy in the United States as to whether instruction for ELLs, particularly the large number of Spanish-speaking ELLs, should be delivered in English, Spanish, or a combination (bilingual). In some states, such as California via its 1998 Proposition 227, educational policy stipulates that English should be the official and only language of instruction. This means that all children, regardless of their English-language skills, must receive instruction using an immersion paradigm in which they are exposed only to English. Regardless of such English-oriented policies, research does not necessarily support the benefits of immersion orientations over bilingual orientations. Generally speaking, an immersion orientation is based on the premise that there is no benefit in delaying English instruction for students who must learn English, whereas a bilingual orientation is based on the premise that children should solidify skills in their native language and then transition to English. This is one area in which educational policy does not seem to reflect research findings, at least for English-only instruction. This is because the accumulated research on the benefits of immersion versus bilingual approaches, at least as applied to ELLs in the United States, indicates that bilingual approaches are more effective (Slavin & Cheung, 2005).

When children who have limited, or no English proficiency arrive in classrooms where English is the language of instruction, they usually progress through four early stages in their L2 development (Tabors, 1997, cited in Genesee et al., 2004).

Some schools have dual language instruction programs in which students are schooled in two or more languages throughout the day.

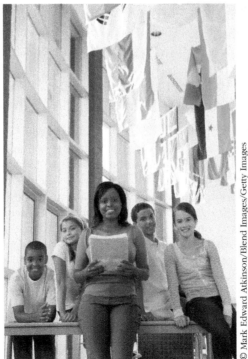

© Mark Edward Atkinson/Blend Images/Getty Images

In the first stage, the home language stage, children use their home language (L1) in the classroom with other children and adults. Children generally do not persist in using their home language for long because they soon realize that doing so does not promote successful communication with other people.

In the second stage, the nonverbal period, children produce little to no language as they begin to acquire their L2 receptively. Some children in the nonverbal period use gestures, such as pointing, to communicate until they have acquired a sufficient number of words in their L2. Older children remain in the nonverbal period from a few weeks to a few months, but younger children usually remain nonverbal for longer periods.

In the third stage, the period of telegraphic and formulaic use, children begin to imitate other people, use single words to label items, and use simple phrases that they memorize. During this period, although children are producing language, they cannot create sentences for a wide variety of communicative functions. Rather, they can express a limited variety of functions, such as requesting ("Please"), negating ("No, I don't know"), affirming ("Yes"), and commenting ("Very good"), among others.

In the fourth stage, the period of language productivity, children are not yet proficient speakers of their L2; however, their communicative repertoire continues to expand. During this stage, children begin to create simple S–V–O (subject–verb–object) sentences, and they rely heavily on the general all-purpose verbs, or GAP verbs, *make*, *do*, and *go*. For example, preschoolers learning ESL may say "I make picture," "I do that too," or "I go home."

English as a Foreign Language

English as a foreign language (EFL) differs from ESL in that children, adolescents, and adults learn English in a non-English-speaking country. Persons learning EFL have a number of reasons for doing so, including establishing oral proficiency in order to engage in business transactions with English-speaking counterparts and establishing grammatical proficiency to increase their chances of being accepted into an English-speaking institution of higher learning. In some countries, native English speakers are employed as EFL teachers, but many teachers have learned EFL themselves. Mixed opinions surround decisions to hire nonnative English speakers as EFL teachers.

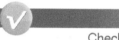

9.3

Check Your Understanding

Click here to gauge your understanding of the concepts in this section.

WHAT ARE SOME THEORIES OF SECOND LANGUAGE ACQUISITION AND THEIR IMPLICATIONS FOR PRACTICE?

As with more general theories about language development, L2 acquisition theories consist of explanatory statements, accepted principles, and methods of analyzing language acquisition. However, L2 acquisition theories differ from L1 development theories in a unique way. Whereas humans begin to acquire their L1 from birth, they may not begin to learn a second language until several years later, possibly even as adults. Thus, theories of L2 acquisition must account for a host of additional variables, both internal to and external to the learner, that influence one's acquisition of second and foreign languages. In this section of the chapter, we provide an overview of some nurture-inspired, nature-inspired, and interactionist theories of L2 acquisition and their implications for second language instruction. Some of these theories were more prominent in the past (and may have only limited relevance to second language instruction today), whereas others have stronger implications for current second language instruction practice. We also discuss more current syntheses of research findings concerning practices for teaching English learner students.

Nurture-Inspired Theories
Contrastive Analysis

Recall that nurture-inspired theories of language development emphasize the notion that humans gain knowledge through experience and exposure to language forms. Following, we detail a nurture-inspired theory of L2 learning, the contrastive analysis hypothesis.

Principles.   Language structures are language units, or forms one can observe directly. The contrastive analysis hypothesis posits that a learner will acquire language structures easily when the structures are similar in the two languages and will experience difficulty acquiring language structures when they differ in the two languages. This process is called L1 interference. Because the contrastive analysis hypothesis is a nurture-inspired theory, proponents believe L1 acquisition and L2 acquisition are similar processes, both of which benefit from imitation, practice, repetition, and reinforcement of language behavior.

Implications for L2 Instruction.   Given that L1 interference makes it difficult for learners to acquire L2 structures, one implication for L2 instruction is a process called contrastive analysis. Contrastive analysis involves performing a structural analysis by identifying aspects of the L1 and L2 that differ. The learner would then focus on practicing the aspects of the L2 that differ so as to avoid reinforcing behaviors or habits from the L1. The learner would also work to replace L1 habits with L2 habits. Contrastive analysis was especially prevalent in the 1950s and 1960s, when behaviorist theories were also more widespread. Another implication for instruction (which may be more common today) is performing contrastive analysis in a more simplified manner to help identify and explain errors in a learner's L2.

Nature-Inspired Theories

Recall that nature-inspired theories of language development assert that an individual's underlying language system is in place at birth and that he or she extracts rules about his or her native language apart from other cognitive abilities. Next, we describe two nature-inspired theories of L2 learning that emphasize how humans have relatively little influence over the process and order by which they learn the rules of their L2, universal grammar and the monitor model.

Universal Grammar
Principles.   Recall from Chapter 4 that universal grammar (UG) is the system of grammatical rules and constraints that are consistent among all world languages. UG is a nature-inspired theory of L2 acquisition because its underlying premise is that an innate, species-specific module is dedicated solely to language and not other forms of learning. Proponents of UG argue that as with L1 acquisition, L2 learners acquire elements of language that other people cannot teach and that input alone cannot provide. For example, native speakers use sentence fragments, false starts, and other forms of language that are "imperfect," yet L2 learners can still demonstrate adequate performance in many cases. UG theory also suggests that adolescents and adults may experience difficulty in acquiring their L2. Lenneberg (1967, as cited in Danesi, 2003) made this claim explicit in his critical period hypothesis, which states that the critical period for language acquisition spans the period between birth and puberty.

Implications for L2 Instruction.   UG probably has the fewest instructional implications of all L2 acquisition theories. Unlike nurture-inspired and interactionist theories of L2 acquisition, UG does not have implications for communication context, student motivation, or external input that is gained through interactions with other people. Instead, UG has implications for understanding the errors L2 learners make as they acquire their second language and for the natural order by which they acquire specific language structures.

Monitor Model

Principles.   The *monitor model* of L2 acquisition (Krashen, 1985) consists of five underlying hypotheses: (a) the acquisition-learning hypothesis, (b) the monitor hypothesis, (c) the natural order hypothesis, (d) the input hypothesis, and (e) the affective filter hypothesis:

1. The *acquisition-learning hypothesis* states that two independent systems are crucial to L2 learning performance: the acquired system and the learned system. The acquired system is an unconscious system by which L2 learners acquire language through natural communicative interactions with other people, similar to the way young children acquire their L1. In comparison, the *learned system* is the result of a conscious process through which L2 learners gain knowledge of the rules of their L2.

2. The *monitor hypothesis* explains the relation of the learned system to the acquired system. The monitor plans, edits, and corrects utterances that the acquired system initiates when the L2 learner has sufficient time to think, focuses on correctness, and knows the rule he or she is trying to express. Krashen (1985) suggested that L2 learners should make only minimal use of the monitor and instead rely as much as possible on the acquired system.

3. The *natural order hypothesis* suggests L2 learners acquire grammatical structures in a natural and predictable sequence. This order does not vary according to instruction but is the result of the acquired system.

4. The *input hypothesis* states that L2 learners move forward in their competence by receiving input that is just slightly ahead of their current state of grammatical knowledge, or comprehensible input. Krashen's (1985) theory suggests language that contains structures an L2 learner has already mastered will not help his or her acquisition, nor will input that is too difficult for him or her. Instead, input should ideally be at the $i + 1$ level, where i = the learner's current state of knowledge.

5. The *affective filter hypothesis* states that "filters" exist that may prevent L2 learners from processing input and thus prevent acquisition. These affective filters include such factors as low motivation, negative attitude, poor self-confidence, and anxiety. The affective filters may account for individual variation in L2 acquisition, and Krashen (1985) contended that young children experience more success with L2 acquisition because they do not have affective filters to inhibit learning.

Implications for L2 Instruction.   The *natural approach* (Terrell, 1977, cited in Danesi, 2003) is an L2 teaching approach that stems from Krashen's (1985) monitor model. To use the natural approach, teachers must help ensure that students' affective filters are "down" and not "up." When students' affective filters are down, they should have more success acquiring comprehensible input from their teacher because they are not thinking about the possibility of failure. Teachers should also introduce grammar and other formal structures only so that students can use this information to "monitor" or make corrections to the output that results from their "acquired" system. Finally, and most important, teachers should ensure that the input they provide is comprehensible in order to push students to increasingly higher levels of competence in their L2.

Interactionist Theories

Recall from Chapter 4, that interactionist theories include characteristics of both nature- and nurture inspired theories. In this section, we describe two interactionist theories of L2 acquisition, one that emphasizes cognitive factors necessary for learning, and one that focuses on the importance of social interactions to L2 learning.

Cognitive Theory with Attention-Processing Model

Principles. The cognitive theory of L2 acquisition rests on five principles that relate to the learner's mental and intellectual functioning (H. D. Brown, 2001). The first principle is that *automaticity* helps account for how L2 learners can acquire language without truly "thinking" about it. According to this principle, L2 learners acquire language subconsciously by using it meaningfully; focusing not on the *forms* of language, but on its *uses*; processing an unlimited number of language forms efficiently and automatically; and resisting the temptation to analyze language forms. Overanalyzing language and consciously lingering on language rules may negatively affect automaticity.

The second principle is that by engaging in *meaningful learning*, L2 learners assimilate new information into their existing memory structures. Engaging in such learning is similar to the cognitive process Piaget called *assimilation*.

The third principle of cognitive theory stems from Skinner's behaviorist principle of operant conditioning (see Chapter 4) and involves the *anticipation of reward*. That is, one factor that drives L2 learners to act or "behave" is anticipation of a reward—either tangible or intangible, and either immediate or long term.

In contrast to the anticipation-of-reward principle, the fourth principle of cognitive theory involves *intrinsic motivation*: The motivation stems from within the L2 learner. In other words, the process of learning an L2 can be rewarding in and of itself, so the learner does not need external rewards.

The fifth, and final, principle concerns *strategic investment*. According to this principle, the L2 learner personally invests time, effort, and attention to L2 learning by using the strategies for understanding and producing language that he or she brings to the learning process.

Implications for L2 Instruction. On the basis of cognitive theory, L2 teachers should consider the following implications (H. D. Brown, 2001):

Principle 1: Automaticity. To foster automaticity in L2 acquisition, teachers should aim to avoid overwhelming students with excess explicit attention to grammar, phonology, and discourse. Teachers need not avoid teaching these formal aspects of language altogether, but when they do provide instruction in these areas, the goal should be to help students process and use language automatically and fluently. As an alternative, teachers should focus much of the lessons on language pragmatics, or how to use language purposefully in genuine contexts and with a variety of functions. Teachers should also recognize that students require time to use language fluently and with automaticity, and exercise patience throughout this process.

Principle 2: Meaningful Learning. To address the principle of meaningful learning, L2 teachers should design instruction to appeal to students' interests and academic and career goals. Teachers should also draw on students' existing background knowledge as a way to facilitate the processes of assimilation and accommodation when introducing new material. Finally, teachers should avoid rote-learning exercises, such as drilling and memorization.

Principle 3: Anticipation of Reward. To address the principle of anticipation of reward, L2 teachers might infuse a liberal amount of oral praise in their instruction so students maintain their confidence. They might also show excitement and enthusiasm in the classroom and encourage students to complement and support one another. Teachers might incorporate short-term reminders of progress (such as progress charts), especially for younger learners, to help students recognize their personal development and achievements. Finally, L2 teachers should help learners understand the long-term benefits of learning their second language.

Principle 4: Intrinsic Motivation. To address the principle of intrinsic motivation, L2 teachers should consider students' intrinsic motives and design activities

Some second language learners are particularly motivated to learn, such as travelers to a foreign country.

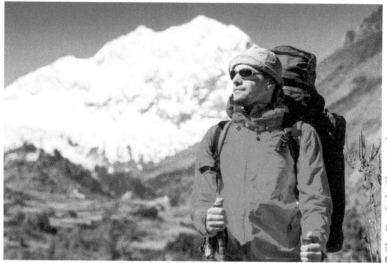

© Olga Danylenko/Shutterstock

that appeal to those motivations. For example, if students derive a great sense of satisfaction from recognizing that they can meet their communication needs in an authentic communication setting, the teacher might structure some activities to promote authentic conversations with native speakers of the language students are learning.

Principle 5: Strategic Investment. To address the principle of strategic investment, teachers should consider students' learning preferences when designing lessons and use variety of techniques (e.g., group work, individual work, visual presentation, auditory presentation) to accommodate all students' learning preferences. For example, some students might benefit from watching videos or movies in the L2 as a way to gain additional language input, whereas other students might benefit from engaging in online discussion forums with native speakers as a way to practice communicating in their L2.

Interaction Hypothesis

Principles.   The *interaction hypothesis* for L2 learning is similar to Vygotsky's social-interactionist theory of L1 development (see Chapter 4) in that it rests on the communicative interactions between an L2 learner and other people. Both the sender and the receiver in communicative interactions are responsible for the success of their communication, and the interaction hypothesis accounts for the importance of this communication dynamic. The interaction hypothesis emphasizes the L2 learner's opportunities to negotiate for meaning during conversations by, for example, making modifications to speech, using repetition, and clarifying often during a conversation.

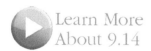

Learn More About 9.14

As you watch the video titled "Total Physical Response", notice how the instructor uses a great deal of repetition, gestures, mimes, and drawings to promote children's comprehension of the phrases that are the target of the lesson. https://www.youtube.com/watch?v=bkMQXFOqyQA

Implications for L2 Instruction.   Advocates of the interaction hypothesis would recommend a focus on communicative strategies that speakers use to carry out specific language functions during interactions with others. Teachers should encourage students to practice selecting and using language forms that are appropriate for specific communicative situations. For example, students could engage in role play to request information ("I'm looking for the art museum. Could you tell me the easiest way to walk there from the train station?"), complain ("This is not what I ordered. Would you exchange it for the correct item?), or share an opinion ("This is one of my favorite restaurants. Let me tell you about it…"), among many other communication functions. Teachers should also have students practice using language with both peers and nonpeers (e.g., adults, teachers) in a range of contexts to support language development.

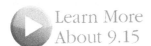

Learn More About 9.15

Watch the video titled "Language Immersion Program", for an example of an immersion program that instructs English-speaking children entirely in Chinese. https://www.youtube.com/watch?v=ZkAXbuNtcmE

Other Theories

Many other theories of L2 acquisition exist, and although we do not discuss them in this book, you should be aware of their considerable influence on L2 teaching approaches, methods, and techniques. For one example, see Theory to Practice: *Suggestopedia*, which describes a neurolinguistic method of L2 teaching. Danesi (2003) aptly summarized the dilemma of bridging the gap between theory and practice in second language instruction:

> Some teachers now reject the reformist theory-into-practice paradigm completely, since no scientifically-designed pedagogical method has ever proven itself to be universally effective. … Yet, despite the many successes that have been documented for contemporary immersion and languages-across-the-curriculum approaches, the search for appropriate classroom pedagogy goes on relentlessly. (p. 3)

What Practices Does Research Support for EL Students?

Given the many theories of second language acquisition and the implications for a number of wide-ranging instructional practices, it may be challenging for practitioners to discern how to best facilitate second language acquisition for students learning English as their second language. As we described in Chapter 4, researchers may test theories of language development repeatedly with an array of scientific methods. Moreover, it is essential to do so before making claims about the efficacy or effectiveness of any instructional methods or strategies stemming from a particular theory. In the field of education, as in the field of medicine, randomized controlled trials (RCTs) are the gold standard for determining the effects of an intervention, program, or policy. RCTs are highly controlled and involve random assignment to treatment and comparison groups. When random assignment to treatment and control groups is not possible, it is important that researchers incorporate other controls to minimize bias and offer a high degree of reliability and validity. In an effort to make practitioners aware of potentially efficacious and effective instructional methods, some organizations and individual researchers evaluate existing high-quality education research and provide recommendations for practitioners to consider when making evidence-based decisions about curricula and programs (e.g., What Works Clearinghouse; http://ies.ed.gov/ncee/wwc/).

In that vein, Coleman and Goldenberg (2012) and Goldenberg (2008) created recommendations for instructing EL students based on two major reviews of EL research completed in 2006 (the National Literacy Panel and the Center for Research on Education, Diversity, and Excellence). They summarize the research findings in three major points: (1) Teaching students to read in their L1 promotes higher levels of reading achievement in English; (2) Principles of good instruction and curriculum for EL students mirror principles of good instruction and curriculum for all students, in general; and (3) When instructing EL students in English, teachers must modify instruction in an effort to address students' language limitations.

It is important that EL students receive two types of instruction in school. The first type of instruction is content area instruction, which L1 English speakers receive as well. The second type of instruction is English language development (ELD) instruction. Coleman and Goldenberg (2012) explain that providing content area instruction for EL students is similar in many ways to providing effective instruction for L1 English speakers. For example, both L1 and L2 speakers presumably benefit from having access to clear goals and objectives for all lessons, well-structured tasks, adequate practice, opportunities to interact with other students, and frequent assessment and reteaching, as a few examples.

Although principles of good instruction apply to both EL students and native English speakers, instructors can also make a number of modifications to content

THEORY TO PRACTICE

Suggestopedia

Suggestopedia is an L2 learning method that emerged during the 1970s (Lozanov, 1979, cited in H. D. Brown, 2001). It stems from learning theories that emphasize optimal conditions for the learner (i.e., relaxed state of consciousness), integration of the five senses in learning, and judicious integration of the right hemisphere of the brain through the use of visual images, color, music, and creativity. Language classes using Suggestopedia include four main stages:

Stage 1. Presentation: In the first stage, the teacher prepares students to relax and to adopt a positive frame of mind for learning.

Stage 2. First Concert—"Active Concert": In this stage, the teacher presents language material for students to learn. For example, the teacher may perform a dramatic reading of text and accompany the reading with classical music.

Stage 3. Second Concert—"Passive Review": In this stage, the teacher invites students to relax and listen to Baroque music. The teacher then reads the text quietly in the background as the music plays. This method is supposed to enable students to acquire new material effortlessly.

Stage 4. Practice: In the final stage, students use games and puzzles to review what they have learned. As a homework assignment, students cursorily read the material from the day's lesson once before going to bed and once again first thing in the morning.

area instruction to assist students learning English, such as (Coleman & Goldenberg, 2012): (1) targeting both language objectives and content objectives in all lessons; (2) employing instruction and expectations that are clear, focused, and systematic; (3) using visuals, charts, and diagrams to promote comprehension; (4) using a student's primary language for support, such as using cognates, or words that appear similar in one's L1 and L2 and mean the same thing (e.g., familia – family); (5) selecting reading material with content familiar to students; and (6) providing opportunities for extra practice and repetition with material.

Coleman and Goldenberg recommend that content area instruction and ELD instruction complement one another. With regard to ELD instruction, they propose a number of practical recommendations, including: (1) providing daily language instruction that includes explicit teaching of English vocabulary, syntax, and conventions, conversational conventions, and language learning strategies (e.g., taking notes; summarizing); (2) providing academic language instruction in vocabulary, syntax, and text structures common to content areas (e.g., the concept of comparing and contrasting); (3) encouraging structured student talk by posing open-ended questions and prompting students to use a specific vocabulary word or sentence structure; (4) allowing sufficient duration of services by continuing ELD instruction until students have reached at least an advanced intermediate level of proficiency (or possibly an advanced or native-like proficiency); (5) grouping EL students carefully and tailoring instruction to their language-learning needs; and (6) encouraging verbal interaction with English speakers, especially within the context of academic tasks and structured practice.

As with children who speak nonmainstream dialects and children learning more than one language at once (i.e., bilingualism), it is important to recognize that language acquisition may vary for children learning English as a second language and that they may differ significantly from native English speakers in their attainment of English language milestones. Factors such age, the age at which a student began instruction in English, and his or her socioeconomic background are also related to an EL student's language skills over time (e.g., Morrow, Goldstein, Gilhool, & Paradis, 2014; Jackson, Schatschneider, & Leacox, 2014). In the final chapter, we discuss the concept of language disorder and describe how professionals differentiate aspects of language diversity from language disorders.

✓ 9.4

Check Your Understanding

Click here to gauge your understanding of the concepts in this section.

SUMMARY

This chapter emphasizes the importance of understanding diversity in language development. The chapter begins with a discussion of the close connection between language and culture. We discuss infant-directed speech as an example of a type of communication accommodation adults make and describe how communicative accommodations range from highly child centered to highly situation centered, according to cultural norms. In the next section, we examine dialects, which are the regional or social varieties of language that differ from one another in terms of pronunciation, vocabulary, and grammar. American English is characterized by a number of dialects, including regional and sociocultural dialects. We also discuss the process of language evolution and change through pidgins and creoles.

Bilingualism is a term that describes the process whereby an individual acquires two or more first languages, either simultaneously or sequentially. We discuss the debate as to whether bilingual individuals have two language systems or a single system. We also distinguish between bilingualism and second language acquisition, describe second language developmental processes and influences, including transfer, interlanguage, overgeneralization, formulaic language, and avoidance, describe code switching, and provide a historical account of attitudes and policies regarding dual language instruction. An examination of research on English as a second language and English as a foreign language completes this section.

Finally, we compare a nurture-inspired theory (contrastive analysis hypothesis), nature-inspired theories (universal grammar and the monitor model), and interactionist theories (the cognitive theory with attention-processing model and the interaction hypothesis) of L2 acquisition. To bridge theory with practice, we also provide some instructional implications for each of these theories and discuss syntheses of research findings concerning practices for teaching English learner students.

 Apply Your Knowledge

Click here to apply your knowledge to practical scenarios.

BEYOND THE BOOK

1. Watch a movie that takes place in the southern part of the United States, such as *Coal Miner's Daughter*, *Bull Durham*, or *Steel Magnolias*. Select a major character and describe the character's dialect.

2. Survey 10 of your friends and relatives from across the United States (and beyond) for what they call a "fizzy drink that comes in a can." List each person's response, identify where he or she lives, and see if you can discern patterns between responses and geography.

3. Collect a brief language sample from two children who are about the same age. Use the same elicitation approach for both children, such as asking each to tell a story about a time he or she had an accident. Record their samples and then compare them for the number of words contained, as well as the number of different words. Examine the two samples for similarities and differences.

4. Identify the dialect of your five closest friends as well as your own. How much variability is there among your friends in the dialect they speak?

5. Have you ever studied a foreign language? If so, are you aware of any errors you make or have made as you have learned the foreign language? Explain why you suppose you make or made specific errors.

 Check Your Understanding

Gauge your understanding of the chapter concepts by taking this self-check quiz.

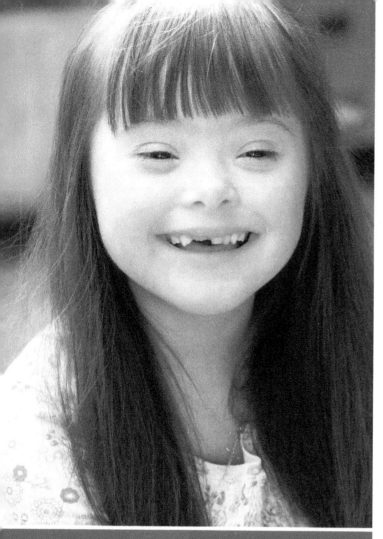

© Denis Kuvaev/Shutterstock

10

Language Disorders in Children

LEARNING OUTCOMES

After completion of this chapter, the reader will be able to:

1. Define a language disorder.

2. Explain who identifies and treats children with language disorders.

3. Identify the major types of child language disorders.

4. Explain how child language disorders are identified and treated.

In many of the preceding chapters, we have discussed major milestones that characterize how most children develop language from infancy to adolescence. However, we have also examined individual differences in language acquisition, such as how girls may develop differently than boys, and how children's experiences can affect their rate of language growth. In Chapter 1, we introduced the concept of *language disorders*, which refers to instances in which children experience significant difficulties in the development of language. In this chapter, we explore language disorders in greater detail and emphasize that variability in language acquisition seems to be the rule rather than the exception. In Chapter 9, we introduced you to Mrs. Riggert's second-grade classroom of twenty-two 7-year-olds at Compass Elementary School. In addition to the children referenced in Chapter 9, who showed an array of language differences, there are several additional children in her classroom who exhibit language disorders. For instance, Brandon has Down syndrome and speaks using only single words supplemented with some simple signs. Aryanna has severe autism spectrum disorder, and the only language she produces involves the repetition of scripts she has heard on television or the radio. Ricardo has a mild language disorder, and omits many verb markers in his sentences, saying things like *I do it* and *He go there*, instead of *I am doing it* and *He is going there.*

WHAT IS A LANGUAGE DISORDER?

Practitioners and researchers use many terms to describe language disorders in children, including *language delay*, *language impairment*, *language disability*, and *language-learning disability*. In general, all of these terms are synonyms used to describe individuals who exhibit significant impairments in the comprehension and/or production of language in form, content, and/or use. Additionally, this impairment must be significant enough to have an adverse impact on an individual's social, psychological, and educational functioning and cannot reflect a language difference, such as dialectical variation.

Distinguishing Between Language Disorders and Language Differences

People who identify and treat language disorders in children recognize that sometimes a fine line exists between a *language difference* and a *language disorder*. These two concepts differentiate between normal variability in language development (e.g., dialectical variations), and variability that reflects an underlying neurological impairment affecting language development. Failure to differentiate correctly between a language difference and a disorder has serious implications for educational practice. For instance, consider an instance in which a 6-year-old child's pragmatic patterns seem very different from those of her peers; perhaps she is slow to initiate conversations with other children or adults, and she never answers a direct question. During conversations, she does not use eye contact and seems unable to take turns. On the one hand, these behaviors could signify the presence of a serious language disorder; perhaps the child does not answer questions because she cannot understand them, for example. On the other hand, these same behaviors could signify a language difference. Perhaps the child comes from a home in which patterns of language use are quite different from mainstream patterns, such that children are considered rude if they initiate conversations with others, converse freely with adults, and use direct eye contact. Failure to differentiate accurately between language disorders and language differences can lead to overidentification of children from minority backgrounds for special education services as well as the opposite (failure to identify children who truly need support for a language disability).

DISCUSSION POINT

In what ways might a language impairment have an adverse impact on an individual's social functioning?

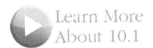

Learn More About 10.1

As you watch the video titled "Difference between a Speech Disorder and a Language Disorder", consider how these two disorders have different impacts on language users. https://www.youtube.com/watch?v=l9a74zGUflo

How do professionals differentiate language differences from language disorders? In large part, such differentiation requires a careful understanding of the cultural context in which a child is learning and applying his or her language abilities. A particular cultural community's approach to socializing children can influence the amount and quality of language children experience in their home and community. In turn, children's exposure to language in the home and in other caregiving contexts is a strong and unique contributor to children's language acquisition. In addition, professionals must be aware of how language acquisition may vary for children who are learning several languages at once (i.e., bilingualism), or who are speaking nonmainstream dialects. Children who are learning English as a second language may differ significantly from native English speakers in their attainment of English-language milestones.

Any two cultural communities can vary substantially in their approaches to child socialization. For instance, adult members of one cultural community may believe children "should be seen but not heard"; therefore, in that community, children may rarely participate in conversations among adults. In another cultural community, adults may believe children should be frequent and active participants in conversations among adults. These differences in socialization practices can affect children's language development. As another example, adults in one cultural community may socialize often with their infants through direct parent–infant talk, whereas in another community adults may rarely speak directly to infants. Again, such variability in the way adults socialize children in their cultural community directly affects the quantity and quality of language children in the community experience. From a cultural perspective, no right or wrong way to socialize children in a cultural community exists, although variability in child socialization practices can readily influence children's rate of language development.

DISCUSSION POINT

In your own words, describe the difference between a language disorder and a language difference.

Prevalence

Language disorders are the most prevalent (common) type of communication impairment affecting children, and often seem to contribute to other issues as well, including problems with social well-being (e.g., making friends with others) and academic achievement, particularly in reading. It is important, therefore, for parents, educators, physicians, and others to be aware of common signs of language disorders, as shown in Table 10.1.

TABLE 10.1

Common Signs of Language Disorders: Preschool to Adolescence

STUDENT'S AGE OR GRADE	LANGUAGE DIFFICULTIES
Preschool	• Omission of grammatical inflections, including present progressive (-*ing*), plural (-*s*), possessive (*'s*), past tense regular and irregular verbs, and auxiliary verbs
	• Slow development of and errors with pronouns
	• Shorter sentence length
	• Problems forming questions with inverted auxiliaries
	• Immature requests (resembling those of younger children)
	• Difficulty with group conversations (conversing with more than one child)
	• Difficulty with oral resolution of conflicts

(continued)

STUDENT'S AGE OR GRADE	LANGUAGE DIFFICULTIES
	• Longer reliance on gesture for meeting needs
	• Difficulty initiating with peers
	• Difficulty sustaining turns in conversation
	• Difficulty comprehending complex directions and narratives
Elementary grades	• Word-finding problems accompanied by pauses and circumlocutions
	• Naming errors (e.g., "shoes" for *pants*)
	• Slower processing speed in language comprehension
	• Difficulty responding to indirect requests
	• Difficulty maintaining topics
	• Difficulty recognizing the need for conversational repair
	• Problems with figurative and nonliteral language
	• Problems with abstract language concepts
	• Problems providing sufficient information to listeners
	• Poor narrative cohesion
	• Difficulty requesting help or clarification
	• Difficulty providing details
Adolescence	• Difficulty expressing ideas about language
	• Inappropriate responses to questions and comments
	• Poor social language
	• Problems providing sufficient information to listeners
	• Redundancy
	• Inadequate sense of limits or boundaries
	• Difficulty expressing needs and ideas
	• Difficulty initiating conversations with peers
	• Immature conversational participation
	• Difficulty requesting help or clarification
	• Difficulty providing details
	• Problems with organizing complex information in oral or written language
	• Word-finding difficulties
	• Socially inappropriate discourse with peers or adults
	• Frequent pauses, hesitations, or repetitions when speaking
	• Delays in responding during conversations or other language tasks

Source: Adapted from "Verb Use in Specific Language Impairment," by G. Conti-Ramsden and M. Jones, 1997, *Journal of Speech, Language, and Hearing Research, 40,* 1298–1313; *Children with Specific Language Impairment,* by L. B. Leonard, 2014, Cambridge: MIT Press; "Intervention for Word-Finding Deficits in Children," by K. K. McGregor and L. B. Leonard, in *Language Intervention: Preschool Through the Elementary Years* (pp. 85–105), edited by M. Fey, J. Windsor, and S. Warren, 1995, Baltimore: Brookes.

Late language emergence (LLE), which generally equates to having a slow start in language, occurs in an estimated one in five children (19%; Zubrick, Taylor, Rice, & Slegers, 2007). Children with LLE, also called *late talkers*, are usually identified at about 2 years of age. Recall that language production really starts to "take off" at around 1 year of age, when many children produce their first word, and that by 18 months or so, children have acquired a productive vocabulary of about 50 words and begin to produce some two-word combinations (*mommy go, want baba*). As a general rule, LLE is identified at the time when the majority of children are commonly using two-word combinations, which occurs around 2 years of age. Therefore, children who do not produce two-word combinations by their second birthday are viewed as late talkers. Many of these children are, as the name implies, simply late talkers who will overcome these early lags within a year or two. A minority of these children do, however, have a significant language disorder that is not readily resolved. These children need to receive intervention to promote their language skills, whether delivered in the home environment or in a clinical/school-based setting (Cable & Domsch, 2011). (See Theory to Practice: *Language Intervention in the Home Environment.*)

Primary language impairment, a significant language impairment in the absence of any other developmental difficulty (e.g., cognitive disability, brain injury), affects about 7%–10% of children older than 4 years (Beitchman

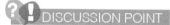

DISCUSSION POINT

About one in five children are slow to develop language in the first 2 years of life and are characterized as late talkers. Many of these children will outgrow these early problems, although some will not. Do you think late talkers should be treated for their delays, or would you advocate for a wait-and-see approach in which treatment is given only to children who have more persistent problems?

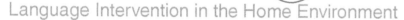

THEORY TO PRACTICE

Language Intervention in the Home Environment

A considerable body of research shows a strong positive relationship between the quality of parent–child conversational interaction and children's early language accomplishments (Levickes, Reilly, Girolametto, Ukoumunne, & Wake, 2014). In one study involving 275 toddlers and preschoolers, researchers studied children's language growth over time in relation to the amount of television viewing and the number of adult–child conversations occurring at home (Zimmerman, Christakis, & Meltzoff, 2009). The most important determinant of children's language abilities was the *number of conversations* that occurred in the home. In fact, the study findings even suggested that adult–child conversations seemed to counter any negative effects of television viewing, leading the authors to conclude: "Parents should be encouraged not merely to provide language input to their children through reading or storytelling, but also to engage their children in two-sided conversations" (p. 346). Given the importance of such findings, how might we translate them into everyday practices within children's homes?

One example of this translation of theory to practice is an intervention approach called parent-child interaction therapy (PCIT; see Falkas et al., 2015). PCIT involves teaching parents optimal ways to interact with their children during conversational exchanges so as to improve their children's language skills. Examples of optimal ways to interact include giving children enough time to talk, following the child's lead during play, and not asking the child an abundance of questions and rather allowing the child to initiate. Typically, a speech–language pathologist or other professional will videotape parents interacting with their children and then the clinician and parent will study the videotapes together to identify specific goals for parents to pursue by which the parent–child interactions can be enhanced. An additional and important feature of PCIT is that parents are asked to set aside special times in which they interact and talk with their children. A recent experiment showed that children with language disorders whose parents used PCIT made greater growth in language skill over a 10-week period (Falkas et al., 2015). Work such as this provides an excellent example of how theories of language development, such as the role of parent input in supporting children's language acquisition, can be used to improve clinical practices with children and their families.

Source: From Teaching by Listening: The Importance of Adult-Child Conversations to Language Development, Pediatrics Vol. 124 No. 1 July 1, 2009 pp. 342–349. Copyright © 2009 by American Academy of Pediatrics. Reprinted by permission.

et al., 1989). Because this disorder is specific to language, it is commonly called specific language impairment (SLI). Many children with SLI have a history of LLE, and also will continue to experience significant problems with the development of language skills well into middle and later adolescence (Durkin, Simkin, Knox, & Conti-Ramsden, 2009; Skibbe et al., 2008). In addition, as they move into adolescence and adulthood, children with LI experience lower levels of educational achievement and occupational success and, by some accounts, high rates of physical health concerns (e.g., Beitchman, Brownlie, & Bao, 2014; St. Clair, Pickles, Durkin, & Conti-Ramsden, 2011).

Certain conditions appear to contribute to a child's risk for SLI, such as preterm birth. Babies are considered preterm when they are born at a low (<37 weeks) gestational age and/or have a very low birth weight (<2500 g; Sansavini et al., 2007). About one-third of preterm children go on to develop SLI (Sansavini et al., 2010). Also, genetic research indicates that the risk for SLI runs in families (Reader, Covill, Nudel, & Newbury, 2014). It may be that SLI is caused by a variety of circumstances, including perinatal complications that impact brain development, as well as genetic vulnerability.

The prevalence of secondary language impairment, language disorders resulting from or secondary to other conditions, is more difficult to estimate. Common types of secondary language impairment include intellectual or cognitive disability and the autism spectrum disorders. Recent estimates from the Centers for Disease Control and Prevention (CDC, 2015), which monitors the prevalence of developmental disabilities in the United States, show that about 12 in 1,000 children exhibit mild to severe intellectual disability. Children with mild disability outnumber those with severe disability by about 3 to 1. These CDC estimates include children who exhibit autism spectrum disorder, which is currently estimated to affect about 1 in 68 children (CDC, 2015). The prevalence of autism spectrum disorder has increased drastically over the last decade. It is unclear whether the actual rates of autism spectrum disorder are on the rise or whether the change in prevalence is driven by an increased awareness of this disorder, improved assessment approaches, and/or other reasons (e.g., increased diagnosis of very mild cases).

WHO IDENTIFIES AND TREATS CHILDREN WITH LANGUAGE DISORDERS?

A variety of professionals are involved with the identification and treatment of language disorders in children. Some professionals provide direct services, whereas others provide indirect services. *Direct services* include diagnosing language disorders and providing treatment to children with disorders through clinical and educational interventions. *Indirect services* include screening children for the possibility of language disorders and referring them for direct services, as well as counseling parents on approaches to supporting language development in the home environment.

The professionals most intimately involved with direct and indirect services include speech-language pathologists, psychologists, general educators, special educators, early interventionists, audiologists, developmental pediatricians, and otorhinolaryngologists.

Speech–Language Pathologists

Speech–language pathologists, or SLPs, are frequently the lead direct service provider for children with language disorders. The scope of practice for SLPs as related to language disorders includes a number of pertinent responsibilities, including

10.1
Check Your Understanding
Click here to gauge your understanding of the concepts in this section.

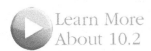
Learn More About 10.2

As you watch the video titled "Expressive and Receptive Language", be aware of the differences between expressive and receptive language and notice how disorders in either area can impact a child's ability to successfully use a language. https://www.youtube.com/watch?v=IdMC1jNf1p4

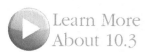

Learn More About 10.3

As you watch the video titled "Speech Language Therapy Pediatrics", notice how an SLP may become involved with a child's intervention and also notice how interconnected an SLP can be to other service providers. Consider how all these connections can positively impact a child's language development. https://www.youtube.com/watch?v=xiKYD9TSDhk

prevention, screening, consultation, assessment and diagnosis, treatment delivery, and counseling. Typical services provided by SLPs therefore include screening children for possible language disorders, conducting evaluations of children with suspected language disorders, diagnosing language disorders, and developing and administering treatments to remediate disorders of language.

SLPs work in many different settings, including public and private schools, hospitals, rehabilitation facilities, home health agencies, community and university clinics, private practices, group homes, state agencies, universities, and corporations. There are currently more than 130,000 SLPs working in the United States; however, there remains a significant shortage of speech–language pathologists in most regions of North America. This shortage of SLPs is not likely to be resolved soon, as the U.S. Department of Labor reports a 20% increase in this job, characteristic of an occupational outlook that is growing "faster than average" (Bureau of Labor Statistics, 2015).

Psychologists

Psychologists also hold important responsibilities in the identification and treatment of child language disorders, and also conduct research important to our understanding of how to identify and treat these disorders. *Cognitive and perceptual psychology* and *developmental psychology* are two branches of psychology that conduct research relevant to child language disorders. These researchers conduct basic and applied research on human perception, thinking, and memory, with developmental psychologists emphasizing growth in these capacities over the lifespan. Their research helps us answer such valuable questions as, "What demographic factors predict whether a child will persist or resolve his/her early language difficulties?" (e.g., Dale, Price, Bishop, & Plomin, 2003), and "How many alphabet letters should children know when they arrive to kindergarten, to be prepared for reading instruction?" (e.g., Piasta, Petscher, & Justice, 2012).

Clinical psychologists, clinical neuropsychologists, rehabilitation psychologists, and *school psychologists* often work more directly with children with language disorders. These professionals work in public and private schools, clinics, and hospitals, with a large number providing services through private practice. Typically, identification and treatment of language disorders is just one small part of what these professionals do.

Clinical psychologists screen for and diagnose impairments of language, often as part of a larger psychoeducational assessment that examines a child's strengths and needs in many areas of development (e.g., nonverbal intelligence, perceptual skills, learning aptitude). Clinical psychologists may offer specialized treatments for various types of language disorders, such as those exhibited by children with autism or those children who have difficulty processing auditory information. Clinical neuropsychologists and rehabilitation psychologists may oversee the diagnosis and treatment of language disorders in children and adolescents resulting from traumatic injuries, such as acquired brain injuries. They may also work with individuals with developmental disabilities (e.g., cerebral palsy, autism) to promote their community involvement and adjustment. School psychologists typically work in private and public schools, and perform essential activities on school-based teams that identify children with language disorders and develop educational programs to remediate or compensate for these disorders.

General Educators

General educators include preschool, elementary, middle school, and high school teachers. General educators have the important role of identifying children in their classrooms who may show signs of difficulty with language within the educational context. General educators must be knowledgeable about the course of typical language development, as well as signs of impaired development. Recall that common signs of language difficulties from preschool into adolescence appear in Table 10.1.

When a general educator suspects a child in his or her classroom may have impaired language abilities, they request that the school's *child study team* (also called the evaluation team) engage in a systematic process that typically involves *pre-referral intervention*, or identification of approaches to support the child's language and communication skills in the classroom environment. General educators are therefore, one of the most important referral sources for children with suspected language disorders. The child study team typically comprises the general educator, the parents of the child with a suspected language difficulty, as well as other professionals (e.g., school psychologist, special educator, speech–language pathologist). The child study team identifies approaches the general educator may use to support the child's language performance in the classroom. If these do not alleviate the general educator's concerns about the child's language performance, a multifactored evaluation (MFE) is then conducted by the child study team to carefully evaluate the child and to determine if a language disorder is present. If the team identifies a language disorder, they also will use the MFE to identify the types of special education services the child should receive to treat her language disorder and to support her academic development.

Whenever possible, children with language disorders receive special education services in the *least restrictive environment* (LRE). LRE is a federal mandate of the Individuals with Disabilities Education Act (IDEA), which stipulates that children with disabilities should receive their education to the maximum extent possible in the same contexts of their peers without disabilities. This means that many children with language disorders will receive their education in the regular classroom with children who do not have disorders of language. It also means that general educators must be skilled at differentiating their instruction to support the academic growth of children with language disorders in the school's curriculum.

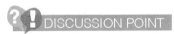

DISCUSSION POINT

A child study team includes people from a variety of disciplines. Why is it important for this team to be multidisciplinary?

Special Educators

Special educators have a critical role to play in supporting the educational progress of children with identified language disorders. The field of special education has grown as a result of federal legislation mandating the free and appropriate education of children with disabilities in our nation's schools. Currently, there are more than 400,000 special educators teaching the nearly 6 million children with disabilities in our nation's schools (Bureau of Labor Statistics, 2015). Nearly one-fourth of these children with disabilities have disabilities of speech and language (U.S. Department of Education, National Center for Education Statistics, 2015).

To meet the needs of students with disabilities, special educators work directly with pupils from preschool through the secondary grades to deliver general and specialized interventions geared toward helping children with disabilities succeed academically. They use a variety of approaches to do this: They may be the lead teacher or co-teacher in classrooms serving primarily children with disabilities; they may consult and collaborate with teachers who have one or several children with disabilities among their pupils; or they may deliver specialized interventions outside of the classroom in pull-out programs. Some special educators serve as *itinerant teachers*; itinerant teachers do not have their own classroom but rather co-teach or collaborate with a number of different teachers. Many itinerant special educators have a special area of expertise, such as the education of children with autism or children who are deaf, and thus go into classrooms in which these children are served to collaborate with teachers and to provide services in the least restrictive classroom environment.

Although special educators may screen and test children for language disorders, their lead responsibility is to design, deliver, and monitor Individualized Education Programs (IEPs) and Individualized Family Service Plans (IFSPs) that specify educational intervention and annual goals for children with identified language disorders receiving special education services in public school programs. IEPs (for 3- to 21-year-olds with disabilities) and IFSPs (for infants to 2-year-olds with disabilities) are required by the U.S. government's, Individuals with Disabilities Education Act (IDEA) and its subsequent amendments. IDEA provides federal funds to the 50 states to provide intervention services to children from infancy through the age of 21 who have identified disabilities or delays in language and other areas of development (e.g., mental and motor development). Organizations may also use federal funds to provide interventions to newborns through 2-year-olds who exhibit significant medical, biological, and environmental risk conditions making them vulnerable for later disability.

Early Interventionists

Early interventionists (sometimes called child development specialists) are professionals with specialization in intervention for infants and toddlers. The field of early intervention is a new one, growing out of the 1986 reauthorization and amendment (P.L. 99-457) of the original 1975 Individuals with Disabilities Education Act. The original act legislated special education services for children ages 6 to 21, with some support available for preschool programs serving children ages 3 to 5. In light of concerns raised about access to services for children who were even younger, the 1986 reauthorization provided federal support to states to implement early intervention services to children with identified or suspected disabilities from birth to age 2. Obviously, states needed well-trained professionals—early interventionists—to support their design and implementation of statewide early intervention systems. P.L. 99–457 provided states with considerable flexibility in determining the credentials early intervention personnel require, and there remains great variability across the nation in the training provided to and required by these professionals.

Early interventionists undoubtedly have one of the most critical roles to play in serving the needs of children with language disorders. Given the importance of the first few years of life to language development, they work with children with language disorders during the best "window of opportunity" for optimizing children's developmental trajectory. In delivering their early intervention services, these professionals often work directly in families' homes, side-by-side with the parents of infants and toddlers to teach them ways to support their children's language learning in the home environment.

Typically, early interventionists work from a clinic, hospital, or community-based organization that has received a grant from the state to provide early intervention services in a particular region. The organization is responsible for serving birth to 2-year-olds in their region who have developmental delays (e.g., slow progress in language development), physical or medical conditions that often result in developmental delays (e.g., low birth weight, HIV), and environmental conditions linked to later developmental problems (e.g., extreme poverty, abuse). For children found eligible for early intervention services, an IFSP is developed to identify the specific early intervention services to be provided, including the intensity, type, and location of services. The IFSP also sets specific objectives for the child and family, and early interventionists oversee progress towards these objectives.

Audiologists

Audiologists are specialists in identifying, assessing, and managing disorders of the auditory, balance, and other neural systems. Audiologists are often involved in the

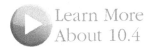

Learn More About 10.4

As you watch the video titled "What is an Audiologist? with Audiologist, Mary Wade", notice how audiologist can be involved with many different areas of a person's communication needs. Additionally, notice how audiologists are also well connected to other professionals that can help with an individual's communication needs. https://www.youtube.com/watch?v=WwOwa8bNNEw

treatment of language disorders when hearing loss is involved, and work closely with SLPs and other professionals in the design of interventions. For instance, for children who are born with profound hearing loss, they might deliver auditory–verbal therapies that simultaneously promote the child's use of residual hearing and her production and comprehension of language. Audiologists also play a critical role in referring children with hearing loss for assessment of language by speech–language pathologists, when they suspect hearing loss may be impacting the child's language development.

Audiologists work in many different settings, to include schools, hospitals, rehabilitation facilities, community and university clinics, private practices, and universities. There are more than 13,000 audiologists currently working in the United States, and the field is expected to expand dramatically in the next decade, with the number of positions increasing by more than 30% over the next decade (Bureau of Labor Statistics, 2015).

Otorhinolaryngologist

Otorhinolaryngologists, or ear–nose–throat physicians (ENTs), are close collaborators in the diagnosis and management of language disorders that result from injury or illness of the ear, nose, or throat. They are a particularly important team member for children who exhibit slow language development as a function of otitis media (OM) or other types of hearing loss. OM is one of the most common causes of hearing loss in children. It results from a viral or bacterial infection of the middle ear space, and in some instances the middle ear space is filled with fluid, which dampens their hearing ability. Some estimates indicate that at any given point, about 10% of children have OM (Monasta et al., 2012). When OM persists either in a single case of the disease or through chronic infections (e.g., five or six in a given year), a child may exhibit delays in the acquisition of language. The ENT has the key role of halting the progress of OM through use of antibiotics and/or the insertion of pressure-equalizing tubes (PE tubes) into the eardrum to equalize pressure between the middle and outer ear and to release any fluids in the middle ear space. ENTs often work closely with speech–language pathologists and audiologists to promote the language and hearing achievements of children with chronic hearing loss.

10.2 Check Your Understanding
Click here to gauge your understanding of the concepts in this section.

Language disorders can occur as a primary impairment or as a function of other developmental disabilities, such as cognitive impairment or autism spectrum disorder.

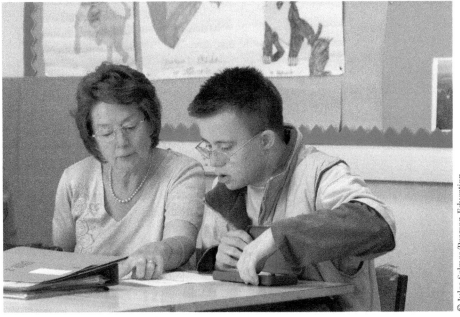

© Jules Selmes/Pearson Education

WHAT ARE THE MAJOR TYPES OF CHILD LANGUAGE DISORDERS?

In this section, we describe the defining characteristics and causes of six conditions typically associated with language disorders among children and adolescents: specific language impairment, autism spectrum disorder, intellectual disability, traumatic brain injury, and hearing loss.

Specific Language Impairment

Defining Characteristics As mentioned previously, SLI (also called *primary language disorder*) is a developmental disability in which an individual shows a significant impairment of expressive or receptive language that cannot be attributed to any other causal condition (Leonard, 2014). Children with SLI have typical hearing skills (although they may have a history of middle-ear infections); normal intelligence; and no obvious neurological, motor, or sensory disturbances, such as seizures or brain injury.

Children are typically diagnosed with SLI after their third birthday (Leonard, 2014). Although signs of language difficulty may be present as early as the first and second years of life, toddlers who are slow to talk are typically classified as late talkers rather than language impaired. Many late talkers overcome their slow start, as we mentioned earlier in this chapter. Therefore, a formal diagnosis of SLI is usually not made until a child is 3 years old or more, when practitioners can more clearly determine whether the child is exhibiting a true language disorder rather than a late start.

Although children with SLI characteristically exhibit a late start in developing language, they differ from late talkers in that most of them have enduring difficulties with language. According to epidemiological research, about 50% of kindergartners with SLI continue to exhibit SLI in fourth grade (Tomblin et al., 2003). Children with SLI whose language impairment affects both expression and comprehension of language show lower remission rates between kindergarten and fourth grade than children with deficits in only language expression or comprehension (Tomblin et al., 2003).

Although children with SLI show considerable individual differences in the domains of language affected and the severity of the disorder, they often share five common traits:

1. Many children with SLI have strengths in some areas of language and weaknesses in others (Tambyraja, Schmitt, Farquharson, & Justice, 2015). For instance, a child may have relatively intact grammatical skills but exhibit poor pragmatic and semantic performance. As another example, a child may have deficits in the expression of language but relatively good comprehension.

2. Many children with SLI have a history of slow vocabulary development. On average, children with SLI produce their first words at about age 2 years (compared with about 1 year for nonimpaired children), and they continue to struggle with learning new words throughout the elementary years (Leonard, 2014). When provided the opportunity to learn a new word, children with SLI learn it more slowly than their nonimpaired same-age peers do (Nash & Donaldson, 2005). Experts attribute these delays in vocabulary learning to a generalized deficit in processing linguistic stimuli (Fernald & Marchman, 2012).

3. Many children with SLI show considerable difficulties with grammatical production and comprehension that begin during toddlerhood and continue through school age (Conti-Ramsden & Jones, 1997). During toddlerhood and the preschool years, children with SLI are likely to omit key grammatical morphemes, such as articles and auxiliary verbs; they produce shorter utterances; and they may have problems with pronoun usage (e.g., substituting object pronouns for subjective pronouns, such as "Her did it"). One area of particular weakness is verb development (Leonard, 2014). Children with SLI use verbs less frequently

than same-age peers do, use fewer types of verbs, and show delayed development of verb morphology, particularly the use of auxiliary verbs (Hansson, 2003).

4. Children with SLI also tend to have difficulty adjusting academically; for example, they may have problems with social skills, behavior, and peer relations (Conti-Ramsden, Mok, Pickles, & Durkin, 2013), as well as with academically oriented skills, such as literacy and mathematics (Justice, Bowles, Pence Turnbull, & Skibbe, 2009). Difficulties with reading development—such as timely development of the alphabetic principle and application of reading comprehension strategies—are strongly associated with SLI (Skibbe et al., 2008; see Research Paradigms: *Prospective and Retrospective Longitudinal Studies*).

5. Most children diagnosed with SLI have long-term difficulties with language achievement. As many as 60% of children who exhibit SLI at kindergarten age continue to show language weaknesses in adolescence and adulthood, and resolution is most unlikely for children who exhibit impairment of both language expression and language comprehension (in contrast, resolution is most likely for children with expressive- and/or receptive-only impairment; Stothard, Snowling, Bishop, Chipchase, & Kaplan, 1998; Tomblin et al., 2003).

RESEARCH **PARADIGMS**

Prospective and Retrospective Longitudinal Studies

The results of a number of studies have revealed that young children with language impairment face significant challenges in the later development of their reading ability (e.g., Catts, Fey, Tomblin, & Zhang, 2002; Skibbe et al., 2008). For instance, Catts and colleagues found that about 50% of kindergartners with language impairment later exhibit poor reading skills in second grade. Some experts contend that preschool language impairment and school-age reading disability are two manifestations of a single underlying developmental language disorder (Scarborough, 2001). Next, we consider two approaches researchers use to study the co-occurrence of early language impairment and later reading disability: prospective and retrospective longitudinal studies.

A *prospective longitudinal study* is a research design in which researchers follow children forward in time as they develop. Researchers test children intermittently (e.g., every 6 months) to track their development. In longitudinal studies, researchers may follow children for several months or for many years. An example of a prospective longitudinal study of reading outcomes for children with language impairment is that of Catts and colleagues (2002). In this study, an initial sample of 7,218 kindergartners was tested using a comprehensive battery of language and cognitive measures. From these children, a subset of children with language impairment (LI, $n = 117$) were identified and tested again in second and fourth grade. The second- and fourth-grade test battery included measures of language, cognition, and reading ability. The researchers used data from the test battery to identify the percentage of children with LI who exhibited

reading disability in second and fourth grade, finding that 53% and 48% of kindergartners with LI had reading disability in second and fourth grade, respectively. (In contrast, about 8% of children with no history of LI had reading disability in second and fourth grade.) This prospective study quantified the increased risk for reading problems among children with LI.

Another way to study the relationship between language impairment and reading disability is a *retrospective longitudinal study*. In such studies, researchers follow children across time to identify those who exhibit a reading disability in the elementary grades, then look backward to determine whether language difficulties were present earlier. An example of this type of research design is Justice and colleagues' retrospective analysis of the early language skills of children who were poor readers in fifth grade: Some poor readers had problems specific to reading comprehension whereas others had problems specific to reading decoding (Justice, Mashburn, & Petscher, 2013). The language skills of these two groups of poor readers, as well as a group of children who were typical readers were examined retrospectively when they were 15, 24, 36, and 54 months of age. These researchers found that even as early as 15 months, children who would have reading-comprehension problems at fifth grade had poorer language skills than the other two groups (children with decoding problems and children who were typical readers). Such work suggests that reading difficulties that interfere with reading comprehension may be the result of long-standing and early-emerging difficulties with language skill.

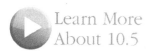

Learn More About 10.5

As you watch the video titled "Signs of SLI", be aware of how an SLI may appear to others and what different areas of language children with an SLI struggle with. https://www.youtube.com/watch?v=JAsf_Wqjz4g For additional material on SLIs, refer to this link titled "What Is SLI" https://www.youtube.com/watch?v=Pqu7w6t3Rmo.

Causes

No known cause for SLI has been identified, although advances in brain-imaging and epidemiological research suggest a strong biological and genetic component to this disorder (O'Brien, Zhang, Nishimura, Tomblin, & Murray, 2003; Reader et al., 2014). Children who have immediate family members with language impairment are more likely than other children to develop SLI, and 20%–40% of children with SLI have a sibling or parent with a language disorder (Rice, Haney, & Wexler, 1998). Current theories on the cause of SLI suggest that biological or genetic factors predispose a child to SLI, which can then interact unfavorably with additional risk factors present in the child's developmental environment. Risk factors that may increase a child's vulnerability to SLI include both environmental (e.g., child neglect and abuse) and physical (e.g., prematurity, malnutrition) health factors.

Autism Spectrum Disorder

Defining Characteristics

Autism spectrum disorder (ASD) is a developmental disability that affects an estimated 1 in 68 children (CDC, 2015), with a higher prevalence among boys and among children with affected family members. Surveillance of ASD in Florida, for instance, found 7 in 1,000 boys affected compared to 1 in 1,000 girls (CDC, 2009). This disability is present at birth, although its signs and symptoms may not be apparent until several years later. Individuals with ASD show persistent and often significant difficulties in using and understanding language in social contexts. Three major areas of difficulty required for an ASD diagnosis include (from American Psychiatric Association, 2013):

1. *Difficulties with social-emotional reciprocity.* Reciprocity as a term refers to exchanges between two entities, and with respect to social-emotional exchanges, it captures the synergies typically evident in communicative exchanges. For instance, when two people have a conversation, they typically offer opportunities to one another to take turns. Likewise, when we converse with one another, we often convey emotional content, such as smiling when a conversational partner shares something funny or frowning at something saddening. Finally, if a friend looks distraught, we might ask her what is wrong or give her a pat on the back. Individuals with ASD have difficulties with these aspects of communication,

2. *Difficulties with nonverbal communicative behaviors.* When individuals communicate, they use a variety of nonverbal communicative behaviors to supplement their verbal behaviors. For instance, we use gestures, eye contact, and facial expressions as a vehicle to communicate. Individuals with ASD show significant difficulties with this aspect of communication. For instance, they may not use gestures or eye gaze when communicating in ways that conform to their cultural norms.

3. *Difficulties developing and maintaining relationships with others.* Individuals with ASD typically have significant difficulties in their relationships with others. They may have no interest in having relationships with others, they may have difficulties engaging in play with others, and they may seldom if ever initiate with peers.

The diagnosis of ASD gives attention to how severe an individual's symptoms are, with severity based on consideration of two issues (American Psychiatric Association, 2013). First, the severity of one's social-communication skills is considered. In the most severe cases, an individual with ASD will have significant deficits in social-communication skill: They may not engage in any way with other people, including responding to social overtures from others. In more mild cases, an individual with ASD will engage with others, but he will show unusual patterns in social communication, such as failing to initiate with others, or to engage in reciprocal conversations. Second, the severity with which an individual shows restricted and repetitive behaviors is considered. Many individuals with ASD have restricted interests and repetitive behaviors, and these can range in severity from mild to severe. For instance, an individual with ASD may show an extreme interest in the sounds of fans and other electrical objects with motors, or have a preoccupation with a certain type of animal. When such preoccupations are severe, an individual with ASD may have extreme difficulty coping when these preoccupations are not present.

The way in which ASD is diagnosed changed in 2013, with the release of the fifth edition of the *Diagnosis and Statistical Manual of Mental Disorders* (American Psychiatric Association, 2013). The DSM-5, as it is called, provides a compendium of all disorders and disabilities and is used by clinicians in many disciplines for diagnosing mental and other disorders. In the prior edition of the DSM, the diagnosis category of *Asperger's Syndrome* was included, but this was removed in the fifth edition. Children with Asperger's syndrome are often referred to as "higher-functioning" children with autism. The language skills of children with Asperger's syndrome are generally well developed and are not viewed as clinically disordered. However, these children may use language in idiosyncratic and unconventional ways. They may also have difficulty using language in social situations and comprehending abstract or figurative language. For instance, they may understand only the literal meaning of idiomatic phrases (e.g., "We really need to *hit the books* to prepare for this test" and "She really is *out of her mind*"). Children with Asperger's syndrome may also have considerable difficulty using language as a social tool, as well as developing and maintaining social relationships. They may have difficulty initiating conversations with peers and using situationally inappropriate language. With the new DSM diagnostic parameters for ASD, an individual would not be diagnosed as having Asperger's; rather, they would be diagnosed as having ASD and severity with respect to social-communication skills, and restricted and repetitive behaviors would likely be documented as relatively mild ("Level 1" in the DSM-5).

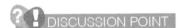

DISCUSSION POINT

The prevalence of autism spectrum disorder seems to be increasing dramatically. What are some possible reasons for this?

Children with autism display an inability to develop, or a lack of interest in developing, relationships with peers and instead participate in social games or routines with other people.

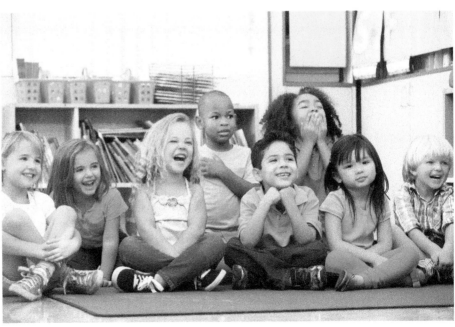

Shutterstock

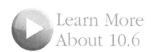

Causes

ASDs are neurobiological disorders that are believed to result from an organic brain abnormality (Hall, 2012). Genetic research showing high rates of co-occurrence between monozygotic twins indicates that there is a strong biological basis of this disability. Some factors may increase a child's risk for developing autism. Certain prenatal and perinatal complications, particularly maternal rubella and anoxia (lack of oxygen to the brain), are associated with an increased risk for autism, as is the presence of some developmental or physical disabilities, such as encephalitis (an inflammation of the brain) and fragile X syndrome (a genetic disorder that results in intellectual disability). Seizure disorder is seen in 25% of children with autism, which suggests a commonality in the brain structures affected by ASD and seizures (Theoharides & Zhang, 2011). Also, extreme sensory deprivation can have a profound impact on communication and social development, and, in severe cases, may result in patterns of development consistent with those of ASD (Kenneally, Bruck, Frank, & Nalty, 1998). Some studies have also shown that parental age is associated with a risk for autism; children who are born to two older parents (mothers >35 years and fathers >40 years) show an elevated risk for ASD (Durkin et al., 2009).

Intellectual Disability

Defining Characteristics

Intellectual disability (ID) is a "condition of arrested or incomplete development of the mind, which is especially characterized by impairment of skills manifested during the developmental period" (American Association on Mental Retardation [AAMR], 2002, p. 103). ID is diagnosed in children younger than age 18 years who meet two criteria: (a) significant limitations in intellectual functioning and (b) significant limitations in adaptive behavior (AAMR, 2002). Thus, children with ID exhibit limitations in intelligence such as difficulty reasoning, planning, solving problems, thinking in abstract terms, comprehending abstract and complex concepts, and learning skills. These children also experience limitations in adaptive behavior and the activities of daily living, including difficulties with conceptual skills (communication, functional academics, self-direction, health and safety), social skills (social relationships, leisure), and practical skills (self-care, home living, community participation, work).

ID ranges from mild to profound (mild cases are more common), and because of the interrelationships among intellectual functioning and language ability, most children with ID have at least mild language impairment (see Table 10.2). In mild cases, the most common type, ID may have only minimal effects, so that the individual exhibits mild language difficulties, yet is able to participate fully in society and to develop strong social relationships with few adaptive limitations. In profound cases, which occur far less frequently, an individual's intellectual and adaptive functioning is severely affected. A person with profound ID may be unable to care for him- or herself, to communicate with other people, or to participate in any community or employment activities.

The language skills of a person with ID usually parallel the degree of intellectual impairment. In general, children with ID show delays in early communicative behaviors (e.g., pointing to request, commenting vocally) and are slow to use their first words and to produce multiword combinations (Paul & Norbury, 2012). Children with mild ID may have well-developed oral language skills, and only minor difficulties with abstract concepts, figurative language, complex syntax, conversational participation, and producing complex narratives (Cleave, Bird, Czutrin, & Smith, 2012). Children and adolescents who have Down syndrome, a relatively common cause of ID, typically produce short sentences use a fairly small expressive vocabulary, and exhibit a slowed rate of speech (Chapman, Seung, Schwartz,

TABLE 10.2
Categories and prevalence of ID

TYPE	PREVALENCE	IQ RANGE	DESCRIPTION
Mild	8.4 in 1,000	50–70	Has mild learning difficulties but can work, maintain good social relationships, and participate in inclusive schooling with academic growth through at least sixth-grade level; shows early lags in language development (form, content, and use) but continues to progress into early adulthood; as an adult, can live somewhat independently (may work in supported employment) but may need supervision and assistance
Moderate	2.1 in 1,000	35–49	Has obvious developmental delays in childhood but can develop some degree of independence in self-care and acquire adequate communication and academic skills; may have significant difficulties in peer interactions and social competence (e.g., using social conventions, participating in conversations); will benefit from targeted vocational training and supported employment opportunities; likely will require supported living arrangements but can work in unskilled and semiskilled positions with supervision
Severe	0.6 in 1,000	20–34	Exhibits early and ongoing significant developmental delays; acquires few or no speech or language skills in preschool years but may later develop minimal communication skills; can master some basic preacademic skills (e.g., reading of some sight words, counting); may benefit from alternative means of communication (e.g., a picture-based system); likely needs continuous levels of support to care for self and participate in the community but can be a full member of the community with supervision
Profound	0.9 in 1,000	<20	Exhibits significant limitations in all aspects of daily living (e.g., self-care, continence); communication is severely affected (the individual may produce no words and understand little); such limitations are usually identified with a neurological condition (e.g., severe brain injury); the individual may be able to communicate using very simple strategies (e.g., pointing to a picture to express a basic need).

Source: Based on information from *Diagnostic and Statistical Manual of Mental Disorders*, Fourth Edition, Text Revision (Copyright 2000, American Psychiatric Association); Murphy, C., Yeargin-Allsopp, M., Decoufle, C., & Drews, P. (1995). The administrative prevalence of mental retardation in 10-year-old children in Metropolitan Atlanta, 1985 through 1987. *American Journal of Public Health*, 85, 319–323.

& Kay-Raining Bird, 1998). Function words, such as copula and auxiliary verbs (*is, were, does*), are frequently omitted, as well as pronouns, conjunctions, and articles. Language comprehension tends to be better than language expression for these children (Næss, Lyster, Hulme, & Melby-Lervåg, 2011). Despite these difficulties, many children with mild ID develop language skills that allow them to participate fully in the academic curricula of their schools, to communicate competently with peers and adults, and to express their needs and interests to other people.

By contrast, children with more severe forms of ID display more significant deficits in language expression and comprehension. Some individuals with ID never learn to express themselves orally. They may produce only a few words or sounds and a few gestures. In addition, they may be able to comprehend only single, simple words representing concrete actions or objects (e.g., *sit*, *cup*). For some individuals with more severe forms of ID, an augmentative and alternative communicative (AAC) system can increase their ability to express themselves. For instance, an individual with profound ID who cannot produce any words may learn to point to pictures representing common actions (e.g., *eat*, *drink*, *walk*, *toilet*) as a means of representing his or her needs and wants.

Causes

ID can occur for many reasons and is typically the result of an injury, brain abnormality, or disease. In about 30%–40% of all cases the cause cannot be identified (American Psychiatric Association, 2013). For the other 60%–70% of cases, in which a cause can be pinpointed, prenatal damage to the developing fetus due to chromosomal abnormalities or maternal ingestion of toxins accounts for the majority of cases (about 30%). These include, for instance, Down syndrome, Cri-du-chat syndrome, and Prader-Willi syndrome, all of which typically result in ID. Pregnancy and perinatal problems—such as fetal malnutrition, prematurity, anoxia (lack of oxygen to the child's brain before, during, or following birth), and viral infections—account for an additional 10% of cases.

Environmental influences and other mental conditions, such as sensory deprivation (e.g., neglect) or the presence of autism, account for about 15%–20% of all cases. Studies of children raised in institutions suggest that many of these children exhibit low intellect (Smyke, Zeanah, Fox, & Nelson, 2009). Medical conditions such as trauma, infection, and poisoning cause about 5% of all cases of ID, and heredity alone accounts for 5% of the cases.

Traumatic Brain Injury
Defining Characteristics

Traumatic brain injury (TBI) refers to damage or injury to an individual's brain tissue sometime after birth. Young children, adolescent males, and older persons have the highest risk, and males are affected twice as often as females (CDC, 2007). Mild injuries, characterized by a concussion and loss of consciousness for 30 min or less, are the most common type of brain injury and usually have few lasting repercussions. In contrast, a severe injury is accompanied by a coma lasting for 6 hr or more. Such injuries can result from infection (e.g., meningitis), disease (e.g., brain tumor), and physical trauma (e.g., gunshot wound). Some of the more common causes of TBI in children include abuse (e.g., shaken baby syndrome), intentional harm (e.g., being hit on the head), accidental poisoning through ingestion of toxic substances (e.g., prescription medications, pesticides), car accidents, and falls.

The most common type of TBI is a closed-head injury (CHI), in which brain matter is not exposed or penetrated. CHI may occur in a car accident, in which a child in the rear seat is thrown forward and then backward with sudden deceleration. Another example of CHI is the brain injury resulting from shaken baby syndrome, in which an infant or a toddler is so violently shaken that the child's brain sustains diffuse injury. In contrast, with open-head injuries (OHIs), the brain matter is exposed through penetration, as would occur with a gunshot wound. OHI tends to cause a more focal brain injury than that resulting from CHI. However, in both CHI and OHI, the immediate injury to the brain—whether diffuse or focal—is often accompanied by secondary brain injuries that result from the primary trauma. For instance, an individual who sustains a CHI may then experience anoxia (lack of oxygen to brain tissue) or edema (swelling of the brain tissue), both of which can cause additional brain damage.

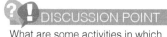

DISCUSSION POINT

What are some activities in which children and adolescents participate that might increase their risk for a traumatic brain injury?

Most children with an acquired brain injury have a history of normal language skills. Injury to the brain typically damages the frontal and temporal lobes of the brain, which house the centers for many of the executive (e.g., reasoning, planning, hypothesizing) and language functions, as we discussed in Chapter 3. Language disorders resulting from brain injury are influenced by the *severity* of the injury, the *site* of damage, and the *characteristics of the child* before the injury occurred. Children with more severe injuries typically have less chance of a full language recovery than do children with more mild injuries. However, even children with more mild cases of TBI may show long-lasting cognitive and language impairments, even though the effects may not be apparent until years later, when damaged areas of the brain are applied to certain skills and activities.

One aspect of language commonly impaired with TBI is language use, or pragmatics. About 75% of all children with severe CHI have problems with discourse; for example, they may produce language that is fragmented and difficult to follow and have difficulty with word retrieval (Chapman, 1997). Brain injury may also affect a child's cognitive, executive, and behavioral skills (Taylor, 2001). Such effects include difficulties with sustained and selective attention (maintaining attention during an ongoing activity, including when distractions are present), storing new information, retrieving known information, planning and setting goals, organizing, reasoning and solving problems, being self-aware, and monitoring behavior (Taylor, 2001). Children and adolescents with brain injury may be more likely to exhibit aggression, irritability, depression, and anxiety. Because the prevalent long-term repercussions of brain injury are more subtle than those of obvious physical manifestations, brain injury is often referred to as an *invisible epidemic* (Brey, 2006).

Causes

The most common causes of brain injuries are falls (28% of injuries), motor vehicle traffic crashes (20%), being struck by or against something (often occurring in sports and recreational activities, 19%), and assaults (11%) (CDC, 2007). For children, recreational and sports injuries, such those sustained while bicycling, playing football, and riding horses, are common causes of brain injury. Risk factors for incurring brain injury include (a) participating in contact sports or other recreational activities that may result in a fall or collision and (b) using drugs or alcohol during these activities or when driving or riding in vehicles.

Hearing Loss
Defining Characteristics

A *hearing loss* is a physical condition in which an individual cannot detect or distinguish the full range of sounds normally available to the human ear. It can result from prenatal, perinatal, or postnatal damage to any of the structures that carry auditory information from the external world to the brain centers that process auditory information. As shown in Figure 10.1, hearing loss resulting from damage to the outer or middle ear is termed conductive loss, whereas hearing loss resulting from damage to the inner ear or auditory nerve is termed sensorineural loss. Conductive and sensorineural loss may occur *bilaterally* (both ears are affected) or *unilaterally* (one ear is affected and the other is intact). Hearing loss that results from damage to the centers of the brain that process auditory information is called auditory-processing disorder (APD).

Individuals with hearing loss compose a heterogeneous group based not only on the type of loss (conductive, sensorineural, APD), but also on the timing and severity of the loss. A hearing loss present at birth is termed a congenital hearing loss. About 50% of all cases of congenital hearing loss occur for unknown reasons (Gallaudet Research Institute, 2001). Several of the more prevalent causes include genetic transmission (i.e., one or both of the child's parents carry a gene for hearing

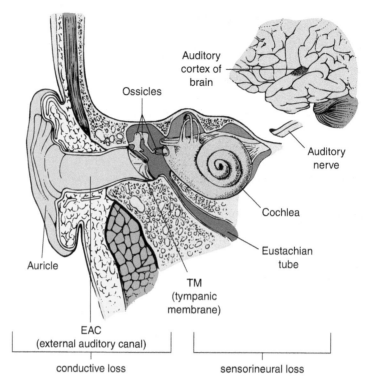

Auditory
cortex of
brain

Ossicles

Auditory
nerve

Cochlea

Eustachian
tube

Auricle

TM
(tympanic
membrane)

EAC
(external auditory canal)

conductive loss   sensorineural loss

FIGURE 10.1

Types of hearing loss based on the location of auditory damage.

Source: Justice, Laura M., Communication Sciences & Disorders: An Introduction, 1st Ed., ©2006.
Reprinted and Electronically reproduced by permission of Pearson Education, Inc., New York,
New York.

loss), in utero infections (e.g., herpes, rubella), prematurity, pregnancy complications, and trauma during the birth process. A hearing loss that occurs after birth is termed an acquired hearing loss. Prominent causes include noise exposure, infection, use of ototoxic medications (i.e., medications that damage the hearing structures), and chronic middle-ear infections (Martin & Greer Clark, 2002). Acquired hearing loss is often differentiated into that acquired after birth but before the child has developed language, termed a prelingual hearing loss, and that acquired sometime after the child has developed language, termed a postlingual hearing loss. Postlingual hearing loss has less of an impact on a child's language development than does prelingual hearing loss.

Whether prelingual or postlingual, hearing loss ranges in severity from mild to profound, as shown in Table 10.3. Professionals typically determine the severity of loss using the *decibel (dB) scale*, which is the standard unit of sound intensity, or loudness. The range of human hearing is from 0 dB (the threshold of sound) to 140 dB, which corresponds to a continuum from the drop of a pin (0 dB) to a fire alarm close to your ear (140 dB). Experts use the decibel scale to identify the threshold at which an individual with hearing loss can hear sound (Pakulski, 2006):

16–25 dB: minimal loss

26–40 dB: mild loss

41–55 dB: moderate loss

56–70 dB: moderately severe loss

71–90 dB: severe loss

91 dB or higher: profound loss

TABLE 10.3

Severity of hearing loss and possible effects

DEGREE OF HEARING IMPAIRMENT (DB HL)	POTENTIAL SPEECH AND LANGUAGE EFFECTS	POTENTIAL EDUCATIONAL EFFECTS
Normal hearing (–10 to +15)	May have difficulty discriminating speech in the presence of background noise	• None
Minimal loss (16–25)	May have difficulty detecting faint and distant speech, listening in a noisy room, and detecting word–sound distinctions (e.g., verb tenses, plural forms, possessives)	• May miss 10% of classroom instruction • May appear inattentive or uninterested • May be more fatigued because of increased listening effort
Mild loss (26–40)	Depending on degree of loss, may miss 25%–50% of speech signals, including many consonants necessary for intelligibility, which will affect language development and articulation	• May appear to daydream or listen only when interested • Likely to be more fatigued or irritable
Moderate loss (41–55)	Without sound amplification, will miss 75% or more of speech signals; thus, will likely have delayed syntax, limited vocabulary, imperfect speech production, and voice-quality issues	• Will have difficulty with receptive and expressive language, reading, spelling, and other school concepts • Will miss most classroom instruction presented orally
Moderately severe loss (56–70)	Will miss as much as 100% of all speech signals, so will have marked difficulty in both one-on-one and group conversations, will have delayed language and syntax and reduced voice quality and speech intelligibility, and will produce unintelligible speech 75% of the time	• Will not be able to keep up with oral instruction and will fall behind academically • All academic subjects likely to be affected
Severe loss (71–90) *and profound loss* (91+)	Without sound amplification, may not develop speech or language, or preexisting skills will deteriorate for acquired conditions	• Without intervention, will not be able to participate in a typical academic setting
Unilateral loss (mild or worse)	May have difficulty hearing faint or distant speech, localizing sounds, and understanding speech in poor listening conditions	• May miss important oral instructions or descriptions (particularly in a noisy room), which will lead to incomplete concept development or misunderstanding

dB HL = decibels hearing level.

Source: Information from *Communication Sciences and Disorders: An Introduction* (p. 260), by L. M. Justice, 2006, Upper Saddle River, NJ: Pearson Education, Inc. Copyright 2006 by Pearson Education, Inc. Reprinted with permission. (Adapted from *Facilitating Hearing and Listening in Young Children*, by C. Flexer, 1994, San Diego, CA: Singular.)

Because audition is the primary way children experience language, the impact of any hearing loss can influence a child's language acquisition profoundly. This is particularly true for children whose hearing loss occurs prelingually (before they have developed language skills). However, the extent to which hearing loss affects a child's language development depends on a number of factors, including the following four:

1. *Timing of the loss:* At what age did the loss occur?
2. *Severity of the loss:* How severe is the loss? Is it unilateral or bilateral?
3. *Age of identification:* At what age was the loss identified?
4. *Exposure to language input:* How much language exposure does the child receive?

Of these factors, the third and fourth are unequivocally the most important because they are most strongly related to whether the child with hearing loss acquires typical or atypical language. A child with even a profound hearing loss, whose loss is identified early and whose exposure to language input is not compromised, can develop language at virtually the same rate as a child without hearing loss. For instance, a child with profound hearing loss who experiences sign language in the home environment because his or her parents are native users of signing, will likely progress at a normal language development rate. Likewise, a child with profound hearing loss whose loss is identified early and soon afterward undergoes cochlear implantation that makes spoken language audible may also progress fairly typically in speech and language acquisition (Niparko et al., 2010; Svirsky, Teoh, & Neuburger, 2004). Cochlear implants serve as an intervention for children ages 12 months and older with severe to profound hearing loss. This intervention is desirable for parents who want their child who is deaf to develop as an oral language user. A cochlear implant requires surgical implantation of a receiver–stimulator (implanted in a hollowed-out portion of the mastoid bone) and an electrode array (implanted in the cochlea), which accompany external hardware worn by the user (microphone, speech processor, transmitter, and power supply). Although children with implants have variable language outcomes (Pisoni, Cleary, Geers, & Tobey, 2000), for many children with profound hearing loss, cochlear implants provide a promising option for accelerating their language growth to approximate that of normal development (e.g., Ertmer, Strong, & Sadagopan, 2003). Recent studies indicate

A cochlear implant involves surgical implantation of a receiver–stimulator and an electrode array. These components process auditory information in the surrounding environment, which makes hearing possible for persons with profound hearing loss.

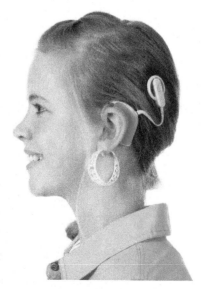

© Elsa Hoffmann/Shutterstock

language outcomes are substantially improved for children who receive implants earlier; in part, this is because children with earlier implants experience a shorter period of hearing deficit (Niparko et al., 2010).

For children whose hearing loss is not identified early, and for whom no consistent avenue to language input (whether signed or spoken) is ensured, the loss can severely compromise their language acquisition. This outcome is true even for relatively mild hearing loss, such as might occur for the child who experiences chronic middle-ear infections accompanied by fluid in the middle ear. For children with mild to more severe hearing loss that is not identified or treated consistently and proactively, language acquisition is often significantly delayed. These children often show language impairment that transcends all five domains of language. With regard to morphology and syntax, children with hearing loss show delays in their acquisition of simple and more complex syntax and their production of grammatical morphemes (Tye-Murray, 2000). In the area of semantics, children with hearing loss show delayed growth in vocabulary and use fewer different words during communication (Coppens et al., 2012). With regard to phonology, children with hearing loss show delays in their acquisition of expressive phonology, including distortions of consonants (Shriberg, Friel-Patti, Flipsen, & Brown, 2000). Finally, in the area of pragmatics, children with hearing loss may communicate less frequently with their peers and show delays in their production of different communicative intentions (e.g., questioning, responding; Most, Shina-August, & Meilijson, 2010).

Causes

Hearing loss is a relatively common condition among children. As many of 50% of young children experience fluctuating hearing loss as a result of chronic otitis media (ASHA, 2005). Although relatively few children exhibit severe or profound permanent hearing loss (about 1%–2%), as many as 8% exhibit hearing loss serious enough to affect their language and educational achievement (ASHA, 2005). The causes of hearing loss are numerous; several of the more prevalent causes are listed in Figure 10.2.

10.3

Check Your Understanding

Click here to gauge your understanding of the concepts in this section.

- Family history of congenital hearing loss

- Congenital infection linked to hearing loss (e.g., herpes, rubella)

- Craniofacial anomaly affecting the ear

- Low birth weight

- Ototoxic medications

- Bacterial meningitis and other infectious diseases associated with hearing loss (e.g., measles)

- Low Apgar scores at birth

- Mechanical ventilation for 10 days or longer

- Presence of a syndrome associated with hearing loss (e.g., Down syndrome)

- Head trauma during or soon after birth

FIGURE 10.2

Prevalent causes of hearing loss.

Source: Based on "1990 Position Statement," by Joint Committee on Infant Hearing, 1991, *ASHA, 33* (Suppl. 5), pp. 3–6; and *Introduction to Audiology* (5th ed.), by F. Martin, 1994, Upper Saddle River, NJ: Prentice Hall.

Identification and Treatment of Language Disorders

Identifying children who exhibit language disorders requires administration of a *comprehensive language evaluation*, most often conducted by a certified SLP. The goal of the evaluation is to determine whether a language disorder is present and, if so, to develop a profile of the child's linguistic strengths and weaknesses and a plan for intervention. The comprehensive language evaluation typically includes a case history and an interview, followed by a comprehensive assessment of language skills.

Case History and Interview

The case history involves administering a questionnaire and interviewing the child's parents; examples of questions appear in Figure 10.3. The case history documents a child's developmental history, general health, medical conditions and allergies, family size and resources, language and communicative history, current skills, interests, and behaviors as well as the parents' and child's perception of suspected problems. Typically, after a parent completes a case history questionnaire, the professional interviews him or her to focus on certain areas, particularly language and communication. For instance, the professional is likely to ask pointed questions about how a child meets his or her needs in the home environment, which words he or she uses often, and when he or she met specific language milestones (e.g., combining two words).

Comprehensive Language Assessment

The SLP designs and administers a comprehensive assessment of a child's language abilities. This assessment is often completed during several hours in a private, quiet location. For young children, the assessment may be administered in several test sessions to prevent fatigue in or frustration of the child. It also often involves observation of the child in different contexts, including the classroom for school-age children. The assessment is designed to analyze both comprehension and production in all language domains. For younger children who are not yet talking, the

---

1. What age was your child when he/she first started to babble?

2. When did your child say his/her first word?

3. What are some examples of words your child used when he/she first started talking?

4. When did your child start to produce short sentences?

5. Do you ever notice occasions when your child has a difficult time expressing him/herself? Can you give me an example of one of these times and what you did in response?

6. How would you describe your child's conversational style? Does he/she often start conversations with you? When you ask him/her questions, does she usually respond?

7. Give me an example of a question you often ask of your child, and how he/she would typically respond.

8. How well does your child communicate with peers who are the same age? How long does a typical conversation last?

9. When eating dinner at your home with your child, what are some typical things he/she might say?

10. Share with me some specific concerns you have about your child's communication, speech, and language. How long have you had these concerns?

FIGURE 10.3

Examples of questions on a case history.

analysis covers the development of critical language precursors, including babbling, gesturing, affect and expression, participation in early communicative routines, and periods of joint attention. For older children, the analysis covers not only oral and written language skills, including reading, writing, and spelling, but also children's performance on classroom- and curriculum-based tasks.

One important characteristic of the comprehensive language assessment is that it focuses on functional aspects of language so that the professional can study the extent to which a child's language skills affect his or her ability to function at home and in school. For young children, the assessment examines children's ability to use language skills in their daily lives to meet their needs through various communicative functions. Such functions include requesting objects and actions; expressing feelings of interest, pleasure, and excitement; responding to other people's questions, requests, and comments; and using social behaviors such as greeting other people. For older children, the analysis examines the extent to which children's language skills affect their ability to participate in the school curriculum and to interact with friends, teachers, and parents effectively.

The professional uses many tests and tasks to conduct the comprehensive language assessment, including criterion-referenced tasks, norm-referenced tests, and observational measures. Criterion-referenced tasks examine a child's performance level for a particular type of language task, such as the percentage of one-step directions (e.g., "Give me the cup") the child can perform correctly. For instance, a professional might use a criterion-referenced task to study a child's understanding of various locational and spatial terms, such as *in, on, under, below, next to, beside, above,* and *behind*. By providing the child with a ball and a box, the professional could assess the child's performance by using a series of directives, such as "Put the ball *under* the box" and "Put the ball *next to* the box." The child's performance on the criterion-referenced task is calculated by dividing the number of items responded to correctly by the number of tasks administered. Criterion-referenced tasks can be used both to provide a baseline examination of a child's skills in a given area and to monitor children's performance gains with time.

Norm-referenced tests compare children's level of language performance to that of a national sample of same-age peers. This type of testing often requires the use of commercially available tests, such as the Clinical Evaluation of Language Fundamentals—Preschool-2 (Wiig, Secord, & Semel, 2004). This norm-referenced test is used with children ages 3–6 years, 11 months and includes six subtests that cover expressive and receptive language skills in the areas of morphology, syntax, and vocabulary. Scores derived from norm-referenced tests show how a child's language skills in different domains of language compare to those of a large population of children at the same age. These scores are often an important aspect of the diagnosis of a language disorder, as the diagnosis is based on showing that a child's language skills are underdeveloped relative to age-based expectations.

Observational measures examine children's language form, content, and use in naturalistic activities with peers or parents. Two types of observational measures are commonly used in language assessment. The first is *conversational analysis*. In conversational analysis, the professional observes a child during interactions with other people to study his or her ability to initiate conversation, to use different communicative intentions, to take turns, to maintain topics, to identify breakdowns in conversation, and to attend to listener needs. The second type is *language sample analysis* (LSA). With LSA, the professional collects a sample of spontaneous language from the child, typically comprising at least 50 utterances, then analyzes the sample for all aspects of language. Some common measures used in LSA are listed in Table 10.4. Various computer programs, such as the Systematic Analysis of Language Transcripts (SALT; Miller & Chapman, 2000), are available for use with LSA. For instance, after inputting a language sample into the SALT computer program, the professional can compute standard statistics on the sample, including the mean length of utterance, the total number of words, the total number of different words, and the use of conjunctions.

TABLE 10.4
Examples of Various Measures Used in Language Sample Analysis

LANGUAGE AREA	MEASURE
Semantics	• Total number of words
	• Number of different words
	• Use of rare words
	• Lexical ties across utterances
	• Naming errors
	• Word-finding problems (e.g., hesitations, circumlocutions)
Phonology	• Percentage of consonants produced correctly
	• Inventory of different consonants used
	• Types of consonant errors (omissions, substitutions, distortions)
	• Consonant use patterns across different syllable structures
Syntax and morphology	• Mean length of utterance
	• Grammatical morpheme use
	• Percentage of grammatically correct utterances
	• Percentage of complex utterances
	• Conjunction use
	• Elaborated noun phrase use
	• Verb phrase use
	• Variety of sentence types
Pragmatics	• Length of conversational turns
	• Number of initiations
	• Contingency of responses
	• Responses to conversational breakdowns
	• Variety of communicative intentions

Diagnosis

Once the professional completes tl
she assesses the findings to determir
if so, to make a diagnosis. The diag
impairment (primary, secondary), a
verity (mild, moderate, severe, profo
prognosis statement. An excellent or
resolve, whereas a poor prognosis m
cases, professionals do not write a
information from other specialists o
responds to treatment has passed.

General Educators
+
Special Educators

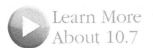

Learn More About 10.7

As you watch the video titled "Speech and Language Disorders", notice the different warning signs of disorders (specifically language disorders). Furthermore, be aware of the different resources caregivers have available to them when faced with helping a child with a speech and/or language disorder.

https://www.youtube.com/watch?v=a43SmCKhfHE

Treatment of Language Disorders

The nature of a child's language disorder drives the course of treatment. For instance, if a child has a severe language disorder, his or her treatment approach will be more intensive than that for a child with mild problems. Likewise, a child whose language disorder is secondary to autism will receive a treatment approach distinct from that of a child whose language disorder is secondary to traumatic brain injury. The professional develops a treatment plan that is unique to the child's needs and strengths. The plan specifies (a) treatment targets, (b) treatment strategies, and (c) treatment contexts.

Treatment Targets

Treatment targets, also called *treatment objectives*, are the aspects of language addressed during treatment. For instance, a treatment target for a 2-year-old might be to produce two-word utterances to communicate needs, whereas a treatment target for an adolescent might be to comprehend figurative language (e.g., jokes heard on the playground). A treatment target for a young child with autism might be to communicate nonverbally for various purposes (request, reject, comment), whereas a treatment target for a first grader with traumatic brain injury might be to answer questions with appropriate, on-topic responses. Some professionals may emphasize only one or two objectives at a time, whereas others may target many objectives simultaneously.

In developing treatment targets, professionals set both long-term and short-term objectives. Long-term objectives specify the long-term goal of treatment, such as "Juan will achieve receptive vocabulary skills commensurate with those of his same-age peers", or "when interacting with other people, Anika will use a full range of communicative intentions to meet her needs." Short-term objectives specify a series of intermediate goals that, when achieved, ultimately lead to the desired long-term objective. For instance, to achieve Anika's long-term objective, a treatment plan for a therapy session might include these two short-term objectives:

1. Anika will use five requests for actions (through gesture, vocalizations, or words) from her peers, given a model by the therapist, during each of three consecutive sessions.

2. Anika will spontaneously use words to pose three requests for actions or objects from her peers during each of three consecutive sessions.

Treatment Strategies

Treatment strategies are the ways in which treatment targets are addressed. There are many strategies available to use to address the language goals for a specific child. One such strategy is called *focused stimulation* (Smith-Lock, Leitao, Lambert, & Nickels, 2013; Solomon-Rice & Soto, 2014). With focused stimulation, the clinician provides multiple and highly salient models of language targets that are goals for the child. For instance, if a child cannot request using the word *want*, the clinician would set up communicative temptations in the context of play-based interactions to entice the child to use the word *want*. The clinician would also repeatedly model use of this word ("I *want* the cookie," "The boy *wants* candy," "The dog *wants* the bone"). To make the word stand out, he or she might say it loudly, slowly, or with dramatic pitch changes. During focused stimulation, the child is not required to respond; however, the parent or professional arranges the environment and uses oral techniques to *entice* the child's oral participation and use of language targets. Focused stimulation and other child-centered strategies are often used with young children (infants and preschoolers) and can be implemented by parents in the home following training by a professional (Girolametto, Pearce, & Weitzman, 1996).

With older children, a more direct approach might be used to teach children with language disorders how to apply specific strategies to compensate for underlying challenges with language comprehension and production. For instance, the clinician might use a barrier game in which he or she places a barrier between himself or herself and the child. The therapist then gives the child an illustration featuring a complex event and asks the child to describe the picture sufficiently so that the therapist can reproduce it. During the barrier task, the therapist coaches the child to use a comprehension monitoring strategy in which the child pauses periodically to check whether the listener is following his or her instructions.

Comprehension monitoring is one strategy children with language disorders can be trained to use to promote more effective communication with other people. A *strategy* is the way an individual approaches a task; it includes both cognitive and behavioral components (i.e., how a person thinks and acts when doing something). Strategy training can be an effective way to improve children's abilities to complete diverse language tasks, such as understanding jokes, initiating conversation with friends or adults, or deciphering unknown words when reading. Strategy instruction focuses on teaching students specific ways to approach a linguistic task by following specific steps. First, the clinician will describe and model the strategy; then, the child will discuss, rehearse, and practice the strategy; finally, the child will be helped to use the strategy in other settings.

Treatment Contexts

Treatment contexts are the settings in which treatment targets and strategies are used. Treatment contexts should include as many settings as possible to promote generalization of skills learned in treatment (i.e., the application of skills to many diverse settings). For instance, children may experience treatment targets and strategies at home with their parents, in the classroom with their teachers, and in the clinic with their SLPs. Clearly, collaboration among parents, teachers, SLPs, and other professionals is critical for ensuring that treatment occurs in many contexts.

For many young children receiving language intervention, treatment is often provided in the home environment. This approach allows parents to observe treatment targets and strategies directly. Home-based interventions are particularly prevalent for children younger than age 3 years who receive language therapy through early intervention services. For older children, treatment usually occurs in the school setting (preschool; elementary, middle, or high school), although parental involvement remains important and should occur at every opportunity. Some children receive language treatment in outpatient hospital clinics or private centers.

In the school setting, treatment contexts can vary. Although historically children received language intervention in a *pullout model*, in which language therapy was provided in a "speech room," there has been a push in recent years to provide children therapy through collaborative classroom-based models, in which teachers and SLPs work together to target language goals within the classroom environment. SLPs may work individually with children in classrooms during small-group or center times, may co-teach or collaborate to develop particular lessons with teachers, or may train teachers to integrate language enhancement techniques into their classroom instruction. However, examination of practices used by school-based SLPs suggest that a majority of children are still served using a pullout model (Brandel & Loeb, 2011), although about 10%–20% of children are served using classroom-based approaches.

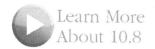

Learn More About 10.8

As you watch the video titled "Speech & Language Therapy: Helping Michael", think about how a child like Michael is identified as having a language disorder, and also think about how treatment for the disorder is implemented in conjunction with the help of many other caregivers (i.e., parents, teacher, etc.). https://www.youtube.com/watch?v=MpdjP0zHeBc

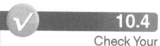

10.4
Check Your Understanding
Click here to gauge your understanding of the concepts in this section.

SUMMARY

A *language disorder* is present when an individual exhibits impaired comprehension or expression of a spoken, written, or other symbol system. Language disorders are the most prevalent type of communication impairment affecting children. When professionals identify a language disorder, they do so by considering the extent to which a child's language difficulties (a) have an adverse impact on social, psychological, and educational functioning; (b) may represent a *language difference* (rather than a disorder); and (c) are significant enough to be considered disordered.

Various professionals are involved with identifying and treating language disorders in children. *Speech–language pathologists* (SLPs) are frequently the lead service providers for children with language disorders. Their responsibilities include prevention, screening, consultation, assessment and diagnosis, and treatment delivery. *Cognitive and developmental psychologists* conduct important basic and applied research relevant to theoretical understanding of language disorders. *Clinical, rehabilitation,* and *school psychologists,* as well as *clinical neuropsychologists,* may work directly with children with language disorders, screening for and identifying the disorders. *General educators* and *special educators* have the important role of supporting the educational achievement of children with language disorders in the school setting. *Early interventionists* specialize in assessment and treatment of developmental disabilities in infants and toddlers; thus, they play a critical role in early identification and intervention for young children with suspected or diagnosed language disorders. *Audiologists*

are specialists in auditory system disorders and are involved with assessing and treating language disorders when the auditory system is involved. *Otorhinolaryngologists* work with children whose language disorders result from disease or infection of the ear, nose, or throat.

Five prevalent developmental conditions associated with language disorder are *specific language impairment* (SLI), *autism spectrum disorder* (ASD), *intellectual disability* (ID), *traumatic brain injury* (TBI), and *hearing loss.* SLI is a primary language impairment in which children show significant challenges with language development in the absence of any other known developmental difficulty. ASD refers to individuals who exhibit disordered social-communication, repetitive behaviors, difficulties with social relationships, and oftentimes restricted interests. ID is a developmental disability associated with language disorders ranging from mild to profound concomitant with intellectual limitations that impair adaptive skills. Language disorders resulting from TBI are typically characterized by discourse problems and additional executive difficulties. Hearing loss may be accompanied by a language disorder if it is not detected and early intervention is not instituted.

Identification of a language disorder requires administration of a *comprehensive language evaluation.* It typically includes a case history, an interview, and completion of a comprehensive language assessment using standardized norm-referenced tasks, criterion-referenced tasks, and observational measures. The treatment of language disorders typically follows a treatment plan that specifies language targets, treatment strategies, and treatment contexts.

 Apply Your Knowledge

Click here to apply your knowledge to practical scenarios.

BEYOND THE BOOK

1. Identify five ways in which an impairment of language might affect an individual's social and educational functioning.

2. Watch a video of a toddler on youtube.com. Document how many different words the child uses in a 2-minute period and how the child uses these words to meet his or her needs. How might a child with language impairment look differently than the child you observed?

3. Look online for a description of the newly revised DSM-5. Study the description of the autism spectrum disorder diagnosis, and compare it to the description of DSM-4. How has the diagnosis of autism changed over time?

4. Watch the movie *Rainman* and observe the language skills of the main character, who has autism spectrum disorder. Would the character be described as having mild, moderate, or a severe disorder of language?

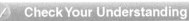 **Check Your Understanding**

Gauge your understanding of the chapter concepts by taking this self-check quiz.

Glossary

accents Varieties of language that vary only in pronunciation, not in vocabulary or grammar. Contrast *dialects*.

acoustics The study of sound.

acquired brain injuries Damage to the brain occurring in utero (before birth) and perinatally (during the birth process), as well as after birth. See also *closed-head injury*; *open-head injuries*; *traumatic brain injury*.

acquired hearing loss Hearing loss that occurs after birth as a result of such factors as noise exposure, infection, use of ototoxic medications, and chronic middle-ear infections. Contrast *congenital hearing loss*. See also *postlingual hearing loss*; *prelingual hearing loss*.

acquisition rate How fast language is learned.

adverse impact An unfavorable or harmful effect.

afferent Used to describe the pathway of information as it moves *toward* the brain. Afferent pathways carry sensory information from the distal body structures to the brain; such pathways are also called *ascending pathways*. Contrast *efferent*.

African American Vernacular English Abbreviated AAVE. A systematic, rule-governed variety of English spoken by African Americans as well as persons of other races and ethnicities. AAVE differs from GAE in many features of form, content, and use.

age of mastery The age by which most children produce a sound in an adultlike manner. See also *customary age of production*.

agent In an event, the entity that performs the action. See also *goal*; *location*; *source*; *theme*.

allocortex In evolutionary terms, the original and older human brain. It and the neocortex compose the cerebrum.

allophones The subtle variations of phonemes that occur as a result of contextual influence on how phonemes are produced in different words. Example: The two /p/ phonemes in *pop* are produced differently and are thus allophones. See also *phonology*.

alphabet knowledge Knowledge about the letters of the alphabet. A type of metalinguistic ability important to emergent literacy development.

alphabetic principle The relationship between letters or combinations of letters (graphemes) and sounds (phonemes).

applied research Studying language development to test different approaches and practices that pertain to real-world settings or to address specific problems in society and to inform practices relevant to language development. Contrast *basic research*.

arachnoid mater The second layer of the meninges. A delicate membrane separated from the pia mater by the subarachnoid space. See also *dura mater*; *pia mater*.

arbitrary A property of human language; describes the notion that there is no relationship between a referent and the language used to describe it.

articulation Manipulation of a breath of air by the oral articulators—including the tongue, teeth, and jaw—so that it comes out as a series of speech sounds that are combined into words, phrases, and sentences. One of four systems involved in speech. See also *phonation*; *resonation*; *respiration*.

assimilation The process by which children change one sound in a syllable so that it takes on the features of another sound in the same syllable. A context-dependent change. Includes velar assimilation.

audition The perception of sound, including general auditory perception and speech perception. See *hearing*.

auditory perception How the brain processes any type of auditory information (e.g., a clap of the hands), not just speech. Contrast *speech perception*.

auditory-processing disorder Abbreviated APD. Hearing loss that results from damage to the centers of the brain that process auditory information. Contrast *conductive loss*; *sensorineural loss*.

avoidance A common developmental process in second language acquisition that describes when a learner avoids using sounds, words, or grammatical constructions he or she finds difficult or does not know.

axon The single efferent nerve extension from the cell body of a neuron. Extends from the cell body for a distance of 1 mm to 1 m, at which point it arborizes into a number of terminal branches. It, along with the dendrites, serves as a vehicle for the cell body to receive and transmit information from other neurons. One of four parts of a neuron. See also *cell body*; *dendrites*; *presynaptic terminal*.

babbling A young child's production of syllables that contain pairs of consonants and vowels (*C–V sequences* when the consonant precedes the vowel). Usually begins between ages 6 and 10 months. See also *jargon*; *marginal babbling*; *nonreduplicated babbling*; *reduplicated babbling*.

basic research Also called *theoretical research*. Studying language development primarily to generate and refine the existing knowledge base. See also *use-inspired basic research*. Contrast *applied research*.

bilingualism Technically, a process by which people acquire *two* first languages. In this text, for the sake of simplicity, a process by which people acquire *two or more* first languages. The two languages can be learned simultaneously or sequentially. A type of language difference (rather than disorder). Contrast *monolingualism*; *second language acquisition*.

bound morphemes   Grammatical morphemes that cannot be freestanding; they must be attached to other morphemes: prefixes and suffixes. Contrast *free morphemes*.

brainstem   One of the three divisions of the brain. Sits directly on top of the spinal cord and serves as a conduit between the rest of the brain and the spinal cord. Comprises the midbrain, the pons, and the medulla oblongata. It has three primary roles: (a) a key transmitter of sensory information to the brain and of motor information away from the brain; (b) a major relay station for the cranial nerves supplying the head and face and for controlling the visual and auditory areas; and (c) a center for metabolic control and arousal. See also *cerebellum*; *cerebrum*.

Broca's area   Named after the French physician Paul Broca. A region of the left frontal lobe of the cerebrum, important for the fine coordination of speech output. See also *premotor cortex*; *primary motor cortex*.

C units   See *communication units*.

categorical perception   An ability that allows humans to categorize speech in ways that highlight differences in meaning and ignore variations that are nonessential or not meaningful in their language.

categorical scope   A principle that builds on the principle of extendibility by limiting the basis for extension to words that are taxonomically similar.

caudal   A positional term that describes the specific nervous system structures along the horizontal and vertical axes of the neuraxis. With regard to the horizontal axis, it means "toward the back of the brain." With regard to the vertical axis, it means "toward the bottom of the spinal cord (near the coccyx, or tailbone)." Contrast *dorsal*; *rostral*; *ventral*.

cell body   The center of a neuron, containing its nucleus. One of four parts of a neuron. See also *axon*; *dendrites*; *presynaptic terminal*.

central nervous system   Abbreviated CNS. The brain and the spinal cord. Contrast *peripheral nervous system*.

cerebellum   One of three major divisions of the brain. Oval-shaped "little brain" that resides posterior to the brainstem. It is primarily responsible for regulating motor and muscular activity and has little to do with the "rational" part of the brain that involves conscious planning responses. It coordinates motor movements, maintains muscle tone, monitors movement range and strength, and maintains posture and equilibrium. See also *brainstem*; *cerebrum*.

cerebrospinal fluid   Abbreviated CSF. Along with bone and the meninges, it shields the central nervous system by circulating between the two innermost layers of the meninges: the pia mater and the arachnoid mater.

cerebrum   Also known as the *cerebral cortex*. The largest of the three major divisions of the brain. Plays roles in language, conceptual thinking, creativity, planning, and the form and substances of human thoughts. Consists of right and left hemispheres and is organized into six lobes of four types: one frontal, one occipital, two temporal, and two

parietal lobes. Comprises the allocortex and the neocortex. See also *brainstem*; *cerebellum*.

child-directed speech   Abbreviated CDS. The talk directed to children by others, including parents and other caregivers.

closed-head injury   Abbreviated CHI. The most common type of traumatic brain injury (TBI), in which brain matter is not exposed or penetrated. One cause in infants is shaken baby syndrome. Usually results in a more diffuse brain injury. Contrast *open-head injuries*.

coarticulation   The overlapping of phonemes during human speech.

code switching   When speakers who have more than one language in common alternate between the languages. Bilingual children may code switch to fill in lexical or grammatical gaps, for pragmatic effect, or to follow the social norms of their community. Example: A child who is bilingual in Spanish and English may produce an English sentence with Spanish syntax. See also *interutterance mixing*; *intrautterance mixing*.

communication breakdowns   Communication problems that occur when receivers do not provide appropriate types or amounts of feedback or when senders do not attend to the feedback. See also *conversational repair*.

communication function   The intention of a communication used in a social context, such as instrumental, regulatory, interactional, personal, heuristic, imaginative, or informative.

communication   The process of sharing information among individuals. Communication can involve only language (e.g., communication in an Internet chat room), or language, hearing, and speech (e.g., a spoken conversation).

communication units (C units)   Each C unit consists of an independent clause and any of its modifiers, such as a dependent clause. Can include incomplete sentences and sentence fragments. C units are coded in transcripts of language samples to assess a student's language form. Contrast *terminable units* (*T units*).

communicative accommodation   The way in which a culture produces infant-directed speech. It can range from highly child centered to highly situation centered.

complex syntax   Grammatically well-formed sentences containing phrases, clauses, and conjunctions, which are used to organize the internal structures of the sentences. Contrast *simple syntax*.

comprehensible input   Language input that is just slightly ahead of a learner's current state of grammatical knowledge. Also known as the *i + 1 level*, where *i* is the learner's current state of knowledge. Part of Krashen's (1985) theory that language that contains structures a second language (L2) learner has already mastered will not help his or her acquisition of the L2, nor will input that is too difficult.

comprehension monitoring   A strategy used during a barrier task, in which the child must pause periodically to check whether the listener is following his or her instructions. Part of a clinician-directed approach to training children with language disorders to communicate more effectively with other people. See also *strategy training*.

comprehensive evaluations   Assessments used to obtain an in-depth probe of a specific child's instructional needs. Such assessments are typically used to identify the presence of a language disability.

conductive loss   Hearing loss resulting from damage to the outer or middle ear. Contrast *auditory-processing disorder; sensorineural loss.*

congenital hearing loss   A hearing loss present at birth. About 50% of all cases occur for unknown reasons. Causes include genetic transmission, in utero infections, prematurity, pregnancy complications, and trauma during the birth process. Contrast *acquired hearing loss.*

connectionist models   Models that attempt to represent the computational architecture of the brain as it processes various types of information, particularly that which is specific to higher-order cognition, such as reasoning and problem solving. According to such models, information processing within the brain involves a network of distributed processors that interact with one another by means of excitatory and inhibitory connections.

content   Synonymous with *semantics.* The meaning of language. The words used and the meaning behind them. One of the three language domains. See also *form; lexicon; use.*

contextualized language   The language used, beginning in infancy, that is grounded in the immediate context, or the here and now. Contrast *decontextualized language.*

contextualized   Relying on the immediate context, or setting, to convey content. Contrast *decontextualized; semanticity.*

contralateral   A feature of the central nervous system whereby the right side of the brain processes information from the left side of the body, and vice versa.

conventionality   A principle stating that for children to communicate successfully, they must adopt the terms people in their language community understand.

conversational repair   When a communication breakdown occurs and the sender or receiver adjusts the exchange to mend the breakdown. It requires the receiver to provide ongoing feedback and the sender to monitor the receiver's feedback closely.

conversations   Exchanges with other people.

corpus callosum   The band of fibers that connects the two hemispheres of the cerebrum. Serves as a conduit for communication between them. See also *longitudinal fissure.*

cranial nerves   The 12 pairs of nerves that emerge from the brain.

criterion-referenced tasks   Tasks used to examine a child's performance level for a particular type of language task, such as understanding locational and spatial terms. Typically used as part of a comprehensive language assessment. See also *dynamic assessment; norm-referenced tests; observational measures.*

critical period   Also called *sensitive period.* The window of opportunity during which children develop language most rapidly and with the most ease.

critical period hypothesis   The theory that the time between birth and puberty is crucial for language acquisition and that adolescents and adults may experience difficulty acquiring a second language.

cultural context   The cultural setting in which a child learns and applies language. Practitioners must take it into account when differentiating between a language difference and a language disorder.

customary age of production   The age by which 50% of all children can produce a given sound in multiple positions in words in an adultlike way. Contrast *age of mastery.*

declarative pointing   Pointing by an infant to call an adult's attention to objects and to comment on objects. Involves a social process between an infant and an adult. Occurs after age 10 months. Contrast *imperative pointing.*

declarative sentences   Sentences that make a statement. Contrast *interrogative sentences; negative sentences.*

decontextualized language   Language that relies heavily on itself in the construction of meaning. Begins to emerge during the preschool period. Contrast *contextualized language.*

decontextualized   Not relying on the immediate context, or setting, to convey content. Contrast *contextualized.*

deep-structure ambiguity   A form of sentential ambiguity in which a noun serves as an agent in one interpretation and as an object in another. Example: *The duck is ready to eat* can mean "The duck is ready to be eaten" or "The duck is hungry." Contrast *surface-structure ambiguity.*

dendrites   The afferent extensions from the single cell body of a neuron. They bring nerve impulses into the cell body from the axonal projections of other neurons. One of four parts of a neuron. See also *axon; cell body; presynaptic terminal.*

dendritic sprouting   The formation of new synaptic connections among neurons. Is necessary for experience dependent plasticity.

derivational morphemes   Prefixes and suffixes added to root words to create derived words. See also *derivational relations.* Contrast *grammatical morphemes.*

derivational relations   The relationship among a corpus of words that share a common root word. Example: *friend, friendless, befriend.* See also *derivational morphemes.*

dialects   Regional or social variations of a language that differ from one another in terms of their pronunciation, vocabulary, and grammar. Dialects can evolve within specific geographic regions or sociocultural communities. A type of language difference (rather than disorder). Example: African American Vernacular English. Contrast *accents.*

dishabituation   Describes a phase in a task used to renew an infant's interest in a stimulus according to a predetermined threshold. Contrast *habituation.*

displacement   The species-specific aspect of language that allows people to represent the world. In particular, it allows people to represent decontextualized events (events that are not immediately present). Also called *semanticity.*

domain general   The same as in other situations. In the context of language development, domain-general language processes are the same as the processes used in other situations, such as solving problems and perceiving objects and events in the environment. Contrast *domain specific.*

domain specific   Dedicated solely to a certain task. In the context of language development, domain-specific language processes are dedicated solely to the tasks of comprehending and producing language. Contrast *domain general*.

dorsal   A positional term experts use when describing the specific nervous system structures along the horizontal and vertical axes of the neuraxis. With regard to the horizontal axis, it means "toward the top of the brain." With regard to the vertical axis, it means "toward the back of the spinal cord (the side nearest the back)." Contrast *caudal; rostral; ventral*.

dual language learners   People who learn two or more languages simultaneously, sequentially, as a second language in school in the United States, or as a foreign language in another country.

dual language system hypothesis   The idea that bilingual children have two separate language systems from the start. According to this theory, bilingual children do not move through stages whereby they eventually differentiate between the two languages. Contrast *unitary language system hypothesis*.

dura mater   Literal meaning is "hard mother." The third and outermost layer of the meninges. Consists of thick, fibrous tissue that completely encases the brain and the spinal cord. See also *arachnoid mater; pia mater*.

duration   In terms of speech, the length of sounds. One of three prosodic characteristics of speech. Contrast *frequency; intensity*.

early consonants   Consonants that emerge early in speech–sound development. Contrast *late consonants*.

ecological validity   The extent to which the data resulting from an assessment or an evaluation can be extended to multiple contexts, including the child's home and day care settings.

efferent   Used to describe the pathway of information as it moves *away* from the brain. Efferent pathways carry motor impulses from the central nervous system to more distal body structures; such pathways are also called *descending pathways*. Contrast *afferent*.

egocentric speech   Speech that describes the worldview from only the speaker's perspective. Self-centered speech. One of the earliest forms of speech; a precursor to true dialogue.

emergent literacy   The earliest period of learning about reading and writing. Children in this stage of literacy are not yet reading and writing in a conventional sense, but their emerging knowledge about print and sounds forms an important foundation for the reading instruction that begins in formal schooling.

English language learner   Abbreviated ELL. A term used in U.S. schools to describe children who are learning English as a second language and have limited English proficiency.

enrichment   The process through which teachers, clinicians, and other adults provide children, adolescents, and adults with an enhanced language-learning environment that builds on existing skills and promotes the development of new and more advanced language skills. One of three direct applications of language theory and research to practice. See also *intervention and remediation; prevention*.

event-related potentials   Abbreviated ERPs. The electrical responses of the brain to particular stimuli, including linguistic stimuli. Used in neuroimaging.

evidence-based practice   Abbreviated EBP. The process of integrating theoretical knowledge with scientific inquiry to inform decision making.

executive functions   Functions that govern the organized, goal-directed, and controlled execution of critical human behaviors, such as monitoring and controlling purposeful behaviors, overriding impulses, and controlling information processing. The frontal lobe of the cerebrum controls these functions.

experience-dependent plasticity   Brain modification that results from highly specific types of experiences. Contrast *experience-expectant plasticity*.

experience-expectant plasticity   Changes in the brain structure that occur as a result of normal experiences. Contrast *experience-dependent plasticity*.

expressive elaboration   When the components of story grammar are combined in an expressive or artful manner of storytelling.

expressive language   The language a person produces spontaneously, without imitating another person's verbalizations. Includes content, form, and use. Contrast *receptive language*.

expressive lexicon   The volume of words a person uses; a "mental dictionary." Contrast *receptive lexicon*.

extended mapping   A full and complete understanding of the meaning of a word.

extendibility   The notion that words label categories of objects, not just the original exemplar.

extralinguistic feedback   See *nonlinguistic feedback*.

fast mapping   A type of task in which the rate at which children map a new word to its referent is determined. Contrast *slow mapping*.

feedback   (a) In models of speech production, information about the timing, delivery, and precision of speech output that is relayed back to the origination of the perceptual target and motor schema. It provides information about what is to come next at the perceptual and motor levels. Speakers are seldom aware of feedback on a conscious level. (b) In models of communication, information provided by the receiver to the sender. The sender responds to this feedback to modulate the flow of communication. See also *linguistic feedback; non-linguistic feedback*.

fictional narrative   A child's spoken or written description of an imaginary event. Contrast *personal narrative*.

figurative language   Language used in nonliteral and often abstract ways. Used to evoke mental images and sense impressions in other people. See also *hyperbole; idioms; irony; metaphor; proverbs; similes*.

follow-in   A way in which children may be exposed to novel words; an adult labels an object or event that is currently the child's attentional focus.

form   How words, sentences, and sounds are organized and arranged to convey content. One of the three language domains. See also *content; use*.

formative evaluations   Assessment of the language process (rather than the products) of language learning and development. Practitioners use these assessments to determine the types of language-learning activities to implement. Contrast *summative evaluations*.

formulaic language   An L2 learner's use of certain language routines or phrases that exist as a unit rather than as individual pieces the learner compiles for meaning (e.g., "How do you say ...?" or "I don't know").

free morphemes   Grammatical morphemes that can stand alone; they include not only words with clear semantic referents (e.g., *dream, dog*) but also words that serve primarily grammatical purposes (e.g., *his, the*). Contrast *bound morphemes*.

frequency   How fast air particles move back and forth during the creation of sound. Pitch. One of three prosodic characteristics of speech. Contrast *duration; intensity*.

frontal lobe   The largest of six lobes in the cerebrum. Resides in the most anterior part of the brain, behind the forehead. Activates and controls both fine and complex motor activities and controls executive functions. Includes the prefrontal cortex, primary motor cortex, and premotor cortex. See also *Broca's area; occipital lobe; parietal lobes; temporal lobes.*

fronting   Replacement of sounds normally produced farther back in the mouth (e.g., /k/) with sounds produced father forward in the mouth (e.g., /t/). A place-of-articulation change that is not context dependent. Example: *Cake* becomes "take."

functional flexibility   The ability to use language for various communicative purposes (e.g., requesting, stating, persuading).

functional magnetic resonance imaging   Abbreviated fMRI. A type of brain imaging that allows researchers and physicians to identify the brain structures involved in specific mental functions. Noninvasive procedure that maps neural activities to specific neural regions according to changes in blood oxygen levels that correspond to changes in neural activity.

gender differences   Language differences relating to gender. Example: Girls usually begin talking before boys do. Usually minor, particularly as children move into the preschool years.

General American English   Abbreviated GAE. Also called *Standard American English*. Dialect used most commonly in the United States (i.e., assigned the highest social status). Includes about 39 phonemes.

genetic epistemology   The study of the development of knowledge. French psychologist Jean Piaget is known for his theories on genetic epistemology.

goal   In an event, the end point for movement. See also *agent; location; source; theme.*

grammatical morphemes   Also called *inflectional morphemes*. Small units of language added to words to allow grammatical inflection of the words. Examples: the plural *-s*, the possessive *'s*, the past tense *-ed*, and the present progressive *-ing*. See also *bound morphemes; free morphemes.* Contrast *derivational morphemes.*

gray matter   Nervous tissue consisting of the cell bodies of neurons and the dendrites. Where information is generated and processed. Contrast *white matter.*

habituation   Describes a task that involves presenting an infant with the same stimulus repeatedly until his or her attention to the stimulus decreases by a predetermined amount. Contrast *dishabituation*.

hearing   The sensory system that allows speech to enter into and be processed by the human brain. See also *communication; speech.*

heritable language impairment   See *primary language impairment.*

Heschl's gyrus   Named after the Austrian anatomist Richard L. Heschl. A small left temporal lobe region that appears to be specialized for processing speech, particularly its temporal aspects.

heterographs   Words that sound alike but have different meanings and are spelled differently (e.g., *brown bear* vs. *bare hands*). A type of lexical ambiguity at the level of the word.

heteronyms   Words that are spelled the same way but have different meanings and different pronunciations (e.g., *record player* vs. *record a movie*). A type of lexical ambiguity at the level of the word. See also *heterphones.*

heterophones   Words that are spelled the same way but have different meanings and different pronunciations (e.g., *record player* vs. *record a movie*). A type of lexical ambiguity at the level of the word. See also *heteronyms.*

home language stage   In this stage of second language acquisition, children use their home language (L1) in the classroom with other children and adults.

homographs   Words that are spelled the same way and may sound alike (e.g., *row a boat* vs. *row of homes*) or may sound different from each other (e.g., *record player* vs. *record a movie*). A type of lexical ambiguity at the level of the word. See also *homonyms; homophones.*

homonyms   Words that are alike in spelling and pronunciation but differ in meaning (e.g., *brown bear* vs. *bear weight*). A specific type of homophone.

homophones   Words that sound alike and may be spelled alike (e.g., *brown bear* vs. *bear weight*) or may be spelled differently (e.g., *brown bear* vs. *bare hands*). A type of lexical ambiguity at the word level. See also *homographs; homonyms.*

horizontal axis   The part of the neuraxis that runs from the anterior (frontal) pole of the brain to the posterior (occipital) pole. See also *vertical axis.*

hyperbole   A type of figurative language that uses exaggeration for emphasis or effect. Example: *I nearly died laughing.*

iconic communication   See *intentional communication.*

idioms   Expressions that contain both literal and figurative language. Two types of idioms are opaque and transparent. Example: *He got out of the wrong side of bed.*

imperative pointing   Pointing by an infant to request an adult to retrieve an object for him or her. Occurs at around age 10 months. Contrast *declarative pointing.*

inflection point   The point in a vocabulary spurt that differentiates between the slow and the rapid stages of vocabulary development.

inner language   Thoughts and ideas that an individual keeps to him- or herself after they are formulated. Contrast *written language.*

innervate   To supply nerves to a particular region or part of the body.

intellectual disability   Abbreviated ID. As defined by the American Association on Mental Retardation, a condition of arrested or incomplete development of the mind, which is especially characterized by impairment of skills manifested during the developmental period. ID was referred to as *mental retardation* (MR) until recently.

intensity   How far apart air particles move when they go back and forth during the creation of sound. Loudness. One of three prosodic characteristics of speech. Contrast *duration*; *frequency.*

intentional communication   Also called *iconic communication.* Communication that is relatively more precise in intent than symbolic communication, but unlike symbolic communication, the relationship between the communicative behavior and its referent is not arbitrary. Rather, it relies on the shared spatial position among the sender, the recipient, and the referent. The relationship between the message and its referent is transparent. Example: When a chimpanzee points to a banana. See also *preintentional communication.* Contrast *symbolic communication.*

intentionality hypothesis   The theory that children's development of language form and content is fostered in part by their experience with other people as they use language to engage with these people.

interlanguage   The language system speakers create during second language (L2) acquisition. It includes elements of the first language (L1) and the L2 as well as elements found in neither of the two languages. Example: L1 phonology combined with L2 syntax, such as "I bring not the children" by a speaker with German as the L1 and English as the L2.

interrogative sentences   Sentences that ask a question. Contrast *declarative sentences*; *negative sentences.*

intersubjective awareness   Recognition of when one person shares a mental focus on some external object or action with another person.

interutterance mixing   When code switching occurs between utterances. Contrast *intrautterance mixing.*

intervention and remediation   Programs or strategies used to help children, adolescents, and adults who exhibit difficulties with some aspect of language development. One of three direct applications of language theory and research to practice. See also *enrichment*; *prevention.*

intonation   The prominence placed on various parts of sentences. Contrast *stress.*

intrautterance mixing   When code switching occurs within a single utterance. Contrast *interutterance mixing.*

irony   A type of figurative language that involves incongruity between what a speaker or writer says and what actually happens. Puns and sarcasm make use of irony. Two types of irony are verbal and dramatic.

jargon   A special type of babbling that contains the true melodic patterns of an infant's native language. Such babbling resembles questions, exclamations, and commands, even in the absence of recognizable words. See also *marginal babbling*; *nonreduplicated babbling*; *reduplicated babbling.*

joint attention   Attention focused on a mutual object. For infants, maintaining joint attention requires them to coordinate their attention between the social partner and the object. Prerequisite to development of a conversational schema.

language   A rule-governed, code-based tool shared by the members of a community. Used to represent thoughts and ideas to other people who know the code.

language acquisition device   Professor of linguistics Noam Chomsky's innate, species-specific module dedicated to language and not other forms of learning.

language comprehension   The ability to understand language. Contrast *language production.*

language difference   The variability among language users. Example: Girls tend to speak earlier than boys do. See also *bilingualism*; *dialects*; *gender differences.* Contrast *language disorder.*

language disorder   A significant difficulty with the development of language. Children with a language disorder typically achieve language milestones more slowly than other children do and exhibit long-standing difficulties with various aspects of language form, content, and use.

language impairment   See *language disorder.*

language production   The ability to use language expressively. Contrast *language comprehension.*

language productivity   In this stage of second language acquisition, children are not yet proficient speakers of their L2; however, their communicative repertoire continues to expand; they begin to create simple S–V–O (subject–verb–object) sentences, and they rely heavily on the general all-purpose verbs, or GAP verbs, *make, do,* and *go.*

language stabilization   In second language (L2) acquisition, when the interlanguage stops evolving and L2 learners reach a plateau in their language development.

late consonants   Consonants emerging later in speech sound development. Contrast *early consonants.*

late language emergence   Abbreviated LLE. Children who have a slow start in language use are generally said to have this condition; it occurs in an estimated one in five children. Children with LLE are also called *late talkers.*

lead-in   A way in which children may be exposed to novel words; an adult labels an object or event that is outside of the child's attentional focus.

left hemisphere   One of two mirror-image halves of the cerebrum. See also *corpus callosum*; *longitudinal fissure.* Contrast *right hemisphere.*

lexical ambiguity   When words or phrases have multiple meanings. Provides the humor in jokes, riddles, comics, and so forth. Example: *That was a real bear* (*bear* has several meanings). See also *sentential ambiguity.*

lexicon   A vocabulary system, or "mental dictionary." Used to convey content. For each word a child learns, he or she creates an entry in the lexicon. The entry contains a series of symbols that compose the word, the sound of the word, the meaning of the word, and its part of speech.

linguistic feedback   The use of speech or vocalizations (e.g., "mm-hmm") to relay information to the sender about his or her message. See also *nonlinguistic feedback*; *paralinguistic feedback*.

literate language   Language used without the aid of context cues to support meaning: highly decontextualized language.

location   In an event, the place where an action occurs. See also *agent*; *goal*; *source*; *theme*.

longitudinal fissure   The long cerebral crevice that separates the two hemispheres of the cerebrum. See also *corpus callosum*.

magnetic resonance imaging   Abbreviated MRI. A technology that allows scientists to obtain detailed images of both the anatomy and the physiology of the nervous system.

majority ethnolinguistic community   A group of people who speak a language that the majority of people in an area (e.g., country, state, province) value and assign high social status. Example: Standard American English (SAE) speakers in the United States. Contrast *minority ethnolinguistic community*.

marginal babbling   An early type of babbling containing short strings of consonant-like and vowel-like sounds. Usually emerges as infants gain control of their articulation, at around age 5–8 months. See also *jargon*; *nonreduplicated babbling*; *reduplicated babbling*.

mean length of utterance   Abbreviated MLU. A calculation of the number of morphemes per utterance used to estimate the syntactic complexity of children's utterances.

meninges   One shield of the central nervous system, comprising three layers that completely encase the CNS. Comprises the pia mater, arachnoid mater, and dura mater.

meningitis   An infection or inflammation of the meninges. Symptoms typically include headache, neck stiffness, high fever, and altered mental state.

mental lexicon   The volume of words a person understands and uses. See also *expressive lexicon*; *receptive lexicon*.

metalinguistic ability   The ability to view language as an object of attention (e.g., preschoolers exhibit metalinguistic ability when they pretend to write or make up rhyming patterns). See also *alphabet knowledge*; *phonological awareness*; *print awareness*.

metalinguistic competence   The ability to think about and analyze language as an object of attention. Acquired mainly in the school-age years.

metaphor   A type of figurative language that conveys similarity through an expression that refers to something it does not denote literally. Components of metaphors are the topic and the vehicle. Two types of metaphors are predictive and proportional.

minimal pairs   Words that differ by only one phoneme, such as *low* and *row*.

minority ethnolinguistic community   A group of people who speak a language that few people in the community speak or value. Example: Japanese speakers in the United States. Contrast *majority ethnolinguistic community*.

model   A representation of an unknown event on the basis of the best current evidence governing the event.

modularity   A cognitive science theory about how the human mind is organized within the brain structures. It contends that the human brain contains a set of highly specific modules—or regions developed to process specific types of information.

modules   Regions of the brain developed to process specific types of information.

monolingualism   Acquisition of only one language. Contrast *bilingualism*.

morphemes   The smallest units of language that carry meaning. They are combined to create words. Example: *pre + school + s = preschools*.

morphology   The rules of language governing the internal organization of words. One of the components of the language domain of form. See also *phonology*; *pragmatics*; *semantics*; *syntax*.

morphophonemic development   When an individual attains the ability to make sound modifications by joining certain morphemes (/əz/ in *matches*), to use vowel shifting (/ai/ to /i/ in *decide–decision*), and to use stress and emphasis to distinguish phrases from compound words (e.g., *green house* vs. *greenhouse*).

myelin   The coating sheathing each neuron. The myelin sheath contributes to the rapid relay of nerve impulses, particularly within white matter, and protects the neuron.

myelinization   The growth of the myelin sheath, a slow process that is not complete until late childhood.

narrative   A child's spoken or written description of a real or a fictional event from the past, the present, or the future. See also *fictional narrative*; *personal narrative*.

negative sentences   Sentences that express negation and rely on such words as *no*, *not*, *can't*, *don't*, and *won't*. Contrast *declarative sentences*; *interrogative sentences*.

neocortex   Means "new cortex" or "new rind." The enlarged outer layers of the brain that, during evolution, grew over the older human brain, or allocortex. The neocortex and the allocortex compose the cerebrum. Controls most of the functions that exemplify human thought and language, including speech, language, reasoning, planning, and problem solving.

neural plasticity   The malleability of the central nervous system, or the ability of the sensory and motor systems to organize and reorganize by generating new synaptic connections or by using existing synapses for alternative means. See also *experience-dependent plasticity*; *experience-expectant plasticity*.

neuraxis   The horizontal and vertical axes along which the human nervous system is organized. See also *horizontal axis*; *vertical axis*.

neuroanatomy   The anatomical structures of the nervous system. See also *neurophysiology*; *neuroscience*.

neurolinguists   Experts who study the structures and functions of the nervous system that relate to language.

neurons   The billions of highly specialized cells that compose the nervous system.

neurophysiology   The way the anatomical structures of the nervous system work together as a complex unit and as separate, distinct biological units. See also *neuroanatomy*; *neuroscience*.

neuroscience   The branch of science involving the study of the anatomy and physiology of the nervous system. See also *neuroanatomy*; *neurophysiology*.

neurotransmitters   Chemical agents that help transmit information across the synaptic cleft between two neurons.

nonlinguistic feedback   The use of eye contact, facial expression, posture, and proximity to relay information to the sender about his or her message. It may supplement linguistic feedback or stand alone. See also *paralinguistic feedback*.

nonostentive word-learning contexts   Also called *inferential contexts*. Situations in which little contextual information is provided about a novel word. Contrast *ostentive word-learning contexts*.

nonreduplicated babbling   Also known as *variegated babbling*. Babbling consisting of nonrepeating consonant–vowel combinations, such as "da ma goo ga." Occurs at around age 6–10 months. See also *jargon*; *marginal babbling*. Contrast *reduplicated babbling*.

nonverbal period   In this stage of second language acquisition, children produce little to no language as they begin to acquire their L2 receptively. Some children use gestures, such as pointing, to communicate until they have acquired a sufficient number of words in their L2.

normative research   Studies in which experts compile data from individuals on a certain aspect of language development and from these data determine and chart the ages (or grades) by which children typically meet certain milestones.

norm-referenced tests   Compare children's level of language performance to that of a national sample of same-age peers.

novel name–nameless category (N3C)   A principle stating that a nameless object included in a group of known objects should be the recipient of a novel label. Supporting the principle of object scope, the principle of N3C is based on the principle of mutual exclusivity but does not presuppose that children avoid attaching more than one label to an object.

object scope   A principle stating that words map to whole objects. See also *whole object assumption*.

obligatory contexts   Situations in which a mature grammar specifies use of a grammatical marker. Example: In the sentence *The girl's hat is lost*, the possessive *'s* is considered obligatory. Used by researchers studying children's achievement of grammatical morphology.

observational measures   Examine children's language form, content, and use in naturalistic activities with peers or parents. Two types are conversational analysis and language sample analysis.

occipital lobe   One of the six lobes of the cerebrum composing the posterior portion of the brain. It is functionally specialized for visual reception and processing. See also *frontal lobe*; *parietal lobes*; *temporal lobes*.

open-head injuries   Abbreviated OHIs. Traumatic brain injuries (TBIs) in which the brain matter is exposed through penetration. One cause is gunshot wounds. Usually result in a more focal brain injury. Contrast *closed-head injury*.

operant conditioning   A concept in B. F. Skinner's behaviorist theory that describes how behaviors are shaped by responses to the behaviors. The result is that behaviors that are reinforced become stronger and those that are punished become suppressed.

oral communication   The combination of speaking and listening.

oral language   Language that is spoken. Comprises three domains: content, form, and use.

ostentive word-learning contexts   Situations in which a lot of contextual information is provided about a novel word, either linguistically or extralinguistically. Contrast *nonostentive word-learning contexts*.

overextension   Three types of overgeneralization that children make: categorical, analogical, and relational (e.g., calling all four-legged animals "dog" after learning the word *dog*, calling the moon "ball," and calling a watering can "flower," respectively). See also *overlap*. Contrast *underextension*.

overgeneralization   A concept in the competition model that describes when children who are learning language make an irregular past tense verb regular by adding a /d/, /t/, or /id/ sound.

overlap   Overextension of a word in certain circumstances and underextension of the same word in other circumstances. Example: Using the word *candy* to refer to jelly beans and grandmother's pills (overextension) but not to chocolate bars (underextension).

paralinguistic   Aspects of communication outside the linguistic information, such as pitch, loudness, posture, and eye contact. With infant-directed speech, paralinguistic features include a high overall pitch, exaggerated pitch contours, and slower tempos than those of adult-directed speech.

paralinguistic feedback   The use of pitch, loudness, and pauses, all of which are superimposed over linguistic feedback, to relay information to a sender about his or her message. See also *nonlinguistic feedback*.

parietal lobes   Two of the six lobes of the cerebrum. They reside posterior to the frontal lobe on the left and right sides (above the ears). Their key functions include perceiving incoming sensory and perceptual information and integrating it with the executive functions of the frontal lobe, comprehending oral and written language, and performing mathematical calculations. Include the primary somatosensory cortex and the sensory association cortex. See also *frontal lobe*; *occipital lobe*; *temporal lobes*.

perceptual narrowing   The process by which infants start to focus more on perceptual differences that are relevant to them (such as the difference between two native phonemes) and focus less on perceptual differences that are not relevant to them or that they encounter less often (such as the difference between two nonnative phonemes).

peripheral nervous system   Abbreviated PNS. The cranial and spinal nerves, which carry information inward to and outward from the brain and spinal cord. Contrast *central nervous system*.

personal narrative   A child's spoken or written description of a factual event. Contrast *fictional narrative*.

phonation   When a breath of air that has been respirated travels over the vocal cords. One of four systems involved in speech. See also *articulation*; *resonation*; *respiration*.

phoneme   The smallest unit of sound that can signal a difference in meaning. In the production of syllables and words, a series of phonemes are strung together. Examples: /m/ + /a/ = "ma."

phonemic awareness   The ability to attend to the phonemic units of words.

phonetic module   According to some experts, a specialized processor that is designed specifically for processing the phonetic segments of speech.

phonetic   Referring to phonemes (speech sounds) and combinations of phonemes. Infants pay close attention to the phonetic details of speech to learn words. Contrast *prosodic*.

phonetically consistent forms   Abbreviated PCFs. The idiosyncratic wordlike productions that children use consistently and meaningfully but that do not approximate adult forms. PCFs have a consistent sound structure, but children may use them to refer to more than a single referent. Example: "aaah" to refer to both water and the desire to be picked up.

phonological ambiguity   A type of sentential ambiguity in which varying pronunciations of a word change the meaning of a sentence. Example: *She needs to visit her psychotherapist* vs. *She needs to visit her psycho therapist*.

phonological awareness   The ability to focus on the sounds that make up syllables and words through implicit or explicit analysis. A type of metalinguistic ability important to emergent literacy. See also *phonemic awareness*.

phonological knowledge   Knowledge of internal representations of the phonemes composing a native language. See also *phonological production*.

phonological processes   The systematic and rule-governed speech patterns that characterize speech, including syllable structure changes, assimilation, place-of-articulation changes, and manner-of-articulation changes.

phonological production   Using the phonemes composing a native language to produce syllables and words. See also *phonological knowledge*.

phonology   The rules of language governing the sounds used to make syllables and words. One of the components of the language domain of form. See also *allophones*; *morphology*; *pragmatics*; *semantics*; *syntax*.

phonotactic cues   Sounds following the phonotactic rules of a native language that allow infants to parse the speech stream. Example: In English, the phoneme sequence /g/ + /z/ does not usually start a word but can end it (*dogs*). Contrast *prosodic cues*.

phonotactic rules   The rules of a person's native language that specify "legal" orders of sounds in syllables and words and the places where specific phonemes can and cannot occur.

phonotactics   How sounds are organized in words. See also *phonology*.

phrasal coordination   The ability to connect phrases, such as with conjunctions. Example: *I'm putting on my coat and my hat*.

pia mater   The inner layer of the meninges. Wraps tightly around the brain and spinal cord. See also *arachnoid mater*; *dura mater*.

postlingual hearing loss   A type of acquired hearing loss that occurs after birth and after a child has developed language. Contrast *prelingual hearing loss*.

pragmatics   Synonymous with *use*. The rules of language governing how language is used for social purposes. See also *morphology*; *phonology*; *semantics*; *syntax*.

prefrontal cortex   The most anterior portion of the frontal lobe of the cerebrum. The part of the brain that evolved most recently, is most developed, and is connected with all other sensory and motor systems of the brain. It regulates the depth of feelings—such as gloom, elation, calmness, and friendliness—and is involved with executive functions.

preintentional communication   Communication in which other people assume the relationship between a communicative behavior and its referent. Example: When an infant cries, the communicative partner must infer the referent or goal of the communication. See also *intentional communication*. Contrast *symbolic communication*.

prelingual hearing loss   A type of acquired hearing loss that occurs after birth but before a child has developed language. Contrast *postlingual hearing loss*.

premotor cortex   One component of the frontal lobe of the cerebrum. Important for speech and other motor functions. Controls musculature and programming patterns and sequences of movements. See also *primary motor cortex*.

prereading stage   Period from birth to the beginning of formal education. Some of children's most critical developments—oral language, print awareness, and phonological awareness—occur during this period.

presynaptic terminal   The distal end of each terminal branch of an axon. A site at which the axonal connection of one neuron corresponds with the dendritic extension of another neuron.

prevention   To inhibit language difficulties from emerging and thus reduce the need to resolve such difficulties later in life. One of three direct applications of language theory and research to practice. See also *enrichment*; *intervention and remediation*.

primary language impairment   Also known as *heritable language impairment* or *specific language impairment* (*SLI*). A significant language impairment in the absence of any other developmental difficulty (e.g., mental retardation, brain injury). Affects approximately 7%–10% of children older than age 5 years. The most common reason for administering early intervention and special education services to toddlers through fourth graders. Contrast *secondary language impairment*.

primary motor cortex   One component of the frontal lobe of the cerebrum. Important for speech and other motor functions. Controls the initiation of skilled, delicate voluntary movements of the extremities and speech. See also *premotor cortex*.

primary somatosensory cortex   Also called the *sensory strip* or *primary sensory cortex*. The region of the parietal lobes that, along with the sensory association cortex, resides just posterior to the primary motor cortex in the frontal lobe. Receives and processes sensory experiences of pain, temperature, touch, pressure, and movement from receptors throughout the body.

print awareness   Understanding of the forms and functions of written language. A type of metalinguistic ability important to emergent literacy.

productivity   The principle of combination whereby small numbers of discrete units are combined into seemingly infinite novel creations. This principle also applies to human activities other than language—such as mathematics and music.

progress monitoring assessments   Used to measure and monitor a child's progress in a certain area of language development (e.g., expressive vocabulary); can be administered multiple times; generally quick and easy to administer.

prosodic bootstrapping   The process by which infants use their sensitivity to the acoustic properties of speech (e.g., pitch, rhythm, pauses, stress) to make inferences about units of language, including clauses, phrases, and words.

prosodic cues   Word and syllable intonation and stress patterns in a language that allow infants to break into the speech stream. Contrast *phonotactic cues*.

prosodic   Referring to the frequency (pitch), duration (length), and intensity (loudness) of sounds. Combinations of prosodic characteristics produce distinguishable stress and intonation patterns that infants can detect to parse the speech stream. Contrast *phonetic*.

proverbs   Statements that express the conventional values, beliefs, and wisdom of a society. A type of figurative language.

receiver   The listener during communication. The person who takes in and then comprehends the information. Contrast *sender*.

receptive language   The language people comprehend. Contrast *expressive language*.

receptive lexicon   The volume of words a person understands. Contrast *expressive lexicon*.

receptive speech area   See *Wernicke's area*.

reduplicated babbling   Babbling that consists of repeating consonant–vowel pairs, such as "da da da." See also *jargon*; *marginal babbling*. Contrast *nonreduplicated babbling*.

reference   A principle stating that words symbolize objects, actions, events, and concepts. Example: The word *Daddy* stands for or symbolizes someone's father.

referent   The aspect of the world to which a word refers. Example: In English, the specific feeling to which the word *happy* refers.

referential communication   See *symbolic communication*.

referential gestures   Gestures such as holding a fist to an ear to indicate *telephone* or waving a hand to indicate *bye-bye*. Used by children beginning to transition from the prelinguistic stage to the one-word stage.

regional dialects   Dialects dating back to colonial America that differ from one another in terms of their pronunciation, vocabulary, and grammar. Examples include Northern and Midwestern dialects.

register   Stylistic variations in language that are used in different situations. Example: How you vary your language form, content, and use when making a request of your best friend versus when making a request of your professor.

resonation   The phase of speech that occurs after a breath of air has been respirated and phonated, when the air travels into and vibrates within the oral and nasal cavities. One of four systems involved in speech. See also *articulation*; *phonation*; *respiration*.

respiration   The act of inspiring a breath of air into the lungs, expiring it from the lungs, and allowing it to travel up through the trachea, or windpipe, before it is phonated. One of four systems involved in speech. See also *articulation*; *phonation*; *resonation*.

responsiveness   How prompt and appropriate a response is. With regard to language development, the promptness, contingency, and appropriateness of caregiver responses to children's bids for communication through words or other means.

right hemisphere   One of two mirror-image halves of the cerebrum. See also *corpus callosum*; *longitudinal fissure*. Contrast *left hemisphere*.

rostral   A positional term used to describe the specific nervous system structures along the horizontal and vertical axes of the neuraxis. With regard to the horizontal axis, it means "toward the front of the brain." With regard to the vertical axis, it means "toward the top of the spinal cord (near the brain)." Contrast *caudal*; *dorsal*; *ventral*.

schema   The building blocks of cognition; internalized representations of the organizational structures of various events.

screenings   Brief assessments used to identify possible areas of difficulty that may signal a need for more in-depth evaluation.

second language acquisition   Also called L2 acquisition or SLA. The process by which children who have already established a solid foundation in their first language (L1) learn an additional language. Contrast *bilingualism*.

secondary language impairment   A language impairment resulting from, or secondary to, conditions such as mental retardation, autism, and traumatic brain injury. Contrast *primary language impairment*.

semantic bootstrapping   The process by which children deduce grammatical structures by using word meanings they acquire by observing events around them. Contrast *syntactic bootstrapping*.

semantic network   A network in which the entries in a person's mental lexicon are stored according to their connective ties. See also *spreading activation*.

semanticity   The species-specific aspect of language that allows people to represent the world. In particular, it allows people to represent decontextualized events (events that are not immediately present). Also called *displacement*.

semantics   Synonymous with *content*. The rules of language governing the meaning of individual words and word combinations. See also *morphology*; *phonology*; *pragmatics*; *syntax*.

sender   The speaker during communication. The person who formulates and then transmits the information he or she wants to convey. Contrast *receiver*.

sensitive period   With regard to the human brain, a time frame of development during which a particular aspect of neuroanatomy or neurophysiology that underlies a given sensory or motoric capacity undergoes growth or change. A critical window of opportunity for development. Example: Deprivation of visual input during the first 6 weeks of the life of a kitten (the critical window) results in permanent blindness.

sensorineural loss   Hearing loss that results from damage to the inner ear or auditory nerve. Contrast *auditory-processing disorder; conductive loss.*

sensory association cortex   The region in the parietal lobes that, along with the primary somatosensory cortex, resides just posterior to the primary motor cortex of the frontal lobe and is involved with processing sensory information.

similes   A type of figurative language, similar to predictive metaphors, in which the comparison between the topic and the vehicle is made explicit by the word *like* or *as.* Examples: *sitting like a bump on a log; flat as a pancake.*

simple syntax   Grammatically well-formed sentences containing simple noun phrases and verb structures. Contrast *complex syntax.*

slow mapping   Gradually refining representations of a word with time and multiple exposures to the word in varying contexts. Occurs after fast mapping. Contrast *fast mapping.*

source   In an event, the starting point for movement. See also *agent; goal; location; theme.*

species specificity   When something pertains to only one species. Language is strictly a human capacity and thus is species specific.

specific language impairment   Abbreviated SLI. See *primary language impairment.*

speech perception   How the brain processes speech and language. The ability to understand the sounds and words of a native language. Studies of speech perception help researchers learn about the kinds of language abilities infants have when they are born and how children use their speech perception to learn language. Contrast *auditory perception.*

speech   The neuromuscular process by which humans turn language into a sound signal that is transmitted through the air (or another medium such as a telephone line) to a receiver. See also *articulation; communication; hearing; phonation; resonation; respiration.*

spinal nerves   The 31 pairs of nerves that emerge from the spinal cord.

spinal tap   Also called a *lumbar puncture;* involves inserting a needle between two of the lower (lumbar) vertebrae and extracting cerebrospinal fluid from the subarachnoid space.

spreading activation   A process in which activation of specific mental lexicon entries spreads across the semantic network according to the strength of connections among the entries.

statistical learning   A domain-general learning mechanism whereby infants compute the statistical properties of the language they hear.

strategy training   Focuses on teaching students specific ways to approach a linguistic task by following specific steps in an effort to improve children's abilities to complete diverse language tasks, such as understanding jokes, initiating conversation with friends or adults, or deciphering unknown words when reading.

stress   In terms of speech, the prominence placed on certain syllables of multisyllabic words. Contrast *intonation.*

subarachnoid space   Separates the arachnoid matter from the pia matter in the central nervous system. It contains cerebrospinal fluid.

summative evaluations   Assessments focused on the products (rather than the process) and final outcomes of language learning and development. Contrast *formative evaluations.*

supported joint engagement   Joint attention in which adults use such techniques as speaking with an animated voice or showing an infant novel objects.

surface-structure ambiguity   A type of sentential ambiguity in which varying the stress and intonation in a sentence changes its meaning. Example: *I fed her bird seed* vs. *I fed her bird seed.* Contrast *deep-structure ambiguity.*

symbolic communication   Also called *referential communication.* When an individual communicates about a specific entity (an object or event), and the relationship between the entity and its referent (e.g., a word) is arbitrary. This type of communication is not limited by space or time. Example: When an infant says "bottle" to request something to drink, the relationship between the word *bottle* and its referent is arbitrary. Contrast *intentional communication; preintentional communication.*

synapse   The site where two neurons meet. For the two neurons to communicate, the nerve impulse must cross the synapse. See also *neurotransmitters; synaptic cleft.*

synaptic cleft   The space between the axon of the transmitting neuron and the dendrite of the receiving neuron. See also *synapse; neurotransmitters.*

synaptic pruning   When excess synapses are pruned after synaptogenesis. Occurs from the end of the first year of life to adolescence.

synaptogenesis   The formation of synaptic connections. Occurs most rapidly during the first year of life, after which excess synapses are pruned (synaptic pruning).

syntactic bootstrapping   The process by which children use the syntactic frames surrounding unknown verbs to successfully constrain the possible interpretations of the verbs. Contrast *semantic bootstrapping.*

syntax   The rules of language governing the internal organization of sentences. One component of the language domain of form. See also *morphology; phonology; pragmatics; semantics.*

T units   See *terminable units (T units).*

telegraphic and formulaic use   In this stage of second language acquisition, children begin to imitate other people, use single words to label items, and use simple phrases that they memorize.

temperament   A person's predominant behavioral style or personality type. Example: bold vs. shy.

temporal lobes   Two of the six lobes of the cerebrum. They sit posterior to the frontal lobe but inferior to the parietal lobes (behind the ears). They contain the functions for processing auditory information and language comprehension. Include Heschl's gyrus and Wernicke's area. See also *frontal lobe; occipital lobe; parietal lobes.*

terminable units (T units) Each T unit consists of an independent clause and any of its modifiers, such as a dependent clause. T units are coded in transcripts of language samples to assess a student's language form. Contrast *communication units (C units)*.

theme In an event, the entity undergoing an action or a movement. See also *agent; goal; location; source*.

theory Descriptive statements that provide stable explanations for a given phenomenon.

theory of mind Abbreviated TOM. One's ability to attribute mental states to others, which is necessary to take the perspective of another.

transfer The influence of one's L1 on his or her L2 development.

traumatic brain injury Abbreviated TBI. Damage or insult to an individual's brain tissue sometime after birth. Ranges from mild (concussion with loss of consciousness for 30 min or less) to severe (accompanied by a coma that lasts for 6 hr or more). Causes include infection, disease, and physical trauma. See also *acquired brain injuries; closed-head injury; open-head injuries*.

treatment plan An approach to helping a child with a language disorder develop language skills. The plan specifies treatment targets, treatment strategies, and treatment contexts.

twin studies Research on identical and monozygotic twins used to estimate the contribution of genetics to language development, as well as the heritability of language disorders.

underextension Using words to refer to only a subset of possible referents. Example: Using the word *bottle* only in reference to baby bottles (and not glass bottles or plastic water bottles). See also *overlap*. Contrast *overextension*.

unitary language system hypothesis The idea that bilingual children have a single language system that eventually splits into two. According to this theory, children are not bilingual until they successfully differentiate between the two languages. Contrast *dual language system hypothesis*.

universal grammar Abbreviated UG. The system of grammatical rules and constraints that are consistent among all world languages. UG, proposed by the linguist Noam Chomsky, is a nature-inspired theory of second language acquisition because it rests on an innate, species-specific module dedicated solely to language acquisition. See also *critical period; language acquisition device*.

universality The idea that all persons around the world have a cognitive infrastructure that they apply to the task of learning language.

use Synonymous with *pragmatics*. How language is used in interactions with other people to express personal and social needs. One of the three domains of language. See also *content; form*.

use-inspired basic research A type of basic research that concentrates on building connections between theory and practice.

variegated babbling See *nonreduplicated babbling*.

ventral A positional term used to describe the specific nervous system structures along the horizontal and vertical axes of the neuraxis. With regard to the horizontal axis, it means "toward the bottom of the brain." With regard to the vertical axis, it means "toward the front of the spinal cord (the side nearest the belly)." Contrast *caudal; dorsal; rostral*.

vertical axis The part of the neuraxis that extends from the superior portion of the brain downward along the entire spinal cord. See also *horizontal axis*.

vocabulary spurt Occurs near the end of the second year of a child's life, when he or she transitions from a slow stage of vocabulary development to a rapid stage of development. See also *inflection point*.

voice onset time The interval between the release of a stop consonant such as *p, b, t,* or *d* and the onset of vocal cord vibrations.

Wernicke's area Named after the German neurologist and psychiatrist Karl Wernicke. Also called the *receptive speech area*. Resides in the superior portion of the left temporal lobe near the intersection of the parietal, occipital, and temporal lobes—or parieto-occipitotemporal junction. Critical for language comprehension.

wh- questions Interrogative sentences that use the *wh* words, such as *who, what, where, when,* and *why*. Contrast *yes–no questions*.

white matter Nervous tissue consisting primarily of axonal fibers that carry information among gray matter tissues. An information conduit. Contrast *gray matter*.

whole object assumption The assumption that words label whole objects and not object parts. See also *object scope*.

written language Thoughts and ideas that an individual writes down after they are formulated. Contrast *inner language*.

Wug Test Elicited production task used to investigate children's acquisition of English morphemes, including the plural marker. Developed by Jean Berko (now Berko Gleason).

yes–no questions Interrogative sentences that require a yes or no response. Contrast *wh- questions*.

zone of proximal development Abbreviated ZPD. A concept in Vygotskian theory that describes the difference between a child's actual developmental level (determined through independent problem solving) and his or her potential developmental level (determined through problem solving in collaboration with a more competent adult or peer).

References

Chapter 1

American Association on Mental Retardation. (2002). *Mental retardation: Definition, classification, and systems of supports* (10th ed.). Washington, DC: Author.

American Psychiatric Association. (2013). *Diagnostic and statistical manual of mental disorders (DSM-5®).* American Psychiatric Pub.

American Speech-Language-Hearing Association (1982). *Language*. Available from www.asha.org/policy.

Beitchman, J., Hood, J., Rochon, J., Peterson, M., Mantini, T., & Majumdar, S. (1989). Empirical classification of speech/language impairment in children: I. Identification of speech/language categories. *Journal of the American Academy of Child & Adolescent Psychiatry, 28*(1), 112–117.

Bickerton, D. (1995). *Language and human behavior.* Seattle: University of Washington Press.

Bookheimer, S. (2002). Functional MRI of language: New approaches to understanding the cortical organization of semantic processing. *Annual Reviews of Neuroscience, 25*, 151–188.

Borden, G. J., Harris, K. S., & Raphael, L. J. (1994). Speech, Language, and Thought. In G. J. Borden, K. S. Harris, & L. J. (Eds.), *Raphael Speech Science Primer: Physiology, Acoustics, and Perception of Speech* (3rd ed., pp. 1-13). Baltimore: Williams and Wilkins.Braisby, N., & Gellatly, A. (Eds.). (2012). *Cognitive psychology*. Oxford University Press.

Brenowitz, E. A., & Beecher, M. D. (2005). Song learning in birds: Diversity and plasticity, opportunities and challenges. *Trends in Neuroscience, 28*, 127–132.

Cabell, S. Q, Justice, L.M., Piasta, S.B., Curenton, S. M., Wiggins, A.K, Turnbull, K.L.P., & Petscher, Y. (2011). The impact of teacher responsivity education on preschoolers' language and literacy skills. American Journal of Speech Language Pathology, 20, 315-330.

Capuron, L., Schroecksnadel, S., Féart, C., Aubert, A., Higueret, D., Barberger-Gateau, P., ... & Fuchs, D. (2011). Chronic low-grade inflammation in elderly persons is associated with altered tryptophan and tyrosine metabolism: Role in neuropsychiatric symptoms. *Biological psychiatry, 70*(2), 175–182.

Cartwright, J. (2000). *Evolution and human behavior.* Cambridge, MA: MIT Press.

Catroppa, C., & Anderson, V. (2009). Neurodevelopmental outcomes of pediatric traumatic injury. *Future Neurology, 4*, 811–821.

Centers for Disease Control and Prevention (2014). *Prevalence of Autism Spectrum Disorder among Children Aged 8 Years*—Autism and Developmental Disabilities Monitoring Network, 11 Sites, United States, 2010. Atlanta, GA: Author.

Champlin, C. (2011). Hearing science. In R. B. Gillam, T. P. Marquardt, & F. N. Martin (Eds.), *Communication sciences and disorders: From science to clinical practice* (2nd ed.) (pp. 295–316). Sudbury, PA: Jones and Bartlett Publishers.

Charity, A. H., Scarborough, H. S., & Griffin, D. M. (2004). Familiarity with School English in African American children and its relation to early reading achievement. *Child Development, 75*, 1340–1356.

Chisholm, N., & Gillett, G. (2005). The patient's journey: Living with locked-in syndrome. *British Medical Journal, 331*, 94–97.

Christiansen, M. H., & Kirby, S. (2003). Language evolution: Consensus and controversies. *Trends in cognitive sciences, 7*(7), 300–307.

Clahsen, H., Rothweiler, M., Sterner, F., & Chilla, S. (2014). Linguistic markers of specific language impairment in bilingual children: The case of verb morphology. *Clinical Linguistics & Phonetics, 28*(9), 709–721.

Conti-Ramsden, G. (2003). Processing and linguistic markers in young children with specific language impairment (SLI). *Journal of Speech, Language, and Hearing Research, 46*, 1029–1037.

Conway, C. M., & Christiansen, M. H. (2001). Sequential learning in non-human primates. *Trends in Cognitive Sciences, 5*(12), 539–546.

Curtiss, S. (2012). Revisiting modularity: Using language as a window to the mind (Chapter 5). In M. Piatelli-Palmerini and R. C. Berwick (Eds), *Rich languages from poor inputs*. Oxford University Press.

Dale, P. S., Price, T. S., Bishop, D. V. M., & Plomin, P. (2003). Outcomes of early language delay: I. Predicting persistent and transient language difficulties at 3 and 4 years. *Journal of Speech, Language, and Hearing Research, 46*, 544–560.

Dunbar, R. I. M., & Aiello, L. C. (1993). Neocortex size, group size, and the evolution of language. *Current Anthropology, 34*, 184–193.

Eden, J., & Stevens, R. (Eds). (2006). *Evaluating the HRSA traumatic brain injury program*. Washington, DC: National Academies Press.

Evans, M. A. (1996). Reticent primary grade children and their more talkative peers: Verbal, nonverbal, and self-concept characteristics. *Journal of Educational Psychology, 88*, 739–749.

Goldstein, B., & Iglesias, A. (2013). Language and dialectal variations. In J. E. Bernthal, N. W. Bankson, & P. Flipsen

(Eds.), *Articulation and phonological disorders* (7th ed). Boston: Allyn & Bacon.

Gopnik, A., Meltzoff, A., & Kuhl, P. (2009). *Scientist in the crib*. New York: Harper Collins.

Halliday, M. A. K. (1975). *Learning how to mean: Exploration in the development of language*. London: Edward Arnold.

Hay, J. F., Pelucchi, B., Estes, K. G., & Saffran, J. R. (2011). Linking sounds to meanings: Infant statistical learning in a natural language. *Cognitive Psychology, 63*(2), 93–106.

Hoff, E. (2013). *Language development*. Cengage Learning.

Huttenlocher, J., Vasilyeva, M., Cymerman, E., & Levine, S. (2002). Language input and child syntax. *Child Psychology, 45*, 337–374.

Kaminski, J., Tempelmann, S., Call, J., & Tomasello, M. (2009). Domestic dogs comprehend human communication with iconic signs. *Developmental Science, 12*(6), 831–837.

Karmiloff, K., & Karmiloff-Smith, A. (2001). *Pathways to language from fetus to adolescent*. Cambridge, MA: Harvard University Press.

Kovas, Y., Hayious-Thomas, M. E., Oliver, B., Bishop, D. V. M., Dale, P. S., & Plomin, R. (2005). Genetic influences in different aspects of language development: The etiology of language skills in 4.5-year-old twins. *Child Development, 76*, 632–651.

Kristal, J. (2005). *The temperament perspective: Working with children's behavioral styles*. Baltimore: Brookes.

Labov, W. (1972). *Language in the inner city: Studies in the Black English Vernacular*. Philadelphia: University of Pennsylvania Press.

Lahey, M. (1988). *Language disorders and language development*. New York: Macmillan.

Lai, C. S., Fisher, S. E., Hurst, J. A., Vargha-Khadem, F., & Monaco, A. P. (2001). A forkhead-domain gene is mutated in severe speech and language disorder. *Nature, 413*, 519–523.

Langlois, J. A., Rutland-Brown, W., & Thomas, K. E. (2007). Traumatic brain injury in the United States: Emergency department visits, hospitalizations, and deaths. Centers for Disease Control and Prevention, Atlanta, GA. Retrieved February 1, 2010, from http://www.cdc.gov/ncipc/pub-res/TBI_in_US_04/TBI_ED.htm

Leavens, D. A., Russell, J. L., & Hopkins, W. D. (2005). Intentionality as measured in the persistence and elaboration of communication by chimpanzees *(Pan troglodytes)*. *Child Development, 76*, 291–306.

Muñoz, M. L., Gillam, R. B., Peña, E. B., & Gulley-Faehnle, A. (2003). Measures of language development in fictional narratives of Latino children. *Language, Speech, and Hearing Services in Schools, 34*, 332–342.

Nelson, C. A., Zeanah, C. H., Fox, N. A., Marshall, P. J., Smyke, A. T., & Guthrie, D. (2007). Cognitive recovery in socially deprived young children: The Bucharest Early Intervention Project. *Science, 318*(5858), 1937–1940.

Okada, R., Okuda, T., Nakano, N., Nishimatsu, K., Fukushima, H., Onoda, M., … & Kato, A. (2013). Brain areas associated with sentence processing: A functional MRI study and a lesion study. *Journal of Neurolinguistics, 26*(4), 470–478.

Pinker, S. (1994). *The language instinct: How the mind creates language*. New York: Morrow.

Rowe, M. L., Raudenbush, S. W., & Goldin-Meadow, S. (2012). The pace of vocabulary growth helps predict later vocabulary skill. *Child Development, 83*(2), 508–525.

Shapiro, K., & Caramazza, A. (2003). Grammatical processing of nouns and verbs in left frontal cortex? *Neuropsychologia, 41*(9), 1189–1198.

Sloutsky, V. M., & Napolitano, A. C. (2003). Is a picture worth a thousand words? Preference for auditory modality in young children. *Child Development, 74*, 822–833.

Smyke, A. T., Koga, S. F., Johnson, D. E., Fox, N. A., Marshall, P. J., Nelson, C. A., & Zeanah, C. H. (2007). The caregiving context in institution-reared and family-reared infants and toddlers in Romania. *Journal of Child Psychology and Psychiatry, 48*(2), 210–218.

Spinath, F. M., Price, T. S., Dale, P. S., & Plomin, R. (2004). The genetic and environmental origins of language disability and ability. *Child Development, 75*, 445–454.

Stromswold, K. (2001). The heritability of language: A review and metaanalysis of twin, adoption, and linkage studies. *Language, 77*, 647–723.

Tamis-LeMonda, C. S., Bornstein, M. H., & Baumwell, L. (2001). Maternal responsiveness and children's achievement of language milestones. *Child Development, 72*, 748–757.

Tomasello, M. (2005). *Constructing a language*. Cambridge, MA: Harvard University Press.

Tomblin, J. B., Records, N. L., Buckwalter, P., Zhang, X., Smith, E., & O'Brien, M. (1997). Prevalence of specific language impairment in kindergarten children. *Journal of Speech, Language, and Hearing Research, 40*, 1245–1260.

Trouton, A., Spinath, F. M., & Plomin, R. (2002). Twins Early Development Study (TEDS): A multivariate, longitudinal genetic investigation of language, cognition, and behaviour problems in childhood. *Twin Research, 5*, 444–448.

Tsao, F. M., Liu, H. M., & Kuhl, P. K. (2004). Speech perception in infancy predicts language development in the second year of life: A longitudinal study. *Child Development, 75*, 1067–1084.

U.S. Census Bureau. (2013). Language use in the United States: 2011. Retrieved April 1, 2015 from https://www.census.gov/prod/2013pubs/acs-22.pdf.

Wang, Q., & Leichtman, M. D. (2000). Same beginnings, different stories: A comparison of American and Chinese children's narratives. *Child Development, 71*, 1329–1346.

Wang, W. S., & Minett, J. W. (2005). The invasion of language: emergence, change and death. *Trends in Ecology & Evolution, 20*(5), 263–269.

Zimmerman, F., Gilkerson, J., Richards, J., Christakis, D., Dongxin, X., Gray, S., & Yapanel, U. (2009). Teaching by listening: The importance of adult–child conversations to language development. *Pediatrics, 124*, 342–349.

Chapter 2

Amayreh, M. M. (2003). Completion of the consonant inventory of Arabic. *Journal of Speech, Language, and Hearing Research, 46,* 517–529.

Andersen, E. (2014). *Speaking with style: The sociolinguistics skills of children.* Routledge.

Anderson, E. (2000). Exploring register knowledge: The value of "controlled improvisation." In L. Menn & N. R. Ratner (Eds.), *Methods for studying language production* (pp. 225–248). Mahwah, NJ: Erlbaum.

Anthony, J. L., Williams, J. M., Durán, L. K., Gillam, S. L., Liang, L., Aghara, R., … & Landry, S. H. (2011). Spanish phonological awareness: Dimensionality and sequence of development during the preschool and kindergarten years. *Journal of Educational Psychology, 103*(4), 857–868.

Atherton, F., & Nutbrown, C. (2013). *Understanding schemas and young children: From birth to three.* New York: Sage.

Becker Bryant, J. (2005). Language in social contexts: Communication competence in preschool years. In J. Berko Gleason (Ed.), *The development of language* (6th ed., pp. 191–229). New York: Allyn & Bacon.

Bellugi, U. (1967). *The acquisition of negation.* Unpublished doctoral dissertation, Harvard University.

Bergelson, E., & Swingley, D. (2013). The acquisition of abstract words by young infants. *Cognition, 127*(3), 391–397.

Bialystok, E., & Miller, B. (1999). The problem of age in second-language acquisition: Influences from language, structure, and task. *Bilingualism: Language and Cognition, 2,* 127–145.

Biemiller, A. (2005). Size and sequence in vocabulary development: Implications for choosing words for primary grade vocabulary instruction. In E. H. Hiebert & M. Kamil (Eds.), *Teaching and learning vocabulary: Bringing research to practice* (pp. 223–245). Mahwah, NJ: Erlbaum.

Bloom, L., & Tinker, E. (2001). The intentionality model and language acquisition. *Monographs of the Society for Research in Child Development, 66*(4), vii–104.

Bornstein, M. H., Hahn, C.-S., & Haynes, O. M. (2004). Specific and general language performance across early childhood: Stability and gender considerations. *First Language, 24,* 267–304.

Brackenbury, T., & Fey, M. E. (2003). Quick incidental verb learning in 4-year-olds: Identification and generalization. *Journal of Speech, Language, and Hearing Research, 46,* 313–327.

Brown, R. (1973). *A first language: The early stages.* Cambridge, MA: Harvard University Press.

Bunce, B. (1995). *Building a language-focused curriculum for the preschool classroom: Volume II: A planning guide.* Baltimore: Brookes.

Charity, A. H., Scarborough, H. S., & Griffin, D. M. (2004). Familiarity with School English in African American children and its relation to early reading achievement. *Child Development, 75,* 1340–1356.

Connor, C. M., & Craig, H. K. (2006). African American preschoolers' language, emergent literacy skills, and use of African American English: A complex relation preschooler' language, emergent literacy, and AAE. *Journal of Speech, Language, and Hearing Research, 49*(4), 771–792.

Conti-Ramsden, G., & Jones, M. (1997). Verb use in specific language impairment. *Journal of Speech, Language, and Hearing Research, 40,* 1298–1313.

Craig, H. K., Zhang, L., Hensel, S. L., & Quinn, E. J. (2009). African American English–speaking students: An examination of the relationship between dialect shifting and reading outcomes. *Journal of Speech, Language, and Hearing Research, 52*(4), 839–855.

Dapretto, M., & Bjork, E. L. (2000). The development of word retrieval abilities in the second year and its relation to early vocabulary growth. *Child Development, 71,* 635–648.

De Deyne, S., Navarro, D. J., & Storms, G. (2013). Better explanations of lexical and semantic cognition using networks derived from continued rather than single-word associations. *Behavior Research Methods, 45*(2), 480–498.

Dixon, J. A., & Marchman, V. A. (2007). Grammar and the lexicon: Developmental ordering in language acquisition. *Child Development, 78,* 190–212.

Eastwood, J., & Mackin, R. (1982). *A basic English grammar.* Oxford, England: Oxford University Press.

Eriksson, M., Marschik, P. B., Tulviste, T., Almgren, M., Pérez Pereira, M., Wehberg, S., … & Gallego, C. (2012). Differences between girls and boys in emerging language skills: Evidence from 10 language communities. *British Journal of Developmental Psychology, 30*(2), 326–343.

Estes, K. G. (2014). Learning builds on learning: Infants' use of native language sound patterns to learn words. *Journal of Experimental Child Psychology, 126,* 313–327.

Evans, M. A. (1996). Reticent primary grade children and their more talkative peers: Verbal, nonverbal, and self-concept characteristics. *Journal of Educational Psychology, 88,* 739–749.

Fenson, L., Dale, P. S., Reznick, J. S., Bates, E., & Thal, D. (1994). Variability in early communicative development. *Monographs of the Society for Research in Child Development, 59*(5), 1–185.

Friedmann, N., Biran, M., & Dotan, D. (2013). Lexical retrieval and its breakdown in aphasia and developmental language impairment. *The Cambridge Handbook of Biolinguistics,* 350–374. New York: Cambridge University Press.

Fuchs, D., Compton, D. L., Fuchs, L. S., Bryant, V. J., Hamlett, C. L., & Lambert, W. (2012). First-grade cognitive abilities as long-term predictors of reading comprehension and disability status. *Journal of Learning Disabilities, 45*(3), 217–231.

Ganger, J., & Brent, M. R. (2004). Reexamining the vocabulary spurt. *Developmental Psychology, 40,* 621–632.

Gerken, L., & Aslin, R. N. (2005). Thirty years of research on infant speech perception: The legacy of Peter W. Jusczyk. *Language Learning and Development, 1,* 5–21.

Gleitman, L. R., Cassidy, K., Nappa, R., Papafragou, A., & Trueswell, J. C. (2005). Hard words. *Language Learning and Development, 1,* 23–64.

Glennen, S. (2002). Language development and delay in internationally adopted infants and toddlers: A review. *American Journal of Speech–Language Pathology, 11,* 333–339.

Goldin-Meadow, S. (2014). In search of resilient and fragile properties of language. *Journal of Child Language, 41*(S1), 64–77.

Goodman, S. H., Rouse, M. H., Connell, A. M., Broth, M. R., Hall, C. M., & Heyward, D. (2011). Maternal depression and child psychopathology: A meta-analytic review. *Clinical Child and Family Psychology Review, 14*(1), 1–27.

Gopnik, A., & Meltzoff, A. N. (1997). *Words, thoughts, and theories.* Cambridge, MA: MIT Press.

Gray, S. (2003). Word learning by preschoolers with specific language impairment: Predictors and poor learners. *Journal of Speech, Language, and Hearing Research, 47,* 1117–1132.

Grunwell, P. (1997). Developmental phonological disability: Order in disorder. In B. W. Hodson & M. L. Edwards (Eds.), *Perspectives in applied phonology* (pp. 61–104). Gaithersburg, MD: Aspect.

Haapala, S., Niemitalo-Haapola, E., Raappana, A., Kujala, T., Suominen, K., Kujala, T., & Jansson-Verkasalo, E. (2014). Effects of recurrent acute otitis media on cortical speech-sound processing in 2-year-old children. *Ear and Hearing, 35*(3), e75–e83.

Harley, T. (2001). *The psychology of language: From data to theory* (2nd ed.). New York: Taylor & Francis.

Hawthorne, K., & Gerken, L. (2014). From pauses to clauses: Prosody facilitates learning of syntactic constituency. *Cognition, 133*(2), 420–428.

Hines, M. (2011). Gender development and the human brain. *Annual Review of Neuroscience, 34,* 69–88.

Hoff, E. (2003). The specificity of environmental influence: Socioeconomic status affects early vocabulary development via maternal speech. *Child Development, 74,* 1368–1378.

Hoff, E. (2013). Interpreting the early language trajectories of children from low-SES and language minority homes: Implications for closing achievement gaps. *Developmental Psychology, 49*(1), 4.

Hollich, G., Newman, R. S., & Jusczyk, P. W. (2005). Infants' use of synchronized visual information to separate streams of speech. *Child Development, 76,* 598–613.

Hurtado, N., Marchman, V. A., & Fernald, A. (2008). Does input influence uptake? Links between maternal talk, processing speed and vocabulary size in Spanish-learning children. *Developmental Science, 11*(6), F31–F39.

Huttenlocher, J., Vasilyeva, M., Cymerman, E., & Levine, S. (2002). Language input and child syntax. *Child Psychology, 45,* 337–374.

Huttenlocher, J., Waterfall, H., Vasilyeva, M., Vevea, J., & Hedges, L. V. (2010). Sources of variability in children's language growth. *Cognitive Psychology, 61*(4), 343–365.

Ingram, D. (1989). *First language acquisition: Method, description, and explanation.* Cambridge: Cambridge University Press.

Jaswal, V. K., & Markman, E. M. (2001a). Learning proper and common names in inferential versus ostensive contexts. *Child Development, 72,* 768–786.

Jaswal, V. K., & Markman, E. M. (2001b). The relative strengths of indirect and direct word learning. *Developmental Psychology, 39,* 745–760.

Jia, G. (2003). The acquisition of the English plural morpheme by native Mandarin Chinese–speaking children. *Journal of Speech, Language, and Hearing Research, 46,* 1297–1311.

Jia, G., Aaronson, D., & Wu, Y. H. (2002). Long-term language attainment of bilingual immigrants: Predictive factors and language group differences. *Applied Psycholinguistics, 23,* 599–621.

Jusczyk, P. W., Luce, P. A., & Charles-Luce, J. (1994). Infants' sensitivity to phonotactic patterns in the native language. *Journal of Memory and Language, 33,* 630–645.

Justice, L. M., Mashburn, A., Pence, K., & Wiggins, A. (2008). Experimental evaluation of a comprehensive language-rich curriculum in at-risk preschools. *Journal of Speech, Language, and Hearing Research, 51,* 1–19.

Kagan, J., & Snidman, N. (2004). *The long shadow of temperament.* Cambridge, MA: Harvard University Press.

Kirjavainen, M. M., Theakston, A. L., & Lieven, E. V. (2009). Can input explain children's me-for-I errors? *Journal of Child Language, 36,* 1091–1140.

Language and Reading Research Consortium. (2015). Learning to read: Should we keep things simple? *Reading Research Quarterly, 50* (2), 151–169.

Laws, G., & Bishop, D. V. M. (2003). A comparison of language abilities in adolescents with Down syndrome and children with specific language impairment. *Journal of Speech, Language, and Hearing Research, 46,* 1324–1339.

Liiva, C. A., & Cleave, P. L. (2005). Roles of initiation and responsiveness in access and participation for children with specific language impairment. *Journal of Speech, Language, and Hearing Research, 48,* 868–883.

Ma, W., Golinkoff, R. M., Hirsh-Pasek, K., McDonough, C., & Tardif, T. (2009). Imageability predicts the age of acquisition of verbs in Chinese children. *Journal of Child Language, 36,* 405–423.

McCune, L., & Vihman, M. M. (2001). Early phonetic and lexical development: A productivity approach. *Journal of Speech, Language, and Hearing Research, 44,* 670–684.

McDowell, K., Lonigan, C., & Goldstein, H. (2007). Relations among SES, age, gender, phonological distinctness, vocabulary, and phonological sensitivity. *Journal of Speech, Language, and Hearing Research, 50,* 1079–1092.

McGregor, K. K., Friedman, R. M., Reilly, R. M., & Newman, R. M. (2002). Semantic representation and naming in young children. *Journal of Speech, Language, and Hearing Research, 45,* 332–346.

Melby-Lervåg, M., Lyster, S. A. H., & Hulme, C. (2012). Phonological skills and their role in learning to read: A meta-analytic review. *Psychological Bulletin, 138*(2), 322.

Metsala, J. L., & Ehri, L. C. (Eds.). (2013). *Word recognition in beginning literacy.* Routledge.

Mistry, R. S., Biesanz, J. C., Taylor, L. C., Burchinal, M., & Cox, M. J. (2004). Family income and its relation to preschool children's adjustment for families in the NICHD study of early child care. *Developmental Psychology, 40,* 727–745.

Moore, C., & Dunham, P. (Eds.). (2014). *Joint attention: Its origins and role in development*. Psychology Press.

Morales, M., Mundy, P., & Rojas, J. (1998). Following the direction of gaze and language development in 6-month-olds. *Infant Behavior and Development, 21*, 373–377.

Nash, M., & Donaldson, M. L. (2005). Word learning in children with vocabulary deficits. *Journal of Speech, Language, and Hearing Research, 48*, 439–458.

Neuman, S. (2006). The knowledge gap: Implications for early education. In D. Dickinson & S. Neuman (Eds.), *Handbook of early literacy research* (Vol. 2, pp. 29–40). New York: Guilford Press.

NICHD Early Child Care Research Network. (1997). Familial factors associated with the characteristics of nonmaternal care for infants. *Journal of Marriage and the Family, 59*, 389–408.

NICHD Early Child Care Research Network. (2005). Duration and developmental timing of poverty and children's cognitive and social development from birth to third grade. *Child Development, 76(4)*, 795–810.

Nelson, K. (1973). Structure and strategy in learning to talk. *Monographs of the Society of Research in Child Development, 38*(1–2), 1–135.

O'Neill, D. K., Main, R. M., & Ziemski, R. A. (2009). "I like Barney": Preschoolers' spontaneous conversational initiations with peers. *First Language, 29*, 401–425.

Pence, K., Justice, L. M., & Wiggins, A. (2008). Preschool teachers' fidelity of Implementation for a language-rich preschool curriculum. *Language, Speech, and Hearing Services in Schools, 39*, 1–14.

Pinker, S. (1994). *The language instinct: How the mind creates language*. New York: Morrow.

Pinker, S. (1999). *Words and rules*. New York: Basic Books.

Rowe, M. L. (2009). Differences in early gesture explain SES disparities in child vocabulary size at school entry. *Science, 323*, 951–953.

Sandler, W., Meir, I., Padden, C., & Aronoff, M. (2005). The emergence of grammar: Systematic structure in a new language. *Proceedings of the National Academy of Sciences of the United States of America, 102*(7), 2661–2665.

Saxton, M. (2008). What's in a name? Coming to terms with the child's linguistic environment. *Journal of Child Language, 35*, 677–686.

Saylor, M. M., & Sabbagh, M. A. (2004). Different kinds of information affect word learning in the preschool years: The case of part-term learning. *Child Development, 75*, 395–408.

Shimpi, P., & Huttenlocher, J. (2007). Maternal labels and infant attention: Relations to early vocabulary development. *Journal of Child Language, 34*, 1–15.

Shukla, M., White, K. S., & Aslin, R. N. (2011). Prosody guides the rapid mapping of auditory word forms onto visual objects in 6-mo-old infants. *Proceedings of the National Academy of Sciences, 108*(15), 6038–6043.

Siegal, M. (2013). *Knowing children: Experiments in conversation and cognition*. Psychology Press.

Storkel, H. L. (2003). Learning new words II phonotactic probability in verb learning. *Journal of Speech, Language, and Hearing Research, 46*(6), 1312–1323.

Suggate, S. P. (2014). A meta-analysis of the long-term effects of phonemic awareness, phonics, fluency, and reading comprehension interventions. *Journal of Learning Disabilities*, 0022219414528540.

Thiessen, E. D., & Saffran, J. R. (2003). When cues collide: Use of stress and statistical cues to word boundaries by 7- to 9-month-old infants. *Developmental Psychology, 39*, 706–716.

Thompson, C. K., Shapiro, L. P., Kiran, S., & Sobecks, J. (2003). The role of syntactic complexity in treatment of sentence deficits in agrammatic aphasia: The complexity account of treatment efficacy (CATE). *Journal of Speech, Language, and Hearing Research, 46*, 591–607.

To, C. K., Cheung, P. S., & McLeod, S. (2013). A population study of children's acquisition of Hong Kong Cantonese consonants, vowels, and tones. *Journal of Speech, Language, and Hearing Research, 56*(1), 103–122.

Tomasello, M. (1988). The role of joint attentional processes in early language development. *Language Sciences, 10*, 69–88.

Tomasi, D., & Volkow, N. D. (2012). Laterality patterns of brain functional connectivity: Gender effects. *Cerebral Cortex, 22*(6), 1455–1462.

Wallace, I. F., Roberts, J. E., & Lodder, D. E. (1998). Interactions of African American infants and their mothers: Relations with development at 1 year of age. *Journal of Speech, Language, and Hearing Research, 41*, 900–912.

Wedel, A., Kaplan, A., & Jackson, S. (2013). High functional load inhibits phonological contrast loss: A corpus study. *Cognition, 128*(2), 179–186.

Wright, V. R., Chau, M., & Aratani, Y. (2010). *Who are America's poor children? The official story*. New York: National Center for Children in Poverty, Mailman School of Public Health, Columbia University.

Zapf, J., & Smith, L. B. (2007). When do children generalize the plural to novel nouns? *First Language, 27*, 53–73.

Chapter 3

Aboitiz, F., & Ricardo, G. V. (1997). The evolutionary origin of the language areas in the brain: A neuroanatomical perspective. *Brain Research Reviews, 25*, 381–396.

Belliveau, J. W., Rosen, B. R., Kantor, H. L., Rzedzian, R. R., Kennedy, D. N., McKinstry, R. C., ... & Brady, T. J. (1990). Functional cerebral imaging by susceptibility-contrast NMR. *Magnetic Resonance in Medicine, 14*(3), 538–546.

Blumstein, S. E., & Amso, D. (2013). Dynamic functional organization of language insights from functional neuroimaging. *Perspectives on Psychological Science, 8*(1), 44–48.

Bookheimer, S. (2002). Functional MRI of language: New approaches to understanding the cortical organization of semantic processing. *Annual Reviews of Neuroscience, 25*, 151–188.

Brennan, J., & Pylkkänen, L. (2012). The time-course and spatial distribution of brain activity associated with sentence processing. *Neuroimage, 60*(2), 1139–1148.

Brown, R. W., Cheng, Y. C. N., Haacke, E. M., Thompson, M. R., & Venkatesan, R. (2014). *Magnetic resonance imaging: Physical principles and sequence design*. John Wiley & Sons.

Bruer, J.T. (2001). A critical and sensitive period primer. In D. Bailey, J. T. Bruer, F. J. Symons, & J. W. Lichtman (Eds.), *Critical thinking about critical periods* (pp. 3–26). Baltimore: Brookes.

Bruer, J.T., & Greenough, W.T (2001). The subtle science of how experience affects the brain. In D. Bailey, J. T. Bruer, F. J. Symons, & J. W. Lichtman (Eds.), *Critical thinking about critical periods* (pp. 209–232). Baltimore: Brookes.

Buchweitz, A., Mason, R. A., Meschyan, G., Keller, T. A., & Just, M. A. (2014). Modulation of cortical activity during comprehension of familiar and unfamiliar text topics in speed reading and speed listening. *Brain and Language, 139*, 49–57.

Carlson, S. M., Koenig, M. A., & Harms, M. B. (2013). Theory of mind. *Wiley Interdisciplinary Reviews: Cognitive Science, 4*(4), 391–402.

Chomsky, N. (1978). *Syntactic structures*. The Hague, The Netherlands: Mouton. (Original work published 1957).

Dennis, M., Simic, N., Bigler, E. D., Abildskov, T., Agostino, A., Taylor, H. G., ... & Yeates, K. O. (2013). Cognitive, affective, and conative theory of mind (ToM) in children with traumatic brain injury. *Developmental Cognitive Neuroscience, 5*, 25–39.

Fernandez-Duque, D., Baird, J., & Posner, M. (2000). Executive attention and metacognitive regulation. *Consciousness and Cognition, 9*, 288–307.

Flege, J. E., Yeni-Komshian, G. H. & Liu, S. (1999). Age constraints on second-language acquisition. *Journal of Memory and Language , 41*, 78-104.

Frackowiak, R. S. J., Friston, K. J., Frith, C. D., Dolan, R. J., Price, C. J., Zeki, S., et al. (2004). *Human brain function* (2nd ed.). San Diego, CA: Academic Press.

Friederici, A. D., Opitz, B., & von Cramon, D. (2000). Segregating semantic and syntactic aspects of processing in the human brain: An fMRI investigation of different word types. *Cerebral Cortex, 10*, 698–705.

Glennen, S. (2015). Internationally adopted children in the early school years: Relative strengths and weaknesses in language abilities. *Language, Speech, and Hearing Services in Schools, 46*(1), 1–13.

Glennen, S., & Masters, M. G. (2002). Typical and atypical language development in infants and toddlers adopted from Eastern Europe. *American Journal of Speech–Language Pathology, 11*, 417–433.

Glezerman, T. B., & Balkoski, V. (1999). *Language, thought, and the brain*. New York: Kluwer Academic.

Glimåker, M., Johansson, B., Grindborg, Ö., Bottai, M., Lindquist, L., & Sjölin, J. (2015). Adult bacterial meningitis: Earlier treatment and improved outcome following guideline revision promoting prompt lumbar puncture. *Clinical Infectious Diseases, 60*(8), 1162–1169.

Golumbic, E. M. Z., Poeppel, D., & Schroeder, C. E. (2012). Temporal context in speech processing and attentional stream selection: a behavioral and neural perspective. *Brain and Language, 122*(3), 151–161.

Groen, W. B., Tesink, C. M. J. Y., Petersson, K. M., Van Berkum, J., Van der Gaag, R. J., Hagoort, P., & Buitelaar, J. K. (2010). Semantic, factual, and social language

comprehension in adolescents with autism: An FMRI study. *Cerebral Cortex, 20*(8), 1937–1945.

Hakuta, K. (2001). A critical period of second language acquisition? In D. Bailey, J. T. Bruer, F. J. Symons, & J. W. Lichtman (Eds.), *Critical thinking about critical periods* (pp. 193–208). Baltimore: Brookes.

Hubel, D. H., & Wiesel, T. N. (1970). The period of susceptibility to the physiological effects of unilateral eye closure in kittens. *Journal of Physiology, 206*, 419–436.

Huttenlocher, P. R. (2002). *Neural plasticity: The effects of environment on the development of the cerebral cortex*. Cambridge, MA: Harvard University Press.

Jerison, H. (2012). *Evolution of the brain and intelligence*. Elsevier.

Kiefer, M., & Pulvermüller, F. (2012). Conceptual representations in mind and brain: Theoretical developments, current evidence and future directions. *Cortex, 48*(7), 805–825.

Kolb, B. (2013). *Brain plasticity and behavior*. Psychology Press.

Lent, R., & Tovar-Moll, F. (2015). How can development and plasticity contribute to understanding evolution of the human brain? *Frontiers in Human Neuroscience, 9*.

Liberman, A. M. (1999). When theories of speech meet the real world. *Journal of Psycholinguistic Research, 27*, 111–122.

Lieberman, P. (1991). *Uniquely human: The evolution of speech, thought, and selfless behavior*. Cambridge, MA: Harvard University Press.

Lieberman, P. (2000). *Human language and our reptilian brain*. Cambridge, MA: Harvard University Press.

Liberman, A. M., & Mattingly, I. G. (2014). Modularity and the effects of experience. *Cognition and the Symbolic Processes: Applied and Ecological Perspectives, 33*.

Matejko, A. A., Price, G. R., Mazzocco, M. M., & Ansari, D. (2013). Individual differences in left parietal white matter predict math scores on the Preliminary Scholastic Aptitude Test. *Neuroimage, 66*, 604–610.

Nelson, C. A., Zeanah, C. H., Fox, N. A., Marshall, P. J., Smyke, A. T., & Guthrie, D. (2007). Cognitive recovery in socially deprived young children: The Bucharest Early Intervention Project. *Science, 318*, 1937–1940.

Newport, E. L., Bavelier, D., & Neville, H. J. (2001). Critical thinking about critical periods: Perspectives on a critical period for language acquisition. *Language, Brain and Cognitive Development: Essays in Honor of Jacques Mehler*, 481–502.

Noback, C. R., Strominger, N. L., Demarest, R. J., & Ruggiero, D. A. (2005). *The human nervous system: Structure and function* (6th ed.). Totowa, NJ: Humana Press.

Office of the Federal Register. (1990). *Presidential Proclamation 6158*. Retrieved December 30, 2005, from http://www.loc.gov/loc/brain/proclaim.html .

Pallier, C., Dehaene, S., Poline, J. B., LeBihan, D., Argenti, A. M., Dupoux, E., et al. (2003). Brain imaging of language plasticity in adopted adults: Can a second language replace the first? *Cerebral Cortex, 13*, 155–161.

Pinker, S. (1994). *The language instinct: How the mind creates language*. New York: Morrow.

Rendall, D., Cheney, D. L., & Seyfarth, R. M. (2000). Proximate factors mediating "contact" calls in adult female and their infants. *Journal of Comparative Psychology, 114*, 36–46.

Schwartz, M. F. (2013). Patterns of speech production deficit within and across aphasia syndromes: Application of a psycholinguistic model. *The Cognitive Neuropsychology of Language (Psychology Revivals), 163.*

Schull, W. J. (1998). The Japanese experience, 1947–1997. *Proceedings of the National Academy of Science, 95,* 5437–5441.

Stoner, R., Chow, M. L., Boyle, M. P., Sunkin, S. M., Mouton, P. R., Roy, S., ... & Courchesne, E. (2014). Patches of disorganization in the neocortex of children with autism. *New England Journal of Medicine, 370* (13), 1209–1219.

Stuss, D. T., & Knight, R. T. (Eds.). (2013). *Principles of frontal lobe function.* Oxford University Press.

Talwar, V., & Lee, K. (2002). Emergence of white-lie telling in children between 3 and 7 years of age. *Merrill-Palmer Quarterly, 48,* 160–181.

U.S. Department of State. (2014). *FY 2014 Annual Report on Intercountry Adoption.* Retrieved March 22, 2015, from http://travel.state.gov/content/dam/aa/pdfs/fy2014_annual_report.pdf.

van Ijzendoorn, M. H., Luijk, M. P. C. M., & Juffer, F. (2008). IQ of children growing up in children's homes: A meta-analysis on IQ delays in orphanages. *Merrill-Palmer Quarterly, 54,* 341–366.

Vorria, P., Papaligoura, Z., Dunn, J., van Ijzendoorn, M. H., Steele, H., Kontopoulou, A., et al. (2003). Early experiences and attachment relationships of Greek infants raised in residential group care. *Journal of Child Psychology and Psychiatry, 44,* 1208–1220.

Weismer, S. E., Plante, E., Jones, M., & Tomblin, J. B. (2005). A functional magnetic resonance imaging investigation of verbal working memory in adolescents with specific language impairment. *Journal of Speech, Language, and Hearing Research, 48,* 405–425.

Weismer, S. E., & Thordardottir, E. (2002). Cognition and language. In P. Accardo, B. Rogers, & A. Capute (Eds.), *Disorders of language development* (pp. 21–37). Timonium, MD: York Press.

Chapter 4

American Speech-Language-Hearing Association. (2005). *Evidence-Based Practice in Communication Disorders* [position statement]. Available from http://www.asha.org/policy.

Aranguri, C., Davidson, B., & Ramirez, R. (2006). Patterns of communication through interpreters: A detailed sociolinguistic analysis. *Journal of General Internal Medicine, 21,* 623–629.

Berko, J. (1958). The child's learning of English morphology. *Word, 14,* 150–177.

Blom-Hoffman, J., O'Neil-Pirozzi, T., Volpe, R., Cutting, J., & Bissinger, E. (2007). Instructing parents to use dialogic reading strategies with preschool children: Impact of a video-based training program on caregiver reading behaviors and children's related verbalizations. *Journal of Applied School Psychology, 23,* 117–131.

Bloom, A. (1979). *Emile: Or, On Education.* New York: Basic Books.

Bloom, L. (2000). The intentionality model of word learning: How to learn a word, any word. In R. M. Golinkoff, K. Hirsh-Pasek, N. Akhtar, L. Bloom, G. Hollich, L. Smith, et al. (Eds.), *Becoming a word learner: A debate on lexical acquisition* (pp. 19–50). New York: Oxford University Press.

Bloom, L., & Tinker, E. (2001). The intentionality model and language acquisition. *Monographs of the Society for Research in Child Development, 66*(4), vii–104.

Brooks, P. J. (2004). Grammatical competence is not a psychologically valid construct. *Journal of Child Language, 31,* 467–470.

Brown, H. D. (2001). *Teaching by principles: An interactive approach to language pedagogy* (2nd ed.). White Plains, NY: Addison Wesley Longman.

Budwig, N. (1995). *A developmental-functionalist approach to child language.* Mahwah, NJ: Erlbaum.

Charity, A. H., Scarborough, H. S., & Griffin, D. M. (2004). Familiarity with School English in African American children and its relation to early reading achievement. *Child Development, 75,* 1340–1356.

Chomsky, N. (1965). *Aspects of the theory of syntax.* Cambridge, MA: MIT Press.

Dale, P. S., & Fenson, L. (1996). Lexical development norms for young children. *Behavior Research Methods, Instruments, & Computers, 28,* 125–127.

Elman, J. L., Bates, E. A., Johnson, M. H., Parisi, D., & Plunkett, K. (1996). *Rethinking innateness: A connectionist perspective on development.* Cambridge, MA: MIT Press.

Fitch, R. H., Miller, S., & Tallal, P. (1997). Neurobiology of speech perception. *Annual Reviews of Neuroscience, 20,* 331–353.

Fodor, J. (1983). *The modularity of mind.* Cambridge, MA: MIT Press.

Galle, M.E., & McMurray, B. (2014). The development of voicing categories: A quantitative review of over 40 years of infant speech perception research. *Psychonomic Bulletin and Review, 21,* 884–906.

Gerken, L., & Aslin, R. N. (2005). Thirty years of research on infant speech perception: The legacy of Peter W. Jusczyk. *Language Learning and Development, 1,* 5–21.

Gleitman, L. (1990). The structural sources of verb meanings. *Language Acquisition, 1,* 3–55.

Hart, B., & Risley, T. (1995). *Meaningful differences in the everyday experiences of young American children.* Baltimore: Brookes.

Heflin, L. J., & Simpson, R. J. (1998). Interventions for children and youth with autism: Prudent choices in a world of exaggerated claims and empty promises. Part 1: Intervention and treatment option review. *Focus on Autism and Other Developmental Disabilities, 13,* 194–211.

Heilmann, J., Weismer, S. E., Evans, J., & Hollar, C. (2005). Utility of the MacArthur–Bates Communicative Development Inventory in identifying language abilities of late-talking and typically developing toddlers. *American Journal of Speech–Language Pathology, 14,* 40–51.

Hirsh-Pasek, K., & Golinkoff, R. M. (1996). *The origins of grammar: Evidence from early language comprehension*. Cambridge, MA: MIT Press.

Hirsh-Pasek, K., Golinkoff, R. M., & Hollich, G. (2000). An emergentist coalition model for word learning: Mapping words to objects is a product of the interaction of multiple cues. In R. M. Golinkoff, K. Hirsh-Pasek, L. Bloom, L. B. Smith, A. L. Woodward, N. Akhtar, et al. (Eds.), *Becoming a word learner: A debate on lexical acquisition* (pp. 136–164). New York: Oxford University Press.

Hollich, G., Hirsh-Pasek, K., & Golinkoff, R. M. (2000). Breaking the language barrier: An emergentist coalition model of the origins of word learning. *Monographs of the Society for Research in Child Development, 65*(3), v–137.

Jusczyk, P. W., & Aslin, R. N. (1995). Infants' detection of sound patterns of words in fluent speech. *Cognitive Psychology, 29*, 1–23.

Jusczyk, P. W., Cutler, A., & Redanz, N. J. (1993). Infants' preference for the predominant stress patterns of English words. *Child Development, 64*, 675–687.

Justice, L. M., Bowles, R. P., Kaderavek, J. N., Ukrainetz, T. A., Eisenberg, S. L., & Gillam, R. B. (2006). The index of narrative microstructure: A clinical tool for analyzing school-age children's narrative performances. *American Journal of Speech Language Pathology, 15*, 177–191.

Karmiloff, K., & Karmiloff-Smith, A. (2001). *Pathways to language from fetus to adolescent*. Cambridge, MA: Harvard University Press.

Kemler Nelson, D. G., Jusczyk, P. W., Mandel, D. R., Myers, J., Turk, A., & Gerken L. (1995). The head-turn preference procedure for testing auditory perception. *Infant Behavior and Development, 18*, 111–116.

Kent, R. D. (1994). *Reference manual for communicative sciences and disorders: Speech and language*. Austin, TX: PRO-ED.

Kita, S., & Özyürek, A. (2003). What does cross-linguistics variation in semantic coordination of speech and gesture reveal? Evidence for an interface representation of spatial thinking and speaking. *Journal of Memory and Language, 48*, 16–32.

Landau, B. (2009). The importance of the nativist-empiricist debate: Thinking about primitives without primitive thinking. *Child Development Perspectives, 3*, 88–90.

Landau, B., & Gleitman, L. R. (1985). *Language and experience: Evidence from the blind child*. Cambridge, MA: Harvard University Press.

Lovaas, O. I. (1987). Behavioral treatment and normal educational and intellectual functioning in young autistic children. *Journal of Consulting and Clinical Psychology, 55*, 3–9.

Luyster, R., Qiu, S., Lopez, K., & Lord, C. (2007). Predicting outcomes of children referred for autism using the MacArthur–Bates Communicative Development Inventory. *Journal of Speech, Language, and Hearing Research, 50*, 667–681.

MacWhinney, B. (1987). The competition model. In B. MacWhinney (Ed.), *Mechanisms of language acquisition* (pp. 249–308). Hillsdale, NJ: Erlbaum.

MacWhinney, B. (2004). A multiple process solution to the logical problem of language acquisition. *Journal of Child Language, 31*, 883–914.

Mattys, S. L., Jusczyk, P. W., Luce, P. A., & Morgan, J. L. (1999). Word segmentation in infants: How phonotactics and prosody combine. *Cognitive Psychology, 38*, 465–494.

Nippold, M. A. (2007). Later *language development: School-Age Children, Adolescents, and Young Adults* (3rd ed.). Austin, TX: PRO-ED.

Pajak, B., & Levy, R. (2014). The role of abstraction in non-native speech perception. *Journal of Phonetics, 46*, 147–160.

Peters-Sheffer, N., Didden, R., Korzilius, H., & Sturmey, P. (2011). A meta-analytic study on the effectiveness of comprehensive ABA-based early intervention programs for children with Autism Spectrum Disorders. *Research in Autism Spectrum Disorders, 5*, 60–69.

Phillips, C. (2001). Levels of representation in the electrophysiology of speech perception. *Cognitive Science, 25*, 711–731.

Piaget, J. (1923). *The language and thought of the child*. London: Kegan Paul.

Pinker, S. (1984). *Language learnability and language development*. Cambridge, MA: Harvard University Press.

Purnell, T., Idsardi, W., & Baugh, J. (1999). Perceptual and phonetic experiments on American English dialect identification. *Journal of Language and Social Psychology, 18*, 10–30.

Rumelhart, D. E., & McClelland, J. L. (1986). On learning the past tenses of English verbs. In D. E. Rumelhart & J. L. McClelland (Eds.), *Parallel distributed processing: Explorations in the microstructure of cognition: Vol. 2. Psychological and biological models* (pp. 216–271). Cambridge, MA: MIT Press.

Saffran, J. R., Aslin, R. N., & Newport, E. L. (1996). Statistical learning by 8-month-old infants. *Science, 274*, 1926–1928.

Sander, E. K. (1972). When are speech sounds learned? *Journal of Speech and Hearing Disorders, 37*, 55–63.

Saylor, M. M., & Sabbagh, M. A. (2004). Different kinds of information affect word learning in the preschool years: The case of part-term learning. *Child Development, 75*, 395–408.

Shavelson, R. J., & Towne, L. (Eds.). (2002). *Scientific research in education*. Washington, DC: National Academy Press.

Sinclair-de-Zwart, H. (1973). Language acquisition and cognitive development. In T. E. Moore (Ed.), *Cognitive development and the acquisition of language* (pp. 9–26). New York: Academic Press.

Skinner, B. F. (1957). *Verbal behavior*. New York: Appleton-Century-Crofts.

Spaulding, T. J., Plante, E., & Farinella, K. A. (2006). Eligibility criteria for language impairment: Is the low end of normal always appropriate? *Language, Speech, and Hearing Services in Schools, 37*, 61–72.

Stokes, D. E. (1997). *Pasteur's quadrant: Basic science and technological innovation*. Washington, DC: Brookings Institution Press.

Thal, D. J., DesJardin, J. L., & Eisenberg, L. S. (2007). Validity of the MacArthur–Bates Communicative Development Inventories for measuring language abilities in children with cochlear implants. *American Journal of Speech–Language Pathology, 16*, 54–64.

Thompson, C. K., Shapiro, L. P., Kiran, S., & Sobecks, J. (2003). The role of syntactic complexity in treatment of sentence deficits in agrammatic aphasia: The complexity account of treatment efficacy (CATE). *Journal of Speech, Language, and Hearing Research, 46*, 591–607.

Throneburg, R. N., Calvert, L. K., Sturm, J. J., Paramboukas, A. A., & Paul, P. J. (2000). A comparison of service delivery models: Effects on curricular vocabulary skills in the school setting. *American Journal of Speech–Language Pathology, 9*, 10–20.

Tomasello, M. (2003). *Constructing a language*. Cambridge, MA: Harvard University Press.

U.S. Department of Education, Institute of Education Sciences, National Center for Education Evaluation and Regional Assistance. (2003). *Identifying and implementing educational practices supported by rigorous evidence: A user friendly guide*. Washington, DC: Author.

Verhaegen, C., & Poncelet, M. (2013). Changes in naming and semantic abilities with aging from 50 to 90 years. *Journal of the International Neuropsychological Society, 19*, 119–126.

Vygotsky, L. S. (1978). *Mind in society: The development of higher psychological processes* (M. Cole, V. John-Steiner, S. Scribner, & E. Souberman, Eds.). Cambridge, MA: Harvard University Press.

Wasik, B. A., Bond, M. A., & Hindman, A. (2006). The effects of a language and literacy intervention on Head Start children and teachers. *Journal of Educational Psychology, 98*, 63–74.

Weitzman, E., & Greenberg, J. (2002). *Learning language and loving it: A guide to promoting children's social, language, and literacy development in early childhood settings* (2nd ed.). Toronto, Ontario, Canada: The Hanen Centre.

Whitehurst, G. J., Falco, F. L., Lonigan, C. J., Fischel, J. E., DeBaryshe, B. D., Valdez-Menchaca, M. C., et al. (1988). Accelerating language development through picture book reading. *Developmental Psychology, 24*, 552–559.

Chapter 5

Adamson, L. B., Bakeman, R., & Deckner, D. F. (2004). The development of symbol-infused joint engagement. *Child Development, 75*, 1171–1187.

Adamson, L. B., & Chance, S. E. (1998). Coordinating attention to people, objects, and language. In A. M. Wetherby, S. F. Warren, & J. Reichle (Eds.), *Transitions in prelinguistic communication: Preintentional to intentional and presymbolic to symbolic* (pp. 15–37). Baltimore: Brookes.

American Academy of Pediatrics. (2012). Kids in U.S. exposed to 4 hours of daily background TV. Retrieved from http://www.aap.org.

American Academy of Pediatrics. (2014). Media and children. Retrieved from http://www.aap.org/en-us/advocacy-and-policy/aap-health-initiatives/Pages/Media-and-Children.aspx.

Baker, S. A., Idsardi, W. J., Golinkoff, R. M., & Petitto, L.-A. (2005). The perception of handshapes in American Sign Language. *Memory & Cognition, 33*(5), 887–904.

Baldwin, D. A. (1991). Infants' contribution to the achievement of joint reference. *Child Development, 62*, 875–890.

Bates, E., Camaioni, L., & Volterra, V. (1975). The acquisition of performatives prior to speech. *Merrill–Palmer Quarterly, 21*, 205–226.

Bates, E., & Carnevale, G. F. (1993). New directions in research on language development. *Developmental Review, 13*, 436–470.

Bates, E., Dale, P. S., & Thal, D. (1995). Individual differences and their implications for theories of language development. In P. Fletcher & B. MacWhinney (Eds.), *Handbook of child language* (pp. 96–151). Oxford, England: Basil Blackwell.

Behl-Chadha, G. (1996). Basic-level and superordinate-like categorical representations early in infancy. *Cognition, 60*, 105–141.

Bernstein Ratner, N. (1986). Durational cues which mark clause boundaries in mother–child speech. *Journal of Phonetics, 14*, 303–309.

Bernstein Ratner, N., & Pye, C. (1984). Higher pitch in BR is not universal: Acoustic evidence from Quiche Mayan. *Journal of Child Language, 11*, 515–522.

Bono, M. A., & Stifter, C. A. (2003). Maternal attention-directing strategies and infant focused attention during problem solving. *Infancy, 4*, 235–250.

Bowerman, M., & Choi, S. (2003). Space under construction: Language-specific spatial categorization in first language acquisition. In D. Gentner & S. Goldin-Meadow (Eds.), *Language in mind: Advances in the study of language and thought* (pp. 387–428). Cambridge, MA: MIT Press.

Burnham, D., Kitamura, C., & Vollmer-Conna, U. (2002). What's new, pussycat? On talking to babies and animals. *Science, 296*, 1435.

Camaioni, L., Perucchini, P., Bellagamba, F., & Colonnesi, C. (2004). The role of declarative pointing in developing a theory of mind. *Infancy, 5*, 291–308.

Casasola, M., Bhagwat, J., & Burke, A. S. (2009). Learning to form a spatial category of tight-fit relations: How experience with a label can give a boost. *Developmental Psychology, 45*, 711–723.

Choi, S., McDonough, L., Bowerman, M., & Mandler, J. M. (1999). Early sensitivity to language-specific spatial categories in English and Korean. *Cognitive Development, 14*, 241–268.

Colombo, J., Shaddy, D. J., Richman, W. A., Maikranz, J. M., & Blaga, O. M. (2004). The developmental course of habituation in infancy and preschool outcome. *Infancy, 5*, 1–38.

Cooper, R. P., & Aslin, R. N. (1990). Preference for infant-directed speech in the first month after birth. *Child Development, 61*, 1584–1595.

Dale, P. S. (1991). The validity of a parent report measure of vocabulary and syntax at 24 months. *Journal of Speech and Hearing Research, 34*, 565–571.

Dale, P. S. (1996). Parent report assessment of language and communication. In K. Cole, P. Dale, & D. Thal (Eds.), *Assessment of communication and language* (Vol. 6, pp. 161–182). Baltimore: Brookes.

Dixon, J. A., & Marchman, V. A. (2007). Grammar and the lexicon: Developmental ordering in language acquisition. *Child Development, 78,* 190–212.

Fenson, L., Bates, E., Dale, P., Goodman, J., Reznick, J. S., & Thal, D. (2000). Measuring variability in early child language: Don't shoot the messenger. *Child Development, 71,* 323–328.

Fenson, L., Dale, P. S., Reznick, J. S., Thal, D., Bates, E., Hartung, J. P., et al. (1993). *The MacArthur Communicative Development Inventories.* San Diego, CA: Singular.

Fenson, L., Pethick, S., Renda, C., Cox, J. L., Dale, P. S., & Reznick, J. S. (2000). Short form versions of the MacArthur Communicative Development Inventories. *Applied Psycholinguistics, 21,* 95–116.

Fernald, A. (1989). Intonation and communicative intent in mothers' speech to infants: Is the melody the message? *Child Development, 60,* 1497–1510.

Fernald, A., & Kuhl, P. (1987). Acoustic determinants of infant preference for motherese speech. *Infant Behavior and Development, 10,* 279–293.

Fernald, A., & Mazzie, C. (1991). Prosody and focus in speech to infants and adults. *Developmental Psychology, 27,* 209–221.

Fernald, A., & Simon, T. (1984). Expanded intonation contours in mothers' speech to newborns. *Developmental Psychology, 20,* 104–113.

Fernald, A., Taeschner, T., Dunn, J., Papousek, M., de Boysson-Bardies, B., & Fukui, I. (1989). A cross-linguistic study of prosodic modifications in mothers' and fathers' speech to preverbal infants. *Journal of Child Language, 16,* 477–501.

Fisher, C., & Tokura, H. (1996). Acoustic cues to grammatical structure in infant-directed speech: Cross-linguistic evidence. *Child Development, 67,* 3192–3218.

Gard, A., Gilman, L., & Gorman, J. (1993). *Speech and language development chart.* Austin, TX: PRO-ED.

Girolametto, L., & Weitzman, E. (2002). Responsiveness of child care providers in interactions with toddlers and preschoolers. *Language, Speech and Hearing Services in Schools, 33,* 268–281.

Girolametto, L., Weitzman, E., Wiigs, M., & Pearce, P. S. (1999). The relationship between maternal language measures and language development in toddlers with expressive vocabulary delays. *American Journal of Speech–Language Pathology, 8,* 354–374.

Goldstein, M. H., Schwade, J. A., & Bornstein, M. H. (2009). The value of vocalizing: Five-month-old infants associate their own noncry vocalizations with responses from adults. *Child Development, 80,* 636–644.

Golinkoff, R. M., & Hirsh-Pasek, K. (1999). *How babies talk: The magic and mystery of language in the first three years of life.* New York: Dutton.

Hart, B., & Risley, T. (1995). *Meaningful differences in the everyday experiences of young American children.* Baltimore: Brookes.

Hart, B., & Risley, T. R. (1999). *The social world of children learning to talk.* Baltimore: Brookes.

Hirsh-Pasek, K., & Golinkoff, R. M. (1996). *The origins of grammar: Evidence from early language comprehension.* Cambridge, MA: MIT Press.

Hollich, G., Golinkoff, R. M., & Hirsh-Pasek, K. (2007). Young children associate novel words with complex objects rather than salient parts. *Developmental Psychology, 43,* 1051–1061.

Hsu, H., Iyer, S.N., & Fogel, A. (2014). Effects of social games on infant vocalizations. *Journal of Child Language, 41,* 132–154.

Irwin, J. R. (2003). Parent and nonparent perception of the multimodal infant cry. *Infancy, 4,* 503–516.

Jusczyk, P. W. (2003). Chunking language input to find patterns. In D. H. Rakison & L. M. Oakes (Eds.), *Early category and concept development: Making sense of the blooming, buzzing confusion* (pp. 27–49). New York: Oxford University Press.Jusczyk, P. W., Cutler, A., & Redanz, N. J. (1993). Infants' preference for the predominant stress patterns of English words. *Child Development, 64,* 675–687.

Jusczyk, P. W., Kennedy, L. J., & Jusczyk, A. M. (1995). Young infants' retention of information about syllables. *Infant Behavior and Development, 18,* 27–42.

Jusczyk, P. W., Luce, P. A., & Charles-Luce, J. (1994). Infants' sensitivity to phonotactic patterns in the native language. *Journal of Memory and Language, 33,* 630–645.

Karrass, J., Braungart-Rieker, J. M., Mullins, J., & Lefever, J. B. (2002). Processes in language acquisition: The roles of gender, attention, and maternal encouragement of attention over time. *Journal of Child Language, 29,* 519–543.

Kent, R. D. (1994). *Reference manual for communicative sciences and disorders: Speech and language.* Austin, TX: PRO-ED.

Kondaurova, M. V., & Bergeson, T.R. (2011). Use of prosodic cues for clause boundaries in speech. *Journal of Speech, Language, and Hearing Research, 54,* 740–754.

Kovelman, I. (2012). Neuroimaging methods. In E. Hoff (Ed.), *Research methods in child language: A practical guide* (pp. 43–59). Malden, MA: Blackwell Publishing Ltd.

Kucirkova, N. (2014, October 24). Is your child under age 2 ? Keep them away from smartphones, tablets and computers. *Washington Post.* Retrieved from http://www.washingtonpost.com.

Kuhl, P. K., & Meltzoff, A. N. (1982). The bimodal perception of speech in infancy. *Science, 218,* 1138–1141.

Laucht, M., Esser, G., & Schmidt, M. H. (1995). Contrasting infant predictors of later cognitive functioning. *Journal of Child Psychology and Psychology and Applied Disciplines, 35,* 649–662.

Liu, J., Golinkoff, R. M., & Sak, K. (2001). One cow does not an animal make: Young children can extend novel words at the superordinate level. *Child Development, 72,* 1674–1694.

Locke, J. L. (1983). *Phonological acquisition and change.* New York: Academic Press.

Mampe, B., Friederici, A. D., Christophe, A., & Wermke, K. (2009). Newborns' cry melody is shaped by their native language. *Current Biology, 19,* 1994–1997.

Mandler, J. (2000). Perceptual and conceptual processes in infancy. *Journal of Cognition and Development, 1,* 3–36.

Marchman, V. A., & Bates, E. (1994). Continuity in lexical and morphological development: A test of the critical mass hypothesis. *Journal of Child Language, 12,* 339–366.

Mattys, S. L., & Jusczyk, P. W. (2001). Phonotactic cues for segmentation of fluent speech by infants. *Cognition, 78,* 91–121.

Meadows, D., Elias, G., & Bain, J. (2000). Mothers' ability to identify infants' communicative acts consistently. *Journal of Child Language, 27,* 393–406.

Mehler, J., Jusczyk, P. W., Lambetz, G., Halsted, N., Bertoncini, J., & Amiel-Tison, C. (1988). A precursor of language acquisition in young infants. *Cognition, 29,* 144–178.

Mervis, C. B., & Crisafi, M. A. (1982). Order of acquisition of subordinate, basic, and superordinate categories. *Child Development, 53,* 258–266.

Miller, C. L. (1988). Parents' perceptions and attributions of infant vocal behaviour and development. *First Language, 8,* 125–141.

Miller, J. L., Ables, E. M., King, A. P., & West, M. J. (2009). Different patterns of contingent stimulation differentially affect attention span in prelinguistic infants. *Infant Behavior and Development, 32,* 254–261.

Nathani, S., Ertmer, D. J., & Stark, R. E. (2006). Assessing vocal development in infants and toddlers. *Clinical Linguistics and Phonetics, 20,* 351–369.

Nelson, K. (1973). Structure and strategy in learning to talk. *Monographs of the Society of Research in Child Development, 38*(1–2), 1–135.

Oller, D.K. (2000). *The emergence of the speech capacity.* Mahwah, NJ: Lawrence Erlbaum Associates.

Papousek, M., Papousek, H., & Symmes, D. (1991). The meanings of melodies in motherese in tone and stress languages. *Infant Behavior and Development, 14,* 415–440.

Parish-Morris, J., Mahajan, N., Hirsh-Pasek, K., Golinkoff, R.M., & Collins, M.F. (2013). Once upon a time: Parent–child dialogue and storybook reading in the electronic era. *Mind, Brain, and Education, 7,* 200–211.

Petitto, L.A., Berens, M.S., Kovelman, I., Dubins, M.H., Jasinska, K, & Shalinsky, M. (2012). The "perceptual wedge" hypothesis as the basis for bilingual babies' phonetic processing advantage: New insights from fNIRS brain imaging. *Brain & Language, 121,* 130–143.

Petitto, L.-A., Holowka, S., Sergio, L. E., & Ostry, S. (2001). Language rhythms in baby hand movements. *Nature, 413,* 35–36.

Pulverman, R., & Golinkoff, R. M. (2004). *Seven-month-olds' attention to potential verb referents in nonlinguistic events.* Paper presented at the 28th annual Boston University Conference on Language Development, Boston, MA.

Quinn, P. C., Eimas, P. D., & Rosenkrantz, S. L. (1993). Evidence for representations of perceptually similar natural categories by 3-month-old and 4-month-old infants. *Perception, 22,* 463–475.

Quenqua, D. (2014, October 11). Is e-reading to your toddler story time, or simply screen time? *The New York Times.* Retrieved from http://www.nytimes.com.

Rescorla, L. (1989). The Language Development Survey: A screening tool for delayed language in toddlers. *Journal of Speech and Hearing Disorders, 54,* 587–599.

Rescorla, L. (1993a). Language Development Survey (LDS): The use of parental report in the identification of communicatively delayed toddlers. *Seminars in Speech and Language, 14,* 264–277.

Rescorla, L. A. (1993b, March). *Outcomes of toddlers with specific expressive language delay (SELD) at ages 3, 4, 5, 6, 7, and 8.* Paper presented at the biennial meeting of the Society for Research in Child Development, New Orleans, LA.

Robertson, S., von Hapsburg, D., & Hay, J.S. (2013). The effect of hearing loss on the perception of infant- and adult-directed speech. *Journal of Speech, Language, and Hearing Research, 56,* 1108–1119.

Robinson, N. M., Dale, P. S., & Landesman, S. (1990). Validity of Stanford–Binet IV with linguistically precocious toddlers. *Intelligence, 14,* 173–186.

Saxton, M. (2008). What's in a name? Coming to terms with the child's linguistic environment. *Journal of Child Language, 35,* 677–686.

Scott, L. S., Pascalis, O., & Nelson, C. A. (2007). A domain-general theory of the development of perceptual discrimination. *Current Directions in Psychological Science, 16,* 197–201.

Slobin, D. I. (2014). Before the beginning: the development of tools of the trade. *Journal of Child Language, 41,* 1–17.

Snow, C. E. (1972). Mothers' speech to children learning language. *Child Development, 43,* 549–565.

Spelke, E. S. (1979). Exploring audible and visual events in infancy. In A. D. Pick (Ed.), *Perception and its development: A tribute to Eleanor J. Gibson* (pp. 221–233). Hillsdale, NJ: Erlbaum.

Stager, C. L., & Werker, J. F. (1997). Infants listen for more phonetic detail in speech perception than in word-learning tasks. *Nature, 388,* 381–382.

Storkel, H. L. (2001). Learning new words I: Phonotactic probability in language development. *Journal of Speech, Language, and Hearing Research, 44,* 1321–1337.

Storkel, H. L. (2003). Learning new words II: Phonotactic probability in verb learning. *Journal of Speech, Language, and Hearing Research, 46,* 1312–1323.

Tamis-LeMonda, C. S., Bornstein, M. H., & Baumwell, L. (2001). Maternal responsiveness and children's achievement of language milestones. *Child Development, 72,* 748–757.

Thal, D. J., Bates, E., Goodman, J., & Jahn-Samilo, J. (1997). Continuity of language abilities: An exploratory study of late- and early-talking toddlers. *Developmental Neuropsychology, 13,* 239–273.

Tomasello, M., & Todd, J. (1983). Joint attention and lexical acquisition style. *First Language, 4,* 197–212.

Trainor, L. J., & Desjardins, R. N. (2002). Pitch characteristics of infant-directed speech affect infants' ability to discriminate vowels. *Psychonomic Bulletin and Review, 9,* 335–340.

Trevarthen, C. (2011). What is it like to be a person who knows nothing? Defining the active intersubjective mind of a newborn human being. *Infant and Child Development, 20,* 119–135.

Trevarthen, C., & Aitken, K.J. (2001). Infant intersubjectivity: Research, theory, and clinical applications. *Journal of Child Psychology and Psychiatry, 42,* 3–48.

van de Weijer, J. (2001). Vowels in infant- and adult-directed speech. In A. Karlsson & J. van de Weijer (Eds.), *Papers from Fonetik 2001 held at Örenäs, May 30–June 1, 2001* (Working Paper 49, pp. 172–175). Lund, Sweden: Lund University.

Weitzman, E., & Greenberg, J. (2002). *Learning language and loving it: A guide to promoting children's social, language, and literacy development in early childhood settings* (2nd ed.). Toronto, Ontario, Canada: The Hanen Centre.

Woodward, A. L. (1998). Infants selectively encode the goal object of an actor's reach. *Cognition, 69,* 1–34.

Woodward, A. L., & Hoyne, K. (1999). Infants' learning about words and sounds in relation to objects. *Child Development, 70,* 65–77.

Yoshida, K. A., Fennell, C. T., Swingley, D., & Werker, J. F. (2009). Fourteen-month-old infants learn similar-sounding words. *Developmental Science, 12,* 412–418.

Zubrick, S. R., Taylor, C. L., Rice, M. L., & Slegers, D. W. (2007). Late language emergence at 24 months: An epidemiological study of prevalence, predictors, and covariates. *Journal of Speech, Language, and Hearing Research, 50,* 1562–1592.

Chapter 6

Akhtar, N. (2005). The robustness of learning through overhearing. *Developmental Science, 8,* 199–209.

Akhtar, N., Jipson, J., & Callanan, M. A. (2001). Learning words through overhearing. *Child Development, 72,* 416–430.

Akhtar, N., & Tomasello, M. (1996). Twenty-four-month-old children learn words for absent objects and actions. *British Journal of Developmental Psychology, 14,* 79–93.

Apel, K., & Masterson, J. J. (2001a). *Beyond baby talk: From sounds to sentences—A parent's complete guide to language development.* Roseville, CA: Prima.

Baldwin, D. A. (1995). Understanding the link between joint attention and language. In C. Moore & P. J. Dunham (Eds.), *Joint attention: Its origins and role in development* (pp. 131–158). Hillsdale, NJ: Erlbaum.

Baldwin, D. A., & Baird, J. A. (1999). Action analysis: A gateway to intentional inference. In P. Rochat (Ed.), *Early social cognition: Understanding others in the first months of life* (pp. 215–240). Mahwah, NJ: Erlbaum.

Bauer, D. J., Goldfield, B. A., & Reznick, J. S. (2002). Alternative approaches to analyzing individual differences in the rate of early vocabulary development. *Applied Psycholinguistics, 23,* 313–335.

Berko, J. (1958). The child's learning of English morphology. *Word, 14,* 150–177.

Bloom, P., & Markson, L. (2001). Are there principles that apply only to the acquisition of words? A reply to Waxman and Booth. *Cognition, 78,* 89–90.

Bradley, R. H., & Corwyn, R. F. (2002). Socioeconomic status and child development. *Annual Review of Psychology, 53,* 371–399.

Brady, N. C., Marquis, J., Fleming, K., & McLean, L. (2004). Prelinguistic predictors of language growth in children with developmental disabilities. *Journal of Speech, Language, and Hearing Research, 47,* 663–677.

Brown, R. (1973). *A first language: The early stages.* Cambridge, MA: Harvard University Press.

Burns, T. C., Yoshida, K. A., Hill, K., & Werker, J. F. (2007). The development of phonetic representation in bilingual and monolingual infants. *Applied Psycholinguistics, 28,* 455–474.

Callanan, M., Akhtar, N., Sussman, L., & Sabbagh, M. (2003). *Learning words in directive and ostensive contexts.* Unpublished manuscript, University of California, Santa Cruz.

Capirci, O., Iverson, J. M., Pizzuto, E., & Volterra, V. (1996). Communicative gestures during the transition to two-word speech. *Journal of Child Language, 23,* 645–673.

Carey, S., & Bartlett, E. (1978). Acquiring a single new word. *Papers and Reports on Child Language Development, 15,* 17–29.

Caselli, M. C. (1983). Communication to language: Deaf children's and hearing children's development compared. *Sign Language Studies, 39,* 113–144.

Caselli, M. C., Volterra, V., & Pizzuto, E. (1984, April). *The relationship between vocal and gestural communication from the one-word to the two-word stage.* Paper presented at the International Conference on Infant Studies, New York, NY.

Clark, E. V. (1993). *The lexicon in acquisition.* New York: Cambridge University Press.

Conboy, B. T., Rivera-Gaxiola, M., Silva-Pereyra, J. F., & Kuhl, P. K. (2008). Event-related potential studies of early language processing: From phonemes, to words, to sentences. In A. D. Friederici & G. Thierry (Eds.), *Early language development: Bridging brain and behaviour, Trends in language acquisition research series* (pp. 23–64). Amsterdam: John Benjamins.

Dollaghan, C. A., Campbell, T. F., Paradise, J. L., Feldman, H. M., Janosky, J. E., Pitcairn, D. N., et al. (1999). Maternal education and measures of early speech and language development. *Journal of Speech, Language, and Hearing Research, 42,* 1432–1443.

Fenson, L., Bates, E., Dale, P., Goodman, J., Reznick, J. S., & Thal, D. (2000). Measuring variability in early child language: Don't shoot the messenger. *Child Development, 71,* 323–328.

Fenson, L., Dale, P. S., Reznick, J. S., Thal, D., Bates, E., Hartung, J. P., et al. (2003). *MacArthur–Bates Communicative Development Inventories.* Baltimore: Brookes.

Fenson, L., Pethick, S., Renda, C., Cox, J. L., Dale, P. S., & Reznick, J. S. (2000). Short form versions of the MacArthur Communicative Development Inventories. *Applied Psycholinguistics, 21,* 95–116.

Fernald, A., Swingley, D., & Pinto, J. P. (2001). When half a word is enough: Infants can recognize spoken words using partial phonetic information. *Child Development, 72,* 1003–1015.

Fisher, C. (2002). Structural limits on verb mapping: The role of abstract structure in 2.5-year-olds' interpretations of novel verbs. *Developmental Science, 5*, 55–64.

Fraser, C., Bellugi, U., & Brown, R. (1963). Control of grammar in imitation, comprehension, and production. *Journal of Verbal Learning and Verbal Behavior, 2*, 121–135.

Gard, A., Gilman, L., & Gorman, J. (1993). *Speech and language development chart*. Austin, TX: PRO-ED.

Gerken, L., & Shady, M. E. (1996). The picture selection task. In D. McDaniel, C. McKee, & H. Smith (Eds.), *Methods for assessing children's syntax* (pp. 125–145). Cambridge, MA: MIT Press.

Gershkoff-Stowe, L. (2001). The course of children's naming errors in early word learning. *Journal of Cognition and Development, 2*, 131–155.

Golinkoff, R. M., Mervis, C. V., & Hirsh-Pasek, K. (1994). Early object labels: The case for a developmental lexical principles framework. *Journal of Child Language, 21*, 125–155.

Golinkoff, R. M., Shuff-Bailey, M., Olguin, R., & Ruan, W. (1995). Young children extend novel words at the basic level: Evidence for the principle of categorical scope. *Developmental Psychology, 31*, 494–505.

Graham, S. A., & Kilbreath, C. S. (2007). It's a sign of the kind: Gestures and words guide infants' inductive inferences. *Developmental Psychology, 43*, 1111–1123.

Halliday, M. A. K. (1978). *Language as a social semiotic: The social interpretation of language and meaning*. Baltimore: University Park Press.

Hoff, E. (2006). How social contexts support and shape language development. *Developmental Review, 26*, 55–88.

Hoff-Ginsberg, E. (1998). The relation of birth order and socioeconomic status to children's language experience and language development. *Applied Psycholinguistics, 19*, 603–629.

Hollich, G., Hirsh-Pasek, K., & Golinkoff, R. M. (2000). Breaking the language barrier: An emergentist coalition model of the origins of word learning. *Monographs of the Society for Research in Child Development, 65*(3), v–137.

Horton-Ikard, R., & Ellis Weismer, S. (2005). *A preliminary examination of vocabulary and word learning in African-American toddlers from low and middle SES homes*. Poster session presented at the 2005 Symposium on Research in Child Language Disorders, Madison, WI.

Huttenlocher, J., Vasilyeva, M., Waterfall, H. R., Vevea, J. L., & Hedges, L. V. (2007). The varieties of speech to young children. *Developmental Psychology, 43*, 1062–1083.

Iverson, J. M., Longobardi, E., & Caselli, M. C. (2003). Relationship between gestures and words in children with Down's syndrome and typically developing children in the early stages of communicative development. *International Journal of Language and Communication Disorders, 38*, 179–197.

Kent, R. D. (1994). *Reference manual for communicative sciences and disorders: Speech and language*. Austin, TX: PRO-ED.

Landau, B., Smith, L., & Jones, S. (1998). Object shape, object function, and object name. *Journal of Memory and Language, 38*, 1–27.

Lust, B., Flynn, S., & Foley, C. (1996). What children know about what they say: Elicited imitation as a research method for assessing children's syntax. In D. McDaniel, C. McKee, & H. Smith (Eds.), *Methods for assessing children's syntax* (pp. 55–76). Cambridge, MA: MIT Press.

Marchman, V. A., & Fernald, A. (2008). Speed of word recognition and vocabulary knowledge infancy predict cognitive and language outcomes in later childhood. *Developmental Science, 11*, F9–F16.

Markman, E. M. (1989). *Categorization and naming in children: Problems of induction*. Cambridge, MA: MIT Press.

Markman, E. M. (1990). Constraints children place on word meanings. *Cognitive Science, 14*, 57–77.

Markman, E. M. (1991). The whole-object, taxonomic, and mutual exclusivity assumptions as initial constraints on word meanings. In S. A. Gelman & J. P. Byrnes (Eds.), *Perspectives on language and thought: Interrelations in development* (pp. 72–106). New York: Cambridge University Press.

Markson, L., & Bloom, P. (1997). Evidence against a dedicated system for word learning in children. *Nature, 385*, 813–815.

McDaniel, D., & Smith Cairns, H. (1998). Eliciting judgments of grammaticality and reference. In D. McDaniel, C. McKee, & H. Smith Cairns (Eds.), *Methods for assessing children's syntax* (pp. 233–254). Boston: MIT Press.

McEachern, D., & Haynes, W. O. (2004). Gesture–speech combinations as a transition to multiword utterances. *American Journal of Speech–Language Pathology, 13*, 227–235.

Meltzoff, A.N. (1999). Origins of theory of mind, cognition, and communication. *Journal of Communication Disorders, 32*, 251–269.

Merriman, W. E., & Bowman, L. (1989). The mutual exclusivity bias in children's early word learning. *Monographs of the Society for Research in Child Development, 54*(3–4), 1–129.

Meyer, M., Leonard, S., Hirsh-Pasek, K., Imai, E., Haryu, E., Pulverman, R., et al. (2003, November). *Making a convincing argument: A cross-linguistic comparison of noun and verb learning in Japanese and English*. Boston: Boston University Conference on Language Development.

Miller, J., & Chapman, R. (1981). The relationship between age and mean length of utterance in morphemes. *Journal of Speech and Hearing Research, 24*, 154–161.

Mills, D. L., Prat, C., Zangl, R., Stager, C. L., Neville, H. J., & Werker, J. F. (2004). Language experience and the organization of brain activity to phonetically similar words: ERP evidence from 14- and 20-month-olds. *Journal of Cognitive Neuroscience, 16*, 1452–1464.

Milligan, K., Astington, J. W., & Dack, L. A. (2007). Language and theory of mind: Meta-analysis of the relation between language ability and false-belief understanding. *Child Development, 78*, 622–646.

National Institute of Child Health and Human Development (NICHD) Early Child Care Research Network. (1996). Characteristics of infant child care: Factors contributing to positive caregiving. *Early Childhood Research Quarterly, 11*, 269–306.

National Institute of Child Health and Human Development (NICHD) Early Child Care Research Network. (2000). The relation of child care to cognitive and language development. *Child Development, 71*, 960–980.

Nelson, P. B., Adamson, L. B., & Bakeman, R. (2008). Toddlers' joint engagement experience facilitates preschoolers' acquisition of theory of mind. *Developmental Science, 11*, 847–852.

O'Grady, W. (1997). Semantics: The analysis of meaning. In W. O'Grady, M. Dobrovolsky, & M. Arnoff (Eds.), *Contemporary linguistics* (3rd ed., pp. 245–287). Boston: Bedford/St. Martin's.

Oller, D. K. (2006). Development and evolution in human vocal communication. *Biological Theory, 1*, 349–351.

Pinker, S. (1999). *Words and rules.* New York: Basic Books.

Raviv, T., Kessenich, M., & Morrison, F. J. (2004). A meditational model of the association between socioeconomic status and three-year-old language abilities: The role of parenting factors. *Early Childhood Research Quarterly, 19*, 528–547.

Rescorla, L. (1980). Overextension in early language development. *Journal of Child Language, 7*, 321–335.

Rizzolatti, G., & Craighero, L. (2004). The mirror-neuron system. *Annual Review of Neuroscience, 27*, 169–192.

Rowe, M. L. (2012). Recording, transcribing, and coding interaction. In E. Hoff, (Ed.), *Research methods in child language: A practical guide* (pp. 193–207). Malden, MA: Wiley-Blackwell.

Rowe, M. L., & Goldin-Meadow, S. (2009). Early gesture selectivity predicts later language learning. *Developmental Science, 12*, 182–187.

Rowe, M. L., Özçaliskan, S., & Goldin-Meadow, S. (2008). Learning words by hand: Gesture's role in predicting vocabulary development. *First Language, 28*, 182–199.

Sabbagh, M. A., & Baldwin, D. A. (2005). Understanding the role of perspective taking in young children's word learning. In N. Eilan, C. Hoerl, T. McCormack, & J. Roessler (Eds.), *Joint Attention: communication and other minds* (pp. 165–184). Oxford: Oxford University Press.

Sander, E. K. (1972). When are speech sounds learned? *Journal of Speech and Hearing Disorders, 37*, 55–63.

Smith, L. B., Jones, S. S., & Landau, B. (1992). Count nouns, adjectives, and perceptual properties in children's novel word interpretations. *Developmental Psychology, 28*, 273–286.

Stoel-Gammon, C., & Dunn, C. (1985). *Normal and disordered phonology in children.* Austin, TX: PRO-ED.

Swingley, D. (2008). The roots of the early vocabulary in infants' learning from speech. *Current Directions in Psychological Science, 17*, 308–312.

Swingley, D., & Aslin, R. N. (2007). Lexical competition in young children's word learning. *Cognitive Psychology, 54*, 99–132.

Van Hulle, C. A., Goldsmith, H. H., & Lemery, K. S. (2004). Genetic, environmental, and gender effects on individual differences in toddler expressive language. *Journal of Speech, Language, and Hearing Research, 47*, 904–912.

Volterra, V., Caselli, M. C., Capirci, O., & Pizzuto, E. (2005). Gesture and the emergence and development of language. In M. Tomasello & D. I. Slobin (Eds.), *Beyond nature–nurture: Essays in honor of Elizabeth Bates* (pp. 3–40). Mahwah, NJ: Erlbaum.

Waxman, S. R., & Booth, A. (2000). Principles that are involved in the acquisition of words, but not facts. *Cognition, 77*, B33–B43.

Waxman, S. R., & Booth, A. E. (2001). On the insufficiency of evidence for a domain-general account of word learning. *Cognition, 78*, 277–279.

Weiss, C. E., Gordon, M. E., & Lillywhite, H. S. (1987). *Clinical management of articulatory and phonologic disorders* (2nd ed.). Baltimore: Williams & Wilkins.

Wiig, E., Secord, W., & Semel, E. (2004). *Clinical evaluation of language fundamentals—preschool 2.* San Antonio, TX: Psychological Corporation.

Wood, J. N., Kouider, S., & Carey, S. (2009) Acquisition of singular-plural morphology. *Developmental Psychology, 45*, 202–206.

Chapter 7

American Academy of Pediatrics. (2014). Literacy promotion: An essential component of primary care pediatric practice. *Pediatrics, 134*, 404–409.

Bagby, J. H., Rudd, L. C., & Woods, M. (2005). The effects of socioeconomic diversity on the language, cognitive, and social-emotional development of children from low-income backgrounds. *Early Child Development and Care, 175*, 395–405.

Biemiller, A. (2005). Size and sequence in vocabulary development: Implications for choosing words for primary grade vocabulary instruction. In E. H. Hiebert & M. Kamil (Eds.), *Teaching and learning vocabulary: Bringing research to practice* (pp. 223–245). Mahwah, NJ: Erlbaum.

Bornstein, M. H., Hahn, C.-S., & Haynes, O. M. (2004). Specific and general language performance across early childhood: Stability and gender considerations. *First Language, 24*, 267–304.

Carey, S. (1978). The child as word learner. In M. Halle, J. Bresnan, & A. Miller (Eds.), *Linguistic theory and psychological reality* (pp. 264–293). Cambridge, MA: MIT Press.

Carey, S., & Bartlett, E. (1978). Acquiring a single new word. *Papers and Reports on Child Language Development, 15*, 17–29.

Carrow-Woolfolk, E. (2011). *Oral and Written Language Scales, Second Edition (OWLS-II).* Torrance, CA: WPS.

Chaney, C. (1994). Language development, metalinguistic awareness, and emergent literacy skills of 3-year-old children in relation to social class. *Applied Psycholinguistics, 15*, 371–394.

Chaney, C. (1998). Preschool language and metalinguistic skills are links to reading success. *Applied Psycholinguistics, 19*, 433–466.

Clark, E. V., & Sengul, C. J. (1978). Strategies in the acquisition of deixis. *Journal of Child Language, 5*, 457–475.

Coyne, M. D., McCoach, D. B., Loftus, S., Zipoli, R., & Kapp, S. (2009). Direct vocabulary instruction in kindergarten: Teaching for breadth versus depth. *The Elementary School Journal, 110*, 1–18.

Dale, E. (1965). Vocabulary measurement: Techniques and major findings. *Elementary English, 42*, 895–901.

Deák, G. O., & Maratsos, M. (1998). On having complex representations of things: Preschoolers use multiple words for objects and people. *Developmental Psychology, 34*, 224–240.

Eskritt, M., Whalen, J., & Lee, K. (2008). Preschoolers can recognize violations of the Gricean maxims. *British Journal of Developmental Psychology, 26*, 435–443.

Ezell, H. K., & Justice, L. M. (2000). Increasing the print focus of shared reading through observational learning. *American Journal of Speech–Language Pathology, 9*, 36–47.

Fey, M. E. (1986). *Language intervention with young children.* Boston: Allyn & Bacon.

Gard, A., Gilman, L., & Gorman, J. (1993). *Speech and language development chart.* Austin, TX: PRO-ED.

Gelman, S. A., & Raman, L. (2007). This cat has nine lives? Children's memory for genericity in language. *Developmental Psychology, 43*, 1256–1268.

Girolametto, L., & Weitzman, E. (2002). Responsiveness of child care providers in interactions with toddlers and preschoolers. *Language, Speech and Hearing Services in Schools, 33*, 268–281.

Graham, S.A., Sedivy, J., & Khu, M. (2014). That's not what you said earlier: Preschoolers expect partners to be referentially consistent. *Journal of Child Language, 41*, 34–50.

Grela, B., Rashiti, L., & Soares, M. (2004). Dative prepositions in children with specific language impairment. *Applied Psycholinguistics, 25*, 467–480.

Grice, H. P. (1989). *Studies in the way of words.* Cambridge, MA: Harvard University Press.

Grice, H.P. (1975). Logic and conversation. In P. Cole & J. L. Morgan (eds.), *Syntax and semantics: Speech acts, Vol. 3* (pp. 41–58). New York: Academic Press.

Gutiérrez-Clellen, V. F., Restrepo, M. A., Bedore, L., Peña, E., & Anderson, R. (2000). Language sample analysis in Spanish-speaking children: Methodological considerations. *Language, Speech, and Hearing Services in Schools, 31*, 88–98.

Haelsig, P. C., & Madison, C. L. (1986). A study of phonological processes exhibited by 3-, 4-, and 5-year-old children. *Language, Speech, and Hearing Services in Schools, 17*, 107–114.

Hage, S. R. V, Resegue, M. M., Viveiros, D. C. S., & Pacheco, E. F. (2007). Analysis of the pragmatic abilities profile in normal preschool children. (original title: Análise do perfil das habilidades pragmáticas em crianças pequenas normais). *Pró-Fono Revista de Atualização Científica, 19*, 49–58.

Hale, C.M., & Tager-Flusberg, H. (2003). The influence of language on theory of mind: A training study. *Developmental Science, 6*, 346–359.

Hall, D. G. (1996). Preschoolers' default assumptions about word meaning: Proper names designate unique individuals. *Developmental Psychology, 32*, 177–186.

Hall, D. G., Burns, T. C., & Pawluski, J. L. (2003). Input and word learning: Caregivers' sensitivity to lexical category distinctions. *Journal of Child Language, 30*, 711–729.

Halliday, M. A. K. (1975). *Learning how to mean: Exploration in the development of language.* London: Edward Arnold.

Halliday, M. A. K. (1977). *Exploration in the functions of language.* New York: Elsevier North-Holland.

Halliday, M. A. K. (1978). *Language as a social semiotic: The social interpretation of language and meaning.* Baltimore: University Park Press.

Haviland, S. E., & Clark, E. V. (1974). This man's father is my father's son: A study of the acquisition of English kin terms. *Journal of Child Language, 1*, 23–47.

Hutchison, J. K. (2001). Telephone communications enhance children's narratives. *Dissertation Abstracts International.* (UMI No. AAT NQ72449).

Huttenlocher, J., Vasilyeva, M., Cymerman, E., & Levine, S. (2002). Language input and child syntax. *Child Psychology, 45*, 337–374.

Invernizzi, M., Sullivan, A., Meier, J., & Swank, L. (2004). *Phonological Awareness Literacy Screening—PreK.* Charlottesville: The Rector and the Board of Visitors of the University of Virginia.

Jaswal, V. K., & Markman, E. M. (2001a). Learning proper and common names in inferential versus ostensive contexts. *Child Development, 72*, 768–786.

Justice, L. M., Bowles, R., Pence, K., & Gosse, C. (2010). A scalable tool for assessing children's language abilities within a narrative context: The NAP (Narrative Assessment Protocol). *Early Childhood Research Quarterly, 25*, 218–234.

Justice, L. M., & Ezell, H. K. (2002a). *The syntax handbook.* Eau Claire, WI: Thinking.

Justice, L. M., & Ezell, H. K. (2002b). Use of storybook reading to increase print awareness in at-risk children. *American Journal of Speech–Language Pathology, 11*, 17–29.

Justice, L. M., & Ezell, H. K. (2004). Print referencing: An emergent literacy enhancement technique and its clinical applications. *Language, Speech, and Hearing Services in Schools, 35*, 185–193.

Justice, L. M., Logan, J. A. R., Lin, T., & Kaderavek, J. N. (2014). Peer effects in early childhood education: Testing the assumptions of special-education inclusion. *Psychological Science, 25*, 1722–1729.

Justice, L. M., Meier, J., & Walpole, S. (2005). Learning new words from storybooks. *Language, Speech, and Hearing Services in Schools, 36*, 17–32.

Justice, L. M., Pence, K., Bowles, R., & Wiggins, A. (2006). An investigation of four hypotheses concerning the order by which 4-year-old children learn the alphabet letters. *Early Childhood Research Quarterly, 21*, 374–389.

Justice, L. M., & Pullen, P. (2003). Promising interventions for promoting emergent literacy skills: Three evidence-based approaches. *Topics in Early Childhood Special Education, 23*, 99–113.

Justice, L. M., Pullen, P., & Pence, K. (2008). Influence of verbal and nonverbal references to print on preschoolers' visual attention to print during storybook reading. *Developmental Psychology, 44*, 855–866.

Justice, L. M., & Schuele, C. M. (2004). Phonological awareness: Description, assessment, and intervention.

In J. E. Bernthal & N. W. Bankson (Eds.), *Articulation and phonological disorders* (5th ed., pp. 376–406). New York: Allyn & Bacon.

Kaderavek, J. N., & Sulzby, E. (2000). Narrative productions by children with and without specific language impairment: Oral narratives and emergent readings. *Journal of Speech, Language, and Hearing Research, 43*, 34–49.

Kelly, S. D. (2001). Broadening the units of analysis in communication: Speech and nonverbal behaviors in pragmatic comprehension. *Journal of Child Language, 28*, 325–349.

Kemler Nelson, D. G., Herron, L., & Holt, M. B. (2003). The sources of young children's name innovations for novel artifacts. *Journal of Child Language, 30*, 823–843.

Khan, K., Nelson, K., & Whyte, E. (2014). Children choose their own stories: The impact of choice on children's learning of new narrative skills. *Journal of Child Language, 41*, 949–962.

Labov, W. (1972). *Language in the inner city: Studies in the Black English Vernacular*. Philadelphia: University of Pennsylvania Press.

Lee, L. L. (1974). *Developmental sentence analysis: A grammatical assessment procedure for speech and language clinicians*. Evanston, IL: Northwestern University Press.

Libby, M. N., & Aries, E. (2006). Gender differences in preschool children's narrative fantasy. *Psychology of Women Quarterly, 13*, 293–306.

Lonigan, C. J., Wagner, R. K., Torgesen, J. K., & Rashotte, C.A. (2007). *TOPEL: Test of Preschool Early Literacy*. Austin, TX: PRO-ED.

McBride-Chang, C. (1999). The ABCs of the ABCs: The development of letter–name and letter–sound knowledge. *Merrill–Palmer Quarterly, 45*, 285–308.

McDaniel, D., & Smith Cairns, H. (1998). Eliciting judgments of grammaticality and reference. In D. McDaniel, C. McKee, & H. Smith Cairns (Eds.), *Methods for assessing children's syntax* (pp. 233–254). Boston: MIT Press.

Miller, J. (1981). *Assessing language production in children: Experimental procedures*. Baltimore: University Park Press.

Miller, J., & Chapman, R. (2000). *SALT: Systematic Analysis of Language Transcripts*. Madison: Language Analysis Laboratory, Waisman Center, University of Wisconsin—Madison.

Miller, P. J., Cho, G. E., & Bracey, J. R. (2005). Working-class children's experience through the prism of personal storytelling. *Human Development, 48*, 115–135.

Mira, W.A., & Schwanenflugel, P.J. (2013). The impact of reading expressiveness on the listening comprehension of storybooks by prekindergarten children. *Language, Speech, and Hearing Services in Schools, 44*, 183–194.

Nittrouer, S. (1996). The relation between speech perception and phonemic awareness: Evidence from low-SES children and children with chronic OM. *Journal of Speech and Hearing Research, 39*, 1059–1070.

Nohara, M. (1996). Preschool boys and girls use no differently. *Journal of Child Language, 23*, 417–429.

O'Grady, W., Dobrovolsky, M., & Arnoff, M. (Eds.). (1997). *Contemporary linguistics* (3rd ed.). Boston: Bedford/St. Martin's.

O'Neill, D. K., Main, R. M., & Ziemski, R. A. (2009). "I like Barney": Preschoolers' spontaneous conversational initiations with peers. *First Language, 29*, 401–425.

Paul, R., & Smith, R. L. (1993). Narrative skills in 4-year-olds with normal, impaired, and late developing language. *Journal of Speech and Hearing Research, 36*, 592–598.

Peterson, C. (1990). The who, when, and where of early narratives. *Journal of Child Language, 17*, 433–455.

Peterson, C.C., Wellman, H.M., & Slaughter, V. (2012). The mind behind the message: Advancing theory of mind scales for typically developing children, and those with deafness, autism, or Asperger syndrome. *Child Development, 83*, 469–485.

Peterson, C., Jesso, B., & McCabe, A. (1999). Encouraging narratives in preschoolers: An intervention study. *Journal of Child Language, 26*, 49–67.

Prime H., Pauker S., Plamondon, A., Perlman, M., & Jenkins, J. (2014), Sibship size, sibling cognitive sensitivity, and children's receptive vocabulary. *Pediatrics, 133*, 394–401.

Reid, D. K., Hresko, W., & Hammill, D. (2002). *Test of early reading ability* (3rd ed.). Austin, TX: PRO-ED.

Robbins, C., & Ehri, L. C. (1994). Reading storybooks to kindergartners helps them learn new vocabulary words. *Journal of Education Psychology, 86*, 54–64.

Sorsby, A. J., & Martlew, M. (1991). Representational demands in mothers' talk to preschool children in two contexts: Picture book reading and a modeling task. *Journal of Child Language, 18*, 373–395.

Speece, D. L., Roth, F. P., Cooper, D. H., & De La Paz, S. (1999). The relevance of oral language skills to early literacy: A multivariate analysis. *Applied Psycholinguistics, 20*, 167–190.

Stanovich, K. E. (2000). *Progress in understanding reading: Scientific foundations and new frontiers*. New York: Guilford Press.

Thomas-Tate, S., Washington, J., Craig, H., & Packard, M. (2006). Performance of African American preschool and kindergarten students on the Expressive Vocabulary Test. *Language, Speech, and Hearing Services in Schools, 37*, 143–149.

Treiman, R., & Broderick, V. (1998). What's in a name? Children's knowledge about the letters in their own names. *Journal of Experimental Child Psychology, 70*, 97–116.

U.S. Department of Education, Office of Planning, Evaluation, and Policy Development, Policy and Program Studies Service. (2005). *Single-sex versus coeducational schooling: A systematic review*. Washington, DC: Author.

Weist, R. M. (2002). Temporal and spatial concepts in child language: Conventional and configurational. *Journal of Psycholinguistic Research, 31*, 195–210.

Wellman, H. M. Fuxi, F., & Peterson, C. C. (2011). Sequential progressions in a theory of mind scale: Longitudinal perspectives. *Child Development, 82*, 780–792.

Whitehurst, G. J., Falco, F. L., Lonigan, C. J., Fischel, J. E., DeBaryshe, B. D., Valdez-Menchaca, M. C., et al. (1988). Accelerating language development through picture book reading. *Developmental Psychology, 24*, 552–559.

Williams, K. T. (2007). *Expressive Vocabulary Test* (2nd ed.). Bloomington, MN: Pearson Assessments.

Zimmerman, I. L., Steiner, V. G., & Pond, R. E. (2011). *Preschool Language Scale* (5th ed.). San Antonio, TX: Psychological Corporation.

Chapter 8

Adams, S., Kuebli, J., Boyle, P. A., & Fivush, R. (1995). Gender differences in parent–child conversations about past emotions: A longitudinal investigation. *Sex Roles, 33*, 309–323.

Ambridge, B. (2012). Assessing grammatical knowledge. In E. Hoff (Ed.), *Research methods in child language: A practical guide* (pp. 113–132). Malden, MA: Blackwell Publishing Ltd.

Ambridge, B., Pine, J. M., Rowland, C. F., & Young, C. R. (2008). The effect of verb semantic class and verb frequency (entrenchment) on children's and adults' graded judgments of argument-structure overgeneralization errors. *Cognition, 106*, 87-129.

Anderson, K. J., & Leaper, C. (1998). Meta-analyses of gender effects on conversational interruption: Who, what, where, when, and how. *Sex Roles, 39*, 225–252.

Anderson, V., & Roit, M. (1996). Linking reading comprehension instruction to language development for language-minority students. *Elementary School Journal, 96*, 295–309.

Apel, K., Brimo, D. Diehm, E., & Apel, L. (2013). Morphological awareness intervention with kindergartners and first- and second-grade students from low socioeconomic status homes: a feasibility study. *Language, Speech, and Hearing Services in Schools, 44*, 161–173.

Apel, K., & Masterson, J. J. (2001b). Theory-guided spelling assessment and intervention: A case study. *Language, Speech, and Hearing Services in Schools, 32*, 182–195.

Apel, K., & Thomas-Tate, S. (2009). Morphological awareness skills of fourth grade African American students. *Language, Speech and Hearing Services in Schools, 40*, 312–324.

Benjamin, B. J. (1997). Speech production of normally aging adults. *Seminars in Speech & Language, 18*, 135–141.

Biemiller, A. (1970). The development of the use of graphic and contextual information as children learn to read. *Reading Research Quarterly, 6*, 75–96.

Bishop, D.V.M. (2003). *The Children's Communication Checklist version 2* (CCC-2). London: Psychological Corporation.

Bosco, F.M., Gabbatore, I., & Tirassa, M. (2014). A broad assessment of theory of mind in adolescence: The complexity of mindreading. *Consciousness and Cognition, 24*, 84–97.

Boudreau, D. M., & Hedberg, N. L. (1999). A comparison of early literacy skills in children with specific language impairment and their typically developing peers. *American Journal of Speech–Language Pathology, 8*, 249–260.

Bowdle, B. F., & Gentner, D. (2005). The career of metaphor. *Psychological Review, 112*, 193–216.

Bryant, G. A., & Tree, J. E. F. (2002). Recognizing verbal irony in spontaneous speech. *Metaphor and Symbol, 17*, 99–119.

Burgess, S. R., Hecht, S. A., & Lonigan, C. J. (2002). Relations of the home literacy environment (HLE) to the development of reading related abilities: A one-year longitudinal study. *Reading Research Quarterly, 37*, 408–426.

Burke, D. M., & Shafto, M. A. (2004). Aging and language production. *Current Directions in Psychological Science, 13*, 21–24.

Bus, A. G., van Ijzendoorn, M. H., & Pellegrini, A. D. (1995). Joint book reading makes for success in learning to read: A meta-analysis on intergenerational transmission of literacy. *Review of Educational Research, 65*, 1–21.

Caccamise, D., & Snyder, L. (2005). Theory and pedagogical practices of text comprehension. *Topics in Language Disorders, 25*, 5–20.

Carson, K. L., Gillon, G. T., & Boustead, T. M. (2013). Classroom phonological awareness instruction and literacy outcomes in the first year of school. *Language, Speech, and Hearing Services in Schools, 44*, 177–160.

Chall, J. S. (1996). *Stages of reading development*. Fort Worth, TX: Harcourt Brace.

Chaney, C. (1998). Preschool language and metalinguistic skills are links to reading success. *Applied Psycholinguistics, 19*, 433–466.

Chapman, A. J., & Foot, H. C. (1996). *Humor and laughter: theory, research, and applications*. Piscataway, NJ: Transaction.

Creusere, M. A. (1999). Theories of adults' understanding and use of irony and sarcasm: Applications to and evidence from research with children. *Developmental Review, 19*, 213–262.

Curenton, S., & Justice, L. M. (2004). Low-income preschoolers' use of decontextualized discourse: Literate language features in spoken narratives. *Language, Speech, and Hearing Services in Schools, 35*, 240–253.

Dixon, J. A., & Foster, D. H. (1997). Gender and hedging: From sex differences to situated practice. *Journal of Psycholinguistic Research, 26*, 89–107.

Dumontheil, I., Apperly, I. A., & Blakemore, S. J. (2010). Online usage of theory of mind continues to develop in late adolescence. *Developmental Science, 13*, 331–338.

Dunn, L., & Dunn, D. (2007). *Peabody Picture Vocabulary Test* (4th ed.). Bloomington, MN: Pearson Assessments.

Dupis, K., & Pichora-Fuller, K. (2010). Use of affective prosody by young and older adults. *Psychology and Aging, 25*, 16–29.

Eisenberg, S. L., Ukrainetz, T. A, Hsu, J. R., Kaderavek, J. N., Justice, L. M., & Gillam, R. B. (2008). Noun phrase elaboration in children's spoken stories. *Language, Speech, and Hearing Services in Schools, 39*, 145–157.

Federmeier, K. D., Van Petten, C., Schwartz, T. J., & Kutas, M. (2003). Sounds, words, sentences: Age-related changes across levels of language processing. *Psychology and Aging, 18*, 858–872.

Gard, A., Gilman, L., & Gorman, J. (1993). *Speech and language development chart*. Austin, TX: PRO-ED.

Gibbs, R. (1987). Linguistic factors in children's understanding of idioms. *Journal of Child Language, 14*, 569–586.

Glenwright, M., & Pexman, P. M. (2010). Development of children's ability to distinguish sarcasm and verbal irony. *Journal of Child Language, 37,* 429–451.

Glenwright, M., Parackel, J. M. Cheung, K. R. J., & Nilsen, E. S. (2014). Intonation influences how children and adults interpret sarcasm. *Journal of Child Language, 41,* 472–484.

Goldman, R., & Fristoe, M. (2000). *Goldman–Fristoe Test of Articulation* (2nd ed.). Circle Pines, MN: American Guidance Services.

Goswami, U., & Mead, F. (1992). Onset and rime awareness and analogies in reading. *Reading Research Quarterly, 27,* 152–162.

Gray, J. (1993). *Men are from Mars, women are from Venus: A practical guide for improving communication and getting what you want in your relationships.* New York: HarperCollins.

Grief, E., & Berko Gleason, J. B. (1980). Hi, thanks, and goodbye: More routine information. *Language in Society, 9,* 159–167.

Hammill, D. D., & Newcomer, P. L. (2008). *Test of Language Development—Primary* (4th ed.). Austin, TX: PRO-ED.

Hannah, A., & Murachver, T. (1999). Gender and conversational style as predictors of conversational behavior. *Journal of Language and Social Psychology, 18,* 153–174.

Ingram, D. (1986). Phonological development: Production. In P. Fletcher & M. Garman (Eds.), *Language acquisition* (2nd ed., pp. 223–239). New York: Cambridge University Press.

Inhelder, B., & Piaget, J. (1958). *The growth of logical thinking from childhood to adolescence.* New York: Basic Books.

James, L. E. (2004). Meeting Mr. Farmer versus meeting a farmer: Specific effects of aging on learning proper names. *Psychology and Aging, 19,* 515–522.

Koike, D. A. (1986). Differences and similarities in men's and women's directives in Carioca Brazilian Portuguese. *Hispania, 69,* 387–394.

Lakoff, R. (1975). *Language and woman's place.* New York: Harper & Row.

Levorato, M. C., Nesi, B., & Cacciari, C. (2004). Reading comprehension and understanding idiomatic expressions: A developmental study. *Brain and Language, 91,* 303–314.

Lund, N. J., & Duchan, J. F. (1993). *Assessing children's language in naturalistic contexts* (3rd ed.). Upper Saddle River, NJ: Prentice Hall.

McCutchen, D., Stull, S., Herrera, B. L., Lotas, S., & & Evans, S. (2013). Putting words to work: Effects of morphological instruction on children's writing. *Journal of Learning Disabilities, 47,* 86–97.

Menyuk, P. (1999). *Reading and linguistic development.* Cambridge, MA: Brookline Books.

Miller, J. F., & Heilmann, J. (2009). New tool assesses narrative structure. *Advance Magazine for Speech–Language Pathologists and Audiologists, 19,* 10.

Nagy, W. E., Carlisle, J.F., & Goodwin, A.P. (2013). Morphological knowledge and literacy acquisition. *Journal of Learning Disabilities, 47,* 3-12.

Nippold, M. A. (1998). *Later language development: The school-age and adolescent years* (2nd ed.). Austin, TX: PRO-ED.

Nippold, M. A. (2000). Language development during the adolescent years: Aspects of pragmatics, syntax, and semantics. *Topics in Language Disorders, 20,* 1528.

Nippold, M. A. (2007). Later *language development: School-age children, adolescents, and young adults* (3rd ed.). Austin, TX: PRO-ED.

Nippold, M. A., Frantz-Kaspar, M. W., Cramond, P. M., Kirk, C., Hayward-Mayhew, C., & MacKinnon, M. (2014). Conversational and narrative speaking in adolescents: Examining the use of complex syntax. *Journal of Speech, Language, and Hearing Research, 57,* 876–886.

Nippold, M. A., Hesketh, L. J., Duthie, J. K., & Mansfield, T. C. (2005). Conversational versus expository discourse: A study of syntactic development in children, adolescents, and adults. *Journal of Speech, Language, and Hearing Research, 48,* 1048–1064.

Nippold, M. A. & Scott, C.M. (2010). Overview of expository discourse. In M.A. Nippold & C.M. Scott (Eds.), *Expository discourse in children, adolescents, and adults* (pp. 1–11). New York: Psychology Press.

Nippold, M. A., Ward-Lonergan, J. M., & Fanning, J. L. (2005). Persuasive writing in children, adolescents, and adults: A study of syntactic, semantic, and pragmatic development. *Language, Speech, and Hearing Services in Schools, 36,* 125–138.

Oliver, B. R., Dale, P. S., & Plomin, R. (2005). Predicting literacy at age 7 from preliteracy at age 4: A longitudinal genetic analysis. *Psychological Science, 16,* 861–865.

Orbelo, D. M., Grim, M. A., Talbott, R. E., & Ross, E. D. (2005). Impaired comprehension of affective prosody in elderly subjects is not predicted by age-related hearing loss or age-related cognitive decline. *Journal of Geriatric Psychiatry and Neurology, 18,* 25–32.

Owens, R. E. (2008). *Language development: An introduction* (7th ed.). Boston: Pearson/Allyn & Bacon.

Paul, R. (1995). *Language disorders from infancy through adolescence: Assessment and intervention.* St. Louis, MO: Mosby–Year Book.

Peterson, C. C., Wellman, H. M., & Slaughter, V. (2012). The mind behind the message: Advancing theory of mind scales for typically developing children, and those with deafness, autism, or Asperger syndrome. *Child Development, 83,* 469–485.

Phelps-Terasaki, D., & Phelps-Gunn, T. (2007). *Test of Pragmatic Language-2 (TOPL-2).* Austin, TX: PRO-ED.

Phillips, B. M., Clancy-Menchetti, J., & Lonigan, C. J. (2008). Successful phonological awareness instruction with preschool children: Lessons learned from the classroom. *Topics in Early Childhood Special Education, 28,* 3–17.

Piaget, J. (1970). *Structuralism.* New York: Basic Books.

Pinker, S. (1994). *The language instinct: How the mind creates language.* New York: Morrow.

Purser, H. R. M., Thomas, M. S. C., Snoxall, S., & Mareschal, D. (2009). The development of similarity: Testing the prediction of a computational model of metaphor comprehension. *Language and Cognitive Processes, 24,* 1406–1430.

Robertson, K., & Murachver, T. (2003). Children's speech accommodation to gendered language styles. *Journal of Language and Social Psychology, 22*, 321–333.

Schuele, C. M., & Boudreau, D. (2008). Phonological awareness intervention: Beyond the basics. *Language, Speech, and Hearing Services in Schools, 39*, 3–20.

Seider, B. H., Hirschberger, G., Nelson, K. L., & Levenson, R. W. (2009). We can work it out: Age differences in relational pronouns, physiology, and behavior in marital conflict. *Psychology and Aging, 24*, 604–613.

Snyder, L. & Caccamise, D. (2010). Comprehension processes for expository text: Building meaning and making sense. In M. A. Nippold & C. M. Scott (Eds.), *Expository discourse in children, adolescents, and adults* (pp. 13–40). New York: Psychology Press.

Spitzberg, B. A., & Adams, T. W. III (2015). *Conversational skills rating scale: An instructional assessment of interpersonal competence.* San Diego, CA: San Diego State University. Retrieved April 25, 2015, from https://www.natcom.org/uploadedFiles/Teaching_and_Learning/Assessment_Resources/PDF-Conversation_Skills_Rating_Scale_2ndEd.pdf.

Talbot, M. (2010). *Language and gender* (2nd ed.). Malden, MA: Polity Press.

Talwar, V., Gordon, H. M., & Lee, K. (2007). Lying in the elementary school years: Verbal deception and its relation to second-order belief understanding. *Developmental Psychology, 43*, 804–810.

Tannen, D. (1991). *You just don't understand: Women and men in conversation.* New York: Ballantine Books.

Tannen, D. (1994). *Talking from 9 to 5: How women's and men's conversational styles affect who gets heard, who gets credit, and what gets done at work.* London: Virago.

Theakston, A. L. (2004). The role of entrenchment on children's and adults' performance on grammaticality judgment tasks. *Cognitive Development, 19*, 15–34.

Tyler, L. K., Shafto, M. A., Randall, B., Wright, P., Marslen-Wilson, W. D., & Stamatakis, E. A. (2010). Preserving syntactic processing across the adult life span: The modulation of the frontotemporal language system in the context of age-related atrophy. *Cerebral Cortex, 20*, 352–364.

Ukrainetz, T. A., Justice, L. M., Kaderavek, J. N., Eisenberg, S. L., Gillam, R. B., & Harm, H. M. (2005). The development of expressive elaboration in fictional narratives. *Journal of Speech, Language, and Hearing Research, 48*, 1363–1377.

Vasilyeva, M., Waterfall, H., & Huttenlocher, J. (2008). Emergence of syntax: Commonalities and differences across children. *Developmental Science, 11*, 84–97.

Verhagen, C. & Poncelet, M. (2013). Changes in naming and semantic abilities with aging from 50 to 90 years. *Journal of the International Neuropsychological Society, 19*, 119–126.

Wellman, H. M., Fuxi, F., & Peterson, C. C. (2011). Sequential progressions in a theory of mind scale: Longitudinal perspectives. *Child Development, 82*, 780–792.

Westby, C. E. (1985). Learning to talk—talking to learn: Oral-literate language differences. In C. S. Simon (Ed.), *Communication skills and classroom success: Therapy methodologies for language-learning disabled students* (pp. 181–218). San Diego, CA: College-Hill Press.

Westby, C. E. (1991). Learning to talk—talking to learn: Oral-literate language differences. In C. S. Simon (Ed.), *Communication skills and classroom success: Assessment and therapy methodologies for language and learning disabled students* (rev. ed., pp. 334–357). Eau Claire, WI: Thinking.

Westby, C. E. (1998). Communicative refinement in school age and adolescence. In W. O. Haynes & B. B. Shulman (Eds.), *Communication development: Foundations, processes, and clinical implications* (pp. 311–360). Baltimore: Williams & Wilkins.

White, T. G., Sowell, J., & Yanagihara, A. (1989). Teaching elementary students to use word-part clues. *Reading Teacher, 42*, 302–308.

Whitehurst, G. J., & Lonigan, C. J. (1998). Child development and emergent literacy. *Child Development, 68*, 848–872.

Wiig, E. H., & Secord, W. (1989). *Test of Language Competence—Expanded.* San Antonio, TX: Psychological Corporation.

Wiig, E. H., & Secord, W. (1992). *Test of Word Knowledge.* San Antonio, TX: Psychological Corporation.

Wolter, J., & & Dilworth, V. (2013). The effects of a multilinguistic morphological awareness approach for improving language and literacy. *Journal of Learning Disabilities, 47*, 76– 85.

Chapter 9

Arias, R., & Lakshmanan, U. (2005). Code-switching in a Spanish-English bilingual child: A communication resource? In J. Cohen, K. McAlister, K. Rolstad, & J. MacSwan (Eds.), *Proceedings of the 4th International Symposium on Bilingualism* (pp. 94–109). Somerville, MA: Cascadilla Press.

Bailey, G., & Tillery, J. (2006). Sounds of the South. In W. Wolfram & B. Ward (Eds.), *American voices: How dialects differ from coast to coast* (pp. 11–16). Malden, MA: Blackwell.

Baker, C. (2000). *A parents' and teachers' guide to bilingualism* (2nd ed.). Tonawanda, NY: Multilingual Matters.

Baugh, J. (2006). Bridging the great divide (African American English). In W. Wolfram & B. Ward (Eds.), *American voices: How dialects differ from coast to coast* (pp. 217–224). Malden, MA: Blackwell.

Bernstein, C. (2006). More than just yada yada yada (Jewish English). In W. Wolfram & B. Ward (Eds.), *American voices: How dialects differ from coast to coast* (pp. 251–257). Malden, MA: Blackwell.

Bernstein Ratner, N. (1986). Durational cues which mark clause boundaries in mother–child speech. *Journal of Phonetics, 14*, 303–309.

Brown, H. D. (2001). *Teaching by principles: An interactive approach to language pedagogy* (2nd ed.). White Plains, NY: Addison Wesley Longman.

Campbell, M. T., & Plumb, G. (n.d.). Generic names for soft drinks by county [Map]. In A. McConchie (Ed.), *The great pop vs. soda controversy.* Retrieved September 26, 2006, from http://www.popvssoda.com/countystats/totalcounty.html

Coleman, R., & Goldenberg, C. (2012). The Common Core challenge for English language learners. *Principal Leadership, 12*, 46–51.

Conn, J. (2006). Dialects in the mist (Portland, OR). In W. Wolfram & B. Ward (Eds.), *American voices: How dialects differ from coast to coast* (pp. 149–155). Malden, MA: Blackwell.

Cooper, R. P., & Aslin, R. N. (1990). Preference for infant-directed speech in the first month after birth. *Child Development, 61*, 1584–1595.

Cross, J. B., DeVaney, T., & Jones, G. (2001). Pre-service teacher attitudes toward differing dialects. *Linguistics and Education, 12*, 211–227.

Danesi, M. (2003). *Second language teaching: A view from the right side of the brain*. Dordrecht, The Netherlands: Kluwer Academic.

Fernald, A. (2000). Speech to infants as hyper-speech: Knowledge-driven processes in early word recognition. *Phonetica, 57*, 242–254.

Fernald, A., & Kuhl, P. (1987). Acoustic determinants of infant preference for motherese speech. *Infant Behavior and Development, 10*, 279–293.

Fernald, A., & Mazzie, C. (1991). Prosody and focus in speech to infants and adults. *Developmental Psychology, 27*, 209–221.

Fitzpatrick, J. (2006). Beantown babble (Boston, MA). In W. Wolfram & B. Ward (Eds.), *American voices: How dialects differ from coast to coast* (pp. 63–69). Malden, MA: Blackwell.

Fletcher, P. (1992). Subgroups in school-age language-impaired children. In P. Fletcher & D. Hall (Eds.), *Specific speech and language disorders in children: Correlates, characteristics, and outcomes* (pp. 152–165). London: Whurr.

Fodor, J. (1983). *The modularity of mind*. Cambridge, MA: MIT Press.

Fought, C. (2003). *Chicano English in context*. New York: Palgrave Macmillan.

Fought, C. (2006). Is Chicano English influencing other dialects? In W. Wolfram & B. Ward (Eds.), *American voices: How dialects differ from coast to coast* (pp. 233–237). Malden, MA: Blackwell.

Frazer, T. C. (1996). Chicano English and Spanish interference in the midwestern United States. *American Speech, 71*, 72–85.

Gass, S. M., & Selinker, L. (2001). *Second language acquisition: An introductory course*. Mahwah, NJ: Erlbaum.

Genesee, F. (1989). Early bilingual development: One language or two? *Journal of Child Language, 16*, 171–179.

Genesee, F., Nicoladis, E., & Paradis, J. (1995). Language differentiation in early bilingual development. *Journal of Child Language, 22*, 611–631.

Genesee, F., Paradis, J., & Crago, M. B. (2004). *Dual language development and disorders: A handbook on bilingualism and second language learning*. Baltimore: Brookes.

Giles, H., & Powesland, P. F. (1975). *Speech style and social evaluation*. London and New York: Academic Press.

Goldenberg, C. (2008). Teaching English language learners: What the research does—and does not—say. *American Educator*, 8–44.

Goldstein, B. (2001). Transcription of Spanish and Spanish-influenced English. *Communication Disorders Quarterly, 23*, 54–60.

Golinkoff, R. M., & Alioto, A. (1995). Infant-directed speech facilitates lexical learning in adults hearing Chinese: Implications for language acquisition. *Journal of Child Language, 22*, 703–726.

Gordon, M. J. (2006). Straight talking from the heartland (Midwest). In W. Wolfram & B. Ward (Eds.), *American voices: How dialects differ from coast to coast* (pp. 106–111). Malden, MA: Blackwell.

Grabe, W. (2002). Applied linguistics: An emerging discipline for the twenty-first century. In R. A. Kaplan (Ed.), *The Oxford handbook of applied linguistics* (pp. 3–12). New York: Oxford University Press.

Gross, T. (2005, December 12). Getting the shmootz on Yiddish [Interview with Michael Wex]. *In Fresh Air from WHYY*. Washington, DC: National Public Radio. Available from http://www.npr.org/templates/story/story.php?storyId=5048943.

Hummel, K. M. (2014). *Introducing second language acquisition: Perspectives and practices*. Malden, MA: Wiley Blackwell.

Jackson, C.W., Schatschneider, C., & Leacox, L. (2014). Vocabulary growth in young Spanish English-speaking children from migrant families. *Language, Speech, and Hearing Services in Schools, 45*, 40–51.

Junker, D. A., & Stockman, I. J. (2002). Expressive vocabulary of German–English bilingual toddlers. *American Journal of Speech–Language Pathology, 11*, 381–394.

Krashen, S. (1985). *The input hypothesis: Issues and implications*. London: Longman.

Kuhl, P., Andruski, J., Chistovich, I., Chistovich, L., Kozhevnikova, E., Ryskina, V., et al. (1997). Cross-language analysis of phonetic units in language addressed to infants. *Science, 277*, 684–686.

Labov, T. G. (1998). English acquisition by immigrants to the United States at the beginning of the twentieth century. *American Speech, 73*, 368–398.

Labov, W., Ash, S., & Boberg, C. (2005). *The atlas of North American English*. New York: Mouton/de Gruyter.

Larsen-Freeman, D., & Long, M. H. (1991). *An introduction to second language acquisition research*. New York: Longman.

Lenneberg, E. H. (1967). *Biological foundations of language*. New York: Wiley.

Lessow-Hurley, J. (1990). *The foundations of dual language instruction*. White Plains, NY: Longman.

Loewen, S. (2015). *Introduction to instructed second language acquisition*. New York: Routledge.

Lozanov, G. (1979). *Suggestology and outlines of suggestopedy*. New York: Gordon and Breach Science.

Lucy, J. A. (1992). *Language diversity and thought: A reformulation of the linguistic relativity hypothesis*. New York: Cambridge University Press.

Luhman, R. (1990). Appalachian English stereotypes: Language attitudes in Kentucky. *Language in Society, 19*, 331–348.

Morrow, A., Goldstein, B. A., Gilhool, A., & Paradis, J. (2014). Phonological skills in English language learners.

Language, Speech, and Hearing Services in Schools, 45, 26–39.

Newman, M. (2006). New York tawk (New York City). In W. Wolfram & B. Ward (Eds.), *American voices: How dialects differ from coast to coast* (pp. 82–87). Malden, MA: Blackwell.

Petitto, L.-A., Katerelos, M., Levy, B. G., Gauna, K., Tétreault, K., & Ferraro, V. (2001). Bilingual signed and spoken language acquisition from birth: Implications for the mechanisms underlying early bilingual language acquisition. *Journal of Child Language, 28,* 453–496.

Roberts, J., Nagy, N., & Boberg, C. (2006). Yakking with the Yankees (New England). In W. Wolfram & B. Ward (Eds.), *American voices: How dialects differ from coast to coast* (pp. 57–62). Malden, MA: Blackwell.

Rosenthal, M. S. (1974). The magic boxes: Pre-school children's attitudes toward Black and Standard English. *The Florida FL Reporter,* spring/fall (pp. 55–62, 92–93).

Ryan, C. (2013). Language use in the United States: 2011. Washington, DC: U.S. Census Bureau. Retrieved January 29, 2015, from https://www.census.gov/prod/2013pubs/acs-22.pdf.

Salvucci, C. (2006). Expressions of brotherly love (Philadelphia, PA). In W. Wolfram & B. Ward (Eds.), *American voices: How dialects differ from coast to coast* (pp. 88–92). Malden, MA: Blackwell.

Sapir, E. (1921). *Language: An introduction to the study of speech.* New York: Harcourt, Brace.

Schieffelin, B. B., & Ochs, E. (1986). Language socialization. *Annual Review of Anthropology, 15,* 163–191.

Senghas, A., & Coppola, M. (2001). Children creating language: How Nicaraguan Sign Language acquired a spatial grammar. *Psychological Science, 12,* 323–328.

Slavin, R. E., & Cheung, A. (2005). A synthesis of research on language of reading instruction for English language learners. *Review of Educational Research, 75,* 247–284.

Southerland, R. H. (1997). Language in social contexts. In W. O'Grady, M. Dobrovolsky, & M. Arnoff (Eds.), *Contemporary linguistics: An introduction* (3rd ed., pp. 509–551). Boston: Bedford/St. Martin's.

Tabors, P. O. (1997). *One child, two languages: A guide for preschool educators of children learning English as a second language.* Baltimore: Brookes.

Terrell, T. D. (1977). A natural approach to second language acquisition and learning. *Modern Language Journal, 61,* 325–337.

Terry, N. P., Connor, C. M., Petscher, Y., & Ross, C. (2012). Dialect variation and reading: Is change in non-mainstream American English use related to reading achievement in first and second grades? *Journal of Speech, Language, and Hearing Research, 55,* 55–69.

U.S. Department of Education, National Center for Education Statistics. (2015). *Local Education Agency Universe Survey, 2011–12.* Retrieved January 31, 2015 from http://nces.ed.gov/programs/coe/indicator_cgf.asp.

U.S. Department of Justice and U.S. Department of Education. (2015). *Fact Sheet, Ensuring English Learner Students Can Participate Meaningfully and Equally in Educational Programs.* Retrieved February 3, 2015 from http://www2.ed.gov/about/offices/list/ocr/docs/dcl-factsheet-el-students-201501.pdf.

Volterra, V., & Taeschner, T. (1978). The acquisition and development of language by bilingual children. *Journal of Child Language, 5,* 311–326.

Watts, G. (2013). *Miami Accents: How 'Miamah' Turned Into A Different Sort Of Twang* Retrieved February 15, 2015, from http://wlrn.org/post/miami-accents-how-miamah-turned-different-sort-twang.

Wolfram, W., & Schilling-Estes, N. (2006). Language evolution or dying traditions? The state of American dialects. In W. Wolfram & B. Ward (Eds.), *American voices: How dialects differ from coast to coast* (pp. 1–7). Malden, MA: Blackwell.

Zentella, A. C. (1997). *Growing up bilingual.* Malden, MA: Blackwell.

Chapter 10

American Association on Mental Retardation. (2002). *Mental retardation: Definition, classification, and systems of supports* (10th ed.). Washington, DC: Author.

American Psychiatric Association. (2013). *Diagnostic and statistical manual of mental disorders,* (*DSM-5®*). American Psychiatric Pub.

American Speech-Language-Hearing Association. (2005). *Causes of hearing loss in children.* Rockville, MD: Author. Retrieved January 5, 2005, from http://www.asha.org/public/hearing/disorders/causes.htm.

Beitchman, J., Hood, J., Rochon, J., Peterson, M., Mantini, T., & Majumdar, S. (1989). Empirical classification of speech/language impairment in children: I. Identification of speech/language categories. *Journal of the American Academy of Child & Adolescent Psychiatry, 28*(1), 112–117.

Beitchman, J. H., Brownlie, E. B., & Bao, L. (2014). Age 31 mental health outcomes of childhood language and speech disorders. *Journal of the American Academy of Child & Adolescent Psychiatry, 53*(10), 1102–1110.

Brandel, J., & Loeb, D. F. (2011). Program intensity and service delivery models in the schools: SLP survey results. *Language, Speech, and Hearing Services in Schools, 42*(4), 461–490.

Brey, R. L. (2006). The silent epidemic: Traumatic brain injury's massive impact on sufferers and society. *Neurology Now, 2*(5), 5.

Bureau of Labor Statistics. (2015). *Occupational outlook handbook.* Retrieved April 2, 2015, from http://www.bls.gov/ooh/healthcare/speech-language-pathologists.htm.

Cable, A. L., & Domsch, C. (2011). Systematic review of the literature on the treatment of children with late language emergence. *International Journal of Language & Communication Disorders, 46*(2), 138–154.

Catts, H. W., Fey, M. E., Tomblin, J. B., & Zhang, X. (2002). Longitudinal investigation of reading outcomes in children with language impairment. *Journal of Speech, Language, and Hearing Research, 45,* 1142–1157.

Centers for Disease Control and Prevention. (2007). *Traumatic brain injury in the United States: Emergency department visits, hospitalizations, and deaths, 2002–2006.* Atlanta: Author.

Centers for Disease Control and Prevention, National Center on Birth Defects and Developmental Disabilities. (2009). *Prevalence of autism spectrum disorders—autism and developmental disabilities monitoring network, United States, 2006.* Atlanta: Author.

Centers for Disease Control and Prevention. (2015). *Autism spectrum disorder: Data and statistics.* Retrieved April 2, 2015, from http://www.cdc.gov/ncbddd/autism/data.html.

Chapman, S. B. (1997). Cognitive–communicative abilities in children with closed head injury. *American Journal of Speech–Language Pathology, 6,* 50–58.

Chapman, R. S., Seung, H. K., Schwartz, S. E., & Kay-Raining Bird, E. (1998). Language skills of children and adolescents with Down syndrome: II. Production deficits. *Journal of Speech, Language, and Hearing Research, 41,* 861–873

Cleave, P., Bird, E. K. R., Czutrin, R., & Smith, L. (2012). A longitudinal study of narrative development in children and adolescents with Down syndrome. *Intellectual and developmental disabilities, 50*(4), 332–342.

Conti-Ramsden, G., & Jones, M. (1997). Verb use in specific language impairment. *Journal of Speech, Language, and Hearing Research, 40,* 1298–1313.

Conti-Ramsden, G., Mok, P. L., Pickles, A., & Durkin, K. (2013). Adolescents with a history of specific language impairment (SLI): Strengths and difficulties in social, emotional and behavioral functioning. *Research in Developmental Disabilities, 34*(11), 4161–4169.

Coppens, K. M., Tellings, A., van der Veld, W., Schreuder, R., & Verhoeven, L. (2012). Vocabulary development in children with hearing loss: The role of child, family, and educational variables. *Research in Developmental Disabilities, 33*(1), 119–128.

Dale, P. S., Price, T. S., Bishop, D. V. M., & Plomin, P. (2003). Outcomes of early language delay: I. Predicting persistent and transient language difficulties at 3 and 4 years. *Journal of Speech, Language, and Hearing Research, 46,* 544–560.

Durkin, K., Simkin, Z., Knox, E., & Conti-Ramsden, G. (2009) Specific language impairment and school outcomes II: Educational context, student satisfaction, and post-compulsory progress. *International Journal of Language and Communication Disorders, 15,* 36–55.

Ertmer, D. J., Strong, L., & Sadagopan, N. (2003). Beginning to communicate after cochlear implantation: Oral language development in a young child. *Journal of Speech, Language, and Hearing Research, 46,* 328–340.

Ewing-Cobbs, L., Fletcher, J. M., Levin, H. S., Francis, D. J., Davidson, K., & Miner, M. E. (1997). Longitudinal neuropsychological outcome in infants and preschoolers with traumatic brain injury. *Journal of the International Neuropsychological Society, 3*(06), 581–591.

Falkus, G., Tilley, C., Thomas, C., Hockey, H., Kennedy, A., Arnold, T., … & Pring, T. (2015). Assessing the effectiveness of parent–child interaction therapy with language delayed children: A clinical investigation. *Child Language Teaching and Therapy.*

Fernald, A., & Marchman, V. A. (2012). Individual differences in lexical processing at 18 months predict vocabulary growth in typically developing and late-talking toddlers. *Child Development, 83*(1), 203–222.

Gallaudet Research Institute. (2001, January). *Regional and national summary report of data from the 1999–2000 Annual Survey of Deaf and Hard of Hearing Children and Youth.* Washington, DC: Gallaudet University.

Girolametto, L., Pearce, P. S., & Weitzman, E. (1996). Interactive focused stimulation for toddlers with expressive vocabulary delays. *Journal of Speech and Hearing Research, 39,* 1274–1283.

Hall, L. J. (2012). *Autism spectrum disorders: From theory to practice.* Pearson Higher Ed.

Hansson, K. (2003). Indefinite articles and definite forms in Swedish children with specific language impairment. *First Language, 23,* 343–362.

Individuals with Disabilities Education Improvement Act of 2004, Pub. L. No. 108–446, 118 Stat. 2647 (2004).

Justice, L. M., Bowles, R. P., Pence Turnbull, K. L., & Skibbe, L. E. (2009). School readiness among children with varying histories of language difficulties. *Developmental Psychology, 45,* 460–476.

Justice, L., Mashburn, A., & Petscher, Y. (2013). Very early language skills of fifth-grade poor comprehenders. *Journal of Research in Reading, 36*(2), 172–185.

Kenneally, S. M., Bruck, G. E., Frank, E. M., & Nalty, L. (1998). Language intervention after thirty years of isolation: A case study of a feral child. *Education and Training in Mental Retardation and Developmental Disabilities, 33,* 13–23.

Leonard, L. B. (2014). *Children with specific language impairment.* Cambridge, MA: MIT press.

Levickis, P., Reilly, S., Girolametto, L., Ukoumunne, O. C., & Wake, M. (2014). Maternal behaviors promoting language acquisition in slow-to-talk toddlers: Prospective community-based study. *Journal of Developmental & Behavioral Pediatrics, 35*(4), 274–281.

Martin, F., & Greer Clark, J. (2002). *Introduction to audiology* (8th ed.). Boston: Allyn & Bacon.

Miller, J., & Chapman, R. (2000). *SALT: Systematic Analysis of Language Transcripts.* Madison: Language Analysis Laboratory, Waisman Center, University of Wisconsin–Madison.

Monasta, L., Ronfani, L., Marchetti, F., Montico, M., Brumatti, L. V., Bavcar, A., … & Tamburlini, G. (2012). Burden of disease caused by otitis media: Systematic review and global estimates. *PLoS One, 7*(4), e36226.

Most, T., Shina-August, E., & Meilijson, S. (2010). Pragmatic abilities of children with hearing loss using cochlear implants or hearing aids compared to hearing children. *Journal of Deaf Studies and Deaf Education,* enq032.

Næss, K. A. B., Lyster, S. A. H., Hulme, C., & Melby-Lervåg, M. (2011). Language and verbal short-term memory skills in children with Down syndrome: A meta-analytic review. *Research in Developmental Disabilities, 32*(6), 2225–2234.

Nash, M., & Donaldson, M. L. (2005). Word learning in children with vocabulary deficits. *Journal of Speech, Language, and Hearing Research, 48,* 439–458.

Niparko, J., Tobey, E., Thal, D., Eisenberg, L., Wang, N., et al. (2010). Spoken language development in children following cochlear implantation. *Journal of the American Medical Association, 303,* 1498–1506.

O'Brien, E. K., Zhang, X., Nishimura, C., Tomblin, J. B., & Murray, J. C. (2003). Association of specific language impairment (SLI) to the region of 7q31. *American Journal of Human Genetics, 72,* 1536–1543.

Pakulski, L. (2006). Pediatric hearing loss. In L. Justice (Ed.), *Communication sciences and disorders: An introduction* (pp. 428–467). Upper Saddle River, NJ: Merrill/Prentice Hall.

Paul, R., & Norbury, C. (2012). *Language disorders from infancy through adolescence: Listening, speaking, reading, writing, and communicating.* Elsevier Health Sciences.

Piasta, S. B., Petscher, Y., & Justice, L. M. (2012). How many letters should preschoolers in public programs know? The diagnostic efficiency of various preschool letter-naming benchmarks for predicting first-grade literacy achievement. *Journal of Educational Psychology, 104*(4), 945.

Pisoni, D., Cleary, M., Geers, A., & Tobey, E. (2000). Individual differences in effectiveness of cochlear implants in children who are prelingually deaf: New process measures of performance. *Volta Review, 10,* 111–164.

Reader, R. H., Covill, L. E., Nudel, R., & Newbury, D. F. (2014). Genome-wide studies of specific language impairment. *Current Behavioral Neuroscience Reports, 1*(4), 242–250.

Rice, M. L., Haney, K. R., & Wexler, K. (1998). Family histories of children with SLI who show extended optional infinitives. *Journal of Speech, Language, and Hearing Research, 41,* 419–432.

Sansavini, A., Guarini, A., Alessandroni, R., Faldella, G., Giovanelli, G., & Salvioli, G. (2007). Are early grammatical and phonological working memory abilities affected by preterm birth? *Journal of Communication Disorders, 40,* 239–256.

Sansavini, A., Guarini, A., Justice, L. M., Savini, S., Alessandroni, R., & Faldella, G. (2010). Does preterm birth increase a child's risk for language impairment? *Early Human Development.*

Scarborough, H. S. (2001). Connecting early language and literacy to later reading (dis)abilities: Evidence, theory, and practice. In S. B. Neuman & D. K. Dickinson (Eds.), *Handbook of early literacy research* (pp. 97–110). New York: Guilford Press.

Shriberg, L. D., Friel-Patti, S., Flipsen, P., Jr., & Brown, R. L. (2000). Otitis media, fluctuant hearing loss and speech–language delay: A preliminary structural equation model. *Journal of Speech, Language, and Hearing Research, 43,* 100–120.

Skibbe, L. E., Grimm, K. J., Stanton-Chapman, T., Justice, L. M., Pence, K. L., & Bowles, R. P. (2008). Reading trajectories of children with language difficulties from preschool through grade five. *Language, Speech, and Hearing Services in Schools, 39,* 475–486.

Smith-Lock, K. M., Leitao, S., Lambert, L., & Nickels, L. (2013). Effective intervention for expressive grammar in children with specific language impairment.

International Journal of Language & Communication Disorders, 48(3), 265–282.

Smyke, A. T., Zeanah, C. H., Fox, N. A., & Nelson, C. A. (2009). A new model of foster care for young children: The Bucharest Early Intervention Project. *Child and Adolescent Psychiatric Clinics of North America, 18*(3), 721–734.

Solomon-Rice, P. L., & Soto, G. (2014). Facilitating vocabulary in toddlers using AAC: A preliminary study comparing focused stimulation and augmented input. *Communication Disorders Quarterly, 35*(4), 204–215.

St. Clair, M. C., Pickles, A., Durkin, K., & Conti-Ramsden, G. (2011). A longitudinal study of behavioral, emotional and social difficulties in individuals with a history of specific language impairment (SLI). *Journal of Communication Disorders, 44*(2), 186–199.

Stothard, S. E., Snowling, M. J., Bishop, D. V. M., Chipchase, B. B., & Kaplan, C. A. (1998). Language-impaired preschoolers: A follow-up into adolescence. *Journal of Speech, Language, and Hearing Research, 41,* 407–418.

Svirsky, M. A, Teoh, S.-W., & Neuburger, H. (2004). Development of language and speech perception in congenitally, profoundly deaf children as a function of age at cochlear implantation. *Audiology & Neuro-Otology, 9,* 224–233.

Tambyraja, S. R., Schmitt, M. B., Farquharson, K., & Justice, L. M. (2015). Stability of Language and Literacy Profiles of Children with Language Impairment in the Public Schools. *Journal of Speech, Language, and Hearing Research.*

Taylor, G. R. (2001). *Educational interventions and services for children with exceptionalities.* Springfield, IL: Charles C Thomas.

Theoharides, T. C., & Zhang, B. (2011). Neuro-inflammation, blood-brain barrier, seizures and autism. *J Neuroinflammation, 8*(1), 168.

Tomblin, J. B., Zhang, X., Buckwalter, P., & O'Brien, M. (2003) The stability of primary language disorder: Four years after kindergarten diagnosis. *Journal of Speech, Language, and Hearing Research, 46,* 1283–1296.

Tye-Murray, N. (2000). The child who has severe or profound hearing loss. In J. B. Tomblin, H. L. Morris, & D. C. Spriestersbach (Eds.), *Diagnosis in speech–language pathology* (2nd ed.). San Diego, CA: Singular.

U.S. Department of Education, National Center for Education Statistics. (2015). *Digest of Education Statistics, 2013* (NCES 2015-011). Retrieved January 17, 2015, from https://nces.ed.gov/fastfacts/display.asp?id=64.

Wiig, E. H., Secord, W., & Semel, E. M. (2004). *CELF preschool 2: Clinical evaluation of language fundamentals preschool.* Pearson/PsychCorp.

Zimmerman, F. J., Christakis, D. A., & Meltzoff, A. N. (2007). Television and DVD/video viewing in children younger than 2 years. *Archives of Pediatrics & Adolescent Medicine, 161,* 473–479.

Zubrick, S. R., Taylor, C. L., Rice, M. L., & Slegers, D. W. (2007). Late language emergence at 24 months: An epidemiological study of prevalence, predictors, and covariates. *Journal of Speech, Language, and Hearing Research, 50,* 1562–1592.

Author Index

Subject Index